History of Blood Donation
and Transfusion Medicine

Zdravko Kvržić

History of Blood Donation and Transfusion Medicine

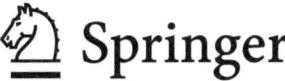
Springer

Zdravko Kvržić
Department of Blood Supply
Blood Transfusion Center of Slovenia
Ljubljana, Slovenia

ISBN 978-3-031-68714-3   ISBN 978-3-031-68715-0 (eBook)
https://doi.org/10.1007/978-3-031-68715-0

© The Editor(s) (if applicable) and The Author(s), under exclusive license to Springer Nature Switzerland AG 2024

This work is subject to copyright. All rights are solely and exclusively licensed by the Publisher, whether the whole or part of the material is concerned, specifically the rights of translation, reprinting, reuse of illustrations, recitation, broadcasting, reproduction on microfilms or in any other physical way, and transmission or information storage and retrieval, electronic adaptation, computer software, or by similar or dissimilar methodology now known or hereafter developed.

The use of general descriptive names, registered names, trademarks, service marks, etc. in this publication does not imply, even in the absence of a specific statement, that such names are exempt from the relevant protective laws and regulations and therefore free for general use.

The publisher, the authors and the editors are safe to assume that the advice and information in this book are believed to be true and accurate at the date of publication. Neither the publisher nor the authors or the editors give a warranty, expressed or implied, with respect to the material contained herein or for any errors or omissions that may have been made. The publisher remains neutral with regard to jurisdictional claims in published maps and institutional affiliations.

This Springer imprint is published by the registered company Springer Nature Switzerland AG
The registered company address is: Gewerbestrasse 11, 6330 Cham, Switzerland

If disposing of this product, please recycle the paper.

Foreword

As a cornerstone of social altruism, blood donation is a sensitive area that requires the careful engagement of relevant institutions and individuals in order to meet the needs of healthcare for blood products. The present work undoubtedly contributes to the reader's wider knowledge of the field of blood donation over time and thereby consolidates the values that are the guiding principles of blood donation in modern times. I can say that it is a contribution that fills a void in the Slovenian space, as both the local and wider history of transfusion medicine are very vividly shown in one place. Just a look at history shows us how strongly the tendency to save lives with transfusion medicine developed both in professional and in the wider society, which laid the foundations for altruistic blood donation. It is interesting to note that, in fact, in all corners of the world, blood donation developed fairly synchronously, and that throughout history, our area did not significantly lag behind pioneering discoveries in transfusion medicine. We can proudly say that Slovenia is one of those countries with voluntary, non-remunerated and anonymous blood donation with a strongly rooted tradition and broader collective pride. The reader, who can also be a blood donor at the same time, quickly comes to the conclusion that blood donation is still often the only way to maintain and save life, or a necessity for healing. At this point, the author definitely wanted to encourage the reader to think about what he can do today and what he can do tomorrow, to contribute his little stone in the mosaic for saving lives and for maintaining the health of people. An extensive review of domestic and foreign literature serves the author as a basis for summarizing the most important milestones for easier orientation for the reader. Confessions and stories from the distant and recent history of blood donation provide a unique contrast to the present work. The author has shown himself in this field to be a thorough and persistent researcher. He also achieves enviable results in his professional field and, above all, has countless satisfied blood donors. The book should encourage the reader to consider how we can help our fellow humans in the most difficult moments of life. All recognition goes to the author for his extremely self-sacrificing and thorough work, which clearly shows the problems of development and practice in the field of blood donation and transfusion medicine. Particularly interesting are the testimonies of individuals in various emergency situations when donated blood, in most cases, helped save lives.

David Pučko
Department of Blood Supply
Blood Transfusion Center of Slovenia
Ljubljana, Slovenia

Preface

Transfusion medicine has a rich and complex history. This book explores the fascinating journey of important milestones and breakthroughs in this honorable field of medicine and its modern-day achievements. The book's main attraction lies in its extensive bibliography, which provides answers to some of the most puzzling questions in the history of blood donation and transfusion medicine. In fact, it took hundreds of years for modern transfusion medicine to develop from humble beginnings, which today ensures the safety of blood and blood products. Blood transfusions have been used in war and peace in the hope of saving lives all around the world. While researching, some historical errors were found in the review of world literature, which are supplemented in the book. The book is undoubtedly useful for different experts, such as doctors, nurses, historians, students, blood donors, and others interested in this noble topic, and is the basis for further research. In addition to the global overview of events, the history of blood donation in the European country of Slovenia is described, along with new findings and descriptions.

Blood Donor and Blood Donation

Blood donation is one of the greatest humanitarian, voluntary, and heartfelt acts for a fellow human being. Blood donors donate part of themselves to restore the health of patients. Blood is needed in everyday life in operation procedures, after transplantation of blood marrow or organs, hemorrhage in trauma, different serious blood disorders, and many other emergency cases. Every century is also marked by different problems; some of them are natural disasters, others are terrible human acts, such as terrorist attacks, which mercilessly destroy lives. In the midst of this helplessness, humanitarians with sincere hearts, true heroes, emerge to help suffering people with their selflessness. One of these heroes with a highly developed sense of helping their fellow human beings is undoubtedly the blood donor. Blood donation is a noble act of solidarity that unites people throughout the world in caring and compassion for one another. Donating blood is safe, and it only takes a couple of minutes for this noble deed. An individual donates blood voluntarily, non-remunerated and anonymously for different reasons, such as altruistic desires for helping others, personal growth, experiences of loved ones who are blood donors or, at some point, needed a transfusion, peer influence, and societal influence. Blood donors can donate whole blood (*blood with all blood components*) or individual blood components with an apheresis procedure. The type of procedure determines the timing of the donation. By donating one unit of whole blood, an individual donates a sufficient amount of blood to save three endangered lives. This is because after the donation, blood is processed into three blood components (*erythrocytes, plasma, and platelets*). Blood is also tested for different impurities, which could endanger the life of a patient. After the blood is processed into different components, it is also stored. The components are stored at a specified temperature before being delivered to hospitals. Blood donors can also donate just one of its components: *plasma, platelets, a concentrated dose of erythrocytes, granulocytes, etc.* From the donated blood components, such as plasma, blood medicines are made. The blood donor must have a healthy lifestyle so that his blood is free of viruses, bacteria, and other harmful impurities that could endanger his life and especially the life of a patient. For a patient to receive healthy blood with a transfusion, the blood must be tested with serological screening tests for HIV, syphilis, and hepatitis B and C. These tests are mandatory under different laws and regulations, especially in developed countries with higher incomes. These countries have developed national blood donor programs. Unfortunately, on the other side, countries that are still developing with low incomes, for example, third-world countries, have a severe blood shortage due to the insufficient number of blood donors. In these cases, it is even more common that a person gives blood only for payment. There is a greater chance that this sort of donated blood contains harmful impurities that can harm the patient. In these countries, the blood is hardly even tested for blood-transmission diseases.

Blood Transfusion and Transfusion Medicine

The patient receives blood through his vein into his circulatory system. The process of receiving blood into the body is professionally called a *"blood transfusion."* There are also specific terms that are used depending on what type of blood transfusion is performed, for example, *"plasma transfusion"* or *"platelet transfusion," "red blood cell transfusion,"* and *"granulocyte transfusion."* Often, to simplify, only the word *"transfusion"* is used. In order to have enough blood available for patients, we need on a daily basis healthy, adult, and altruistically motivated blood donors around the world who are always ready to help patients by donating their precious blood. Every second, there is someone in the world who needs blood to survive, and blood transfusions around the world save millions of precious lives. Transfusion medicine is a significant area of medicine that deals with all aspects of providing patients with safe blood, including other scientific topics.

Ljubljana, Slovenia   Zdravko Kvržić

Acknowledgments

For all of the support that has been given to me for my writing and research, I am thankful to my dear family. For all of the support and for believing in me, I am also sincerely grateful to my editor, Marie Come-Garry, Clinical Medicine, Nursing, and Midwifery Books. For giving his professional opinion about Chap. 7: The Discovery of Blood Groups in the Twentieth Century, for providing a photo of a Scannell apparatus, and for other information, I am sincerely thankful to Mr. Steven Pierce, a co-author of the book *Bloody Brilliant! A History of Blood Groups and Blood Groupers*, and an immunohematology historian. I am also sincerely thankful to Mr. Phil Learoyd, British Blood Transfusion Society archivist and historian, for answering my key questions regarding the early history of English transfusion medicine. I am also sincerely grateful to many other experts worldwide for providing me with the essential information and permission to use their images. I am also sincerely grateful to my allies and colleagues for their permission to use different images and for all of their support. Peter Kavčič, Lara Miholič Ilc, Rok Zabukovec, Lev Arnejšek, Simona and Primož Hozjan, Valerija Zupan, Miro Brus, Bogdan Fludernik, Romana Lesjak, Alenka Kryštufek, Marko Gomišček, Gabrijel "Elko" Borko, Borut Banič, Zvonka Zupanič Slavec Institute for the History of Medicine of the Faculty of Medicine in Ljubljana, Anna Stow Konservator Medicinhistoriska museet, Jelena Jovanović Simić Serbian Medical Society, Charles C. Thomas publisher, Elsevier publisher, BMJ publisher, Dulwich Society, King's College Hospital NHS Foundation Trust, Willy Toiviainen Finnish Red Cross Blood Service, Nurses and Midwives Association of Slovenia, Center for Public Relations and Marketing of the University Clinical Center Maribor, and the Archives of the Republic of Slovenia.

Ethics Approval For this research on history, informed consent to participate was obtained from individual participants. This research was also performed in line with the principles of the Declaration of Helsinki.

Contents

1 **Blood and the Circulatory System**......................... 1
   1.1 The Circulatory System............................... 1
   References.. 7

2 **The View and Study of Blood through History and its Impact on Blood Donation and Transfusion Medicine**................ 9
   2.1 The View on Blood in Ancient Times 9
   2.2 Scientific Debates and Discoveries 10
   2.3 The Discovery of Different Cells and Platelets in the Human Body 14
   References... 15

3 **The Curious Case of Pope Innocent VIII** 19
   3.1 The Origin of the Story and Later Impact 19
   3.2 Conclusion 23
   References... 23

4 **Animal Blood Donors for Human Patients**.................... 25
   4.1 Early Experiments 25
   4.2 Jean Denys Xenotransfusion 26
   References... 29

5 **The First Human to Human Blood Transfusion in 1818**......... 31
   5.1 James Blundell and His Fascination with Blood Transfusion Medicine 31
   5.2 The Impellor and the Gravitator......................... 35
   5.3 Influence of James Blundell on Blood Transfusion Medicine...... 37
   References... 38

6 **Interesting Cases of Blood Transfusion in the Nineteenth Century** 41
   6.1 Blood Transfusion Medicine in the Nineteenth Century.......... 41
   6.2 Nurse Tender in Ireland Gives Blood to Save a Woman 48
   6.3 Women as a Blood Donor for Patients with Hemophilia.......... 48
   6.4 A Blood Transfusion for a Boy with Hemophilia 49
   6.5 Blood Donation for Sister 50

	6.6	Early Case of a Successful Autotransfusion During an Operation in Europe	50
	6.7	Blood Transfusions in the USA	52
		6.7.1 Early Case of Autotransfusion in USA	53
	References		54
7	**The Discovery of Blood Groups in the Twentieth Century**		**57**
	7.1	The Discovery of Blood Groups and Later Achievements	57
		7.1.1 Some Early Observations on Hemolysis and Agglutination	58
		7.1.2 The Discovery of ABO Blood Group System by Karl Landsteiner 1900–1901	59
		7.1.3 Further Discoveries on ABO Blood Group System by Other Experts	60
		7.1.4 Some Interesting Facts About ABO Blood Group System	61
		7.1.5 Blood Grouping	62
	7.2	The Discovery of Rh Blood Group System	63
	7.3	Erythroblastosis Fetalis	64
	7.4	Discovery of Other Blood Group Systems	67
	7.5	Compatibility of Blood Donors and Patients Cross-Match Testing	69
	7.6	Definition of Universal Blood Donor and Patient	70
	7.7	Coombs Tests	70
	7.8	Important Events in Immunohematology and Serology	71
		7.8.1 Some Important Achievements in Serology in the 1950s	71
		7.8.2 Some Important Achievements in Immunohematology from the 1950s to 1970s	71
	7.9	Organ Transplantation	72
	7.10	Hematopoietic Stem Cell Transplantation	73
	References		74
8	**New Developments During World War I**		**79**
	8.1	Arteriovenous Anastomosis	79
	8.2	Anastomosis with Paraffin Wax Methods	81
	8.3	Syringe Methods During the War	87
	8.4	Introduction of Sodium Citrate as an Anticoagulant	89
	8.5	Interesting Cases of Blood Donation during World War I	100
		8.5.1 Blood Transfusion on the Battlefield	100
		8.5.2 Remarkable Operation	100
		8.5.3 A Courageous Wife	101
		8.5.4 Heroic Soldier	101
		8.5.5 Blood Transfusion for a Wounded Captain	101
	References		102

9 Different Methods of Blood Transfusion by the Twentieth Century ... 107
- 9.1 Difference Between Direct and Indirect Blood Transfusion ... 107
  - 9.1.1 Classification of Blood Transfusion Methods (1929–1949) ... 108
- 9.2 Blood Transfusion Apparatuses for Direct Blood Transfusion in the Twentieth Century ... 110
  - 9.2.1 The Images of Different Apparatuses for Direct Blood Transfusion (1920–1941) ... 114
- 9.3 Indirect Methods of Blood Transfusion ... 117
  - 9.3.1 Defibrinated Blood for Blood Transfusion ... 117
  - 9.3.2 Sodium Citrate for Blood Transfusion ... 118
- 9.4 Venesection and Venipuncture Technique ... 120
  - 9.4.1 Venesection Procedure ... 122
- 9.5 Dosage and Rate of Blood Transfusion ... 125
- References ... 139

10 The First Voluntary Blood Transfusion Service in the World ... 143
- 10.1 Percy Lane Oliver ... 143
- 10.2 Organization of the First Voluntary Blood Transfusion Service ... 144
- References ... 147

11 The First Blood Banks ... 149
- 11.1 Blood Bank ... 149
- 11.2 Early Blood Banks ... 150
  - 11.2.1 The First Blood Bank in the Soviet Union ... 150
  - 11.2.2 The First Blood Bank in Spain ... 151
  - 11.2.3 The First Blood Bank in the USA ... 152
- References ... 153

12 Blood Organization During the Spanish Civil War ... 155
- References ... 157

13 Transfusion Medicines During World War II ... 159
- 13.1 The United Kingdom ... 159
- 13.2 The United States of America ... 160
  - 13.2.1 Liquid and Dried Plasma and Serum ... 163
  - 13.2.2 Plasma for Britain ... 168
  - 13.2.3 Race Segregation of Blood Products ... 169
- 13.3 The Soviet Union ... 170
- 13.4 The Third Reich ... 170
- References ... 171

14 Equipment and Technology for Collection of Whole Blood and Blood Components 175
14.1 Equipment and Material for Whole Blood Collection.......... 175
14.2 Equipment and Material Standards 181
    14.2.1 Plastic Bags in Transfusion Medicine 184
    14.2.2 Whole Blood and Apheresis Technology.............. 188
References.. 200

15 Anticoagulants and Additive Solutions.......................... 205
15.1 Important Facts About Anticoagulants and Additive Solutions.................................... 205
    15.1.1 Some Important Events for Storing Red Blood Cells................................. 208
References.. 210

16 Processing and Storage of Blood Components................... 213
16.1 Processing of Whole Blood 213
16.2 Storage of Blood Components............................ 215
References.. 216

17 Blood Donor Screening....................................... 219
17.1 Syphilis 220
17.2 Hepatitis B 221
17.3 Hepatitis C 222
17.4 HIV and AIDS 223
    17.4.1 LGBTQ+ Community and Blood Donation 224
17.5 Interesting Facts About Different Tests 226
References.. 228

18 Blood Donors: The Past and the Present 231
18.1 Blood Donors... 231
    18.1.1 Blood Donor Eligibility........................... 233
    18.1.2 Variant Creutzfeldt-Jakob Disease (vCJD) as a Deferral for Blood Donation.................... 235
18.2 Some Important Events for Blood Donors and for Blood Donation 237
18.3 Establishment of Different Worldwide Organizations for Promotion of Blood Donation and Blood Transfusion Medicine 238
    18.3.1 The International Federation of Red Cross and Red Crescent Societies (IFRC).................. 239
    18.3.2 International Society of Blood Transfusion (ISBT)...... 239
    18.3.3 The Association for the Advancement of Blood and Biotherapies (AABB).................. 240
    18.3.4 The World Health Organization (WHO) 240
    18.3.5 The International Federation of Blood Donor Organizations (IFBDO) 240

		18.3.6	The European Blood Alliance (EBA) 241
		18.3.7	The Council of Europe. 241
		18.3.8	International Plasma and Fractionation Association (IPFA). 242
		18.3.9	Plasma Protein Therapeutics Association (PPTA). 242
	18.4	Young Blood Donor Associations 243	
	18.5	Presented Cases of Altruistic Worldwide Blood Donation in Different Tragedies 244	
	References. 245		
19	**Plasma Fractionation** 249		
	19.1	Important Milestones in Plasma Fractionation 249	
	19.2	The Shortage of Plasma Products 251	
	References. 253		
20	**COVID-19 Pandemic** 255		
	References. 257		

Appendix A: History of Transfusion Medicine in Slovenia from 1875 to 1945 259

Appendix B: History of Transfusion Medicine in Slovenia from 1945 to 2023 277

References 305

About the Author

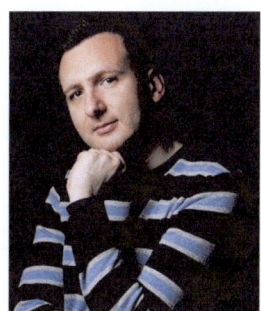

Zdravko Kvržić was born on November 27, 1987, in Ljubljana, Slovenia. After successfully completing primary school at "Osnovna šola Vide Pregarc," he enrolled in the four-year program to become a practical nurse at the secondary school of nursing, which he successfully completed in 2006. After that, he enrolled in a three-year first-cycle professional higher education study program in nursing at the Faculty of Health Sciences of the University of Ljubljana, where he graduated on time in 2010. The title of his graduation thesis is *"Nursing care of a patient after implantation of a total hip endoprothesis in the intensive care unit."* Kvržić has been a member of the *"Nurses and Midwives Association of Slovenia"* since 2011. He is a licensed registered nurse with many years of professional experience in the field of transfusion medicine, as he has been working at the *"Blood Transfusion Center of Slovenia"* since 2011. He works there as the head registered nurse of the plasmapheresis section, which is an organizational unit of the Center for Blood Donor Selection and Blood Collection of the Department of Blood Supply. Kvržić loves history and transfusion medicine as an important field in medicine, and therefore has thoroughly researched the extremely important and extensive history of blood donation and transfusion medicine within this book.

Blood and the Circulatory System 1

Contents

1.1 The Circulatory System.. 1
References... 7

1.1 The Circulatory System

Through an interconnected network of veins and arteries, our heart circulates blood throughout the body (Image 1.1). Another way to think about our circulatory system is to consider it our cardiovascular system. Vascular refers to blood vessels, while cardio indicates the heart.[1] The heart, arteries, capillaries, and veins are the system's main components.[2] The human body has two interconnected blood circulation systems, not just one. Blood is supplied to organs, tissues, and cells through systemic circulation, enabling them to absorb oxygen and other essential nutrients. The blood absorbs fresh oxygen through the pulmonary circulation. At the same time, the blood releases carbon dioxide.[3] The peripheral vessels transport deoxygenated blood back to the heart through the capillaries to the venules, out to the right side of the heart, and then to the lungs. The lungs transport oxygenated blood from the left

---

[1] Cleveland Clinic: Circulatory sytem. https://my.clevelandclinic.org/health/body/21775-circulatory-system (2023). Accessed 3 Dec 2023.

[2] Vascular Society: Circulatory system. https://www.vascularsociety.org.uk/patients/vascular_health/the_circulatory_system.aspx (2023). Accessed 3 Dec 2023.

[3] InformedHealth.org, Cologne, Germany: Institute for Quality and Efficiency in Health Care (IQWiG); 2006-. How does the blood circulatory system work? https://www.ncbi.nlm.nih.gov/books/NBK279250/. (2010). Accessed 3 Dec 2023.

© The Author(s), under exclusive license to Springer Nature
Switzerland AG 2024
Z. Kvržić, *History of Blood Donation and Transfusion Medicine*,
https://doi.org/10.1007/978-3-031-68715-0_1

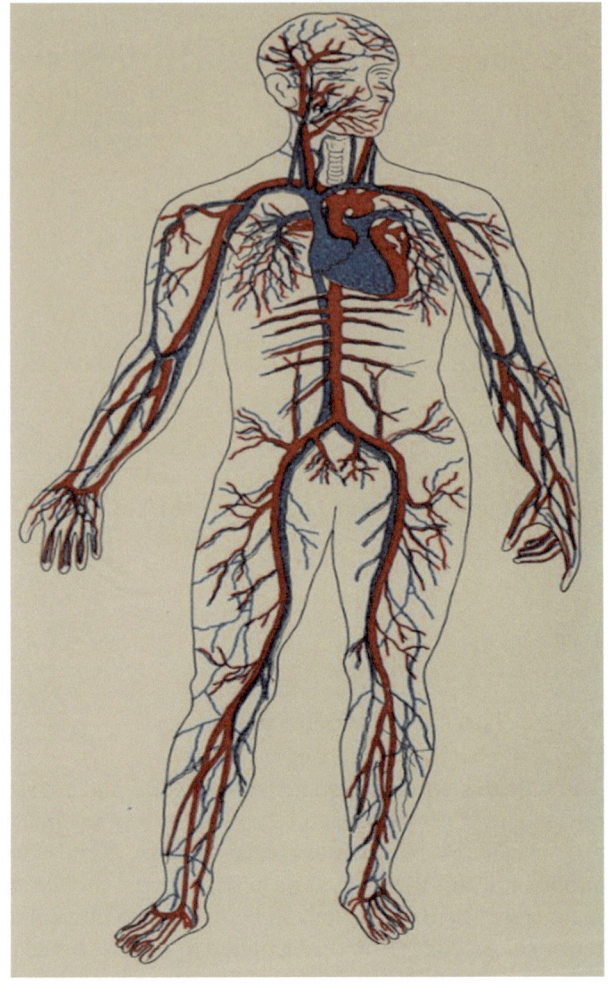

Image 1.1 The circulatory system. (Source: Brands, O. M., Van Gieson H. C. The circulatory system. An Academic Physiology and Hygiene. Boston, B. H. Sanborn & co, 1903. Retrieved from the Library of Congress, public domain. www.loc.gov/item/03014869/. Accessed 7 Dec 2023)

side of the heart to the aorta, then to the arteries, arterioles, and finally to the capillaries, where nutrient exchange takes place. Oxygen and nutrients are mainly stored and unloaded in the capillaries.[4] One of the major differences between arteries and veins is that from our heart, the arteries carry oxygenated blood through our body, and veins carry deoxygenated blood back to our heart. The valves of veins, with hard work against gravity, ensure blood flows toward the heart.[5] The blood vessels that carry blood out of the heart (arteries) and those that return blood to the heart

---

[4] Tucker WD, Arora Y, Mahajan K. Anatomy, Blood Vessels. In: StatPearls. Treasure Island (FL): StatPearls Publishing; 2023. https://www.ncbi.nlm.nih.gov/books/NBK470401/. Accessed 3 Dec 2023.

[5] USA Vein Clinics: Understanding vein valves: importance and function. https://www.usaveinclinics.com. /blog/what-are-vein-valves/ (2023). Accessed 3 Dec 2023.

(veins) are connected by capillaries, the smallest and most common type of blood vessel. The exchange of materials between tissue cells and blood is the capillaries' main purpose.[6] Regarding other small blood vessels, such as venules and arterioles, venules receive blood from the capillaries. They are involved in the exchange of nutrients and oxygen for water products as well.[7] Connectors between our arteries and capillaries are arterioles, small blood channels that transport blood away from our heart. Their muscles change their diameter, which allows them to regulate our blood pressure and blood flow throughout our body. To exchange waste, nutrients, and oxygen, they link with capillaries.[8]

Blood is a unique kind of bodily fluid. Red blood cells (erythrocytes), white blood cells (leukocytes), platelets (thrombocytes), and plasma make up its four primary constituent parts. Blood serves a variety of purposes, such as delivering nutrition and oxygen to the tissues and lungs; creating clots of blood to stop excessive bleeding; containing antibodies and cells to combat infection; delivering waste materials to the liver and kidneys, which clean and filter the blood; and controlling the body temperature.[9] This is also important for maintaining homeostasis.

Homeostasis is the ability to sustain the internal environment without giving way to outside factors that could upset the state of balance.[10]

Whole blood is composed of roughly 45% red cells.[11] Approximately 55% of our blood is made up of plasma, which has antibodies called immunoglobulins that help fight infection. These antibodies are used to create medications that treat immune disorders, genetic conditions, and rare diseases.[12] The body produces antibodies, also known as immunoglobulins, which are Y-shaped molecules of proteins that aid in the defense against foreign substances known as antigens. Any material that triggers the immune system to create antibodies is considered an antigen. The bacteria, viruses, or fungi that cause illness and infection are known as antigens.[13]

Occasionally misconstrued as a synonym for plasma, serum is actually plasma without fibrinogen. In plasma, there are 8–9% solids and 91–92% water. It is primarily made up of proteins like albumin and globulin, coagulants like fibrinogen,

---

[6] National Cancer Institute, seer training modules: Classification and structure of blood vessels. https://training.seer.cancer.gov/anatomy/cardiovascular/blood/classification.html (2023). Accessed 3 Dec 2023.

[7] Tucker WD, Arora Y, Mahajan K. 2023.

[8] Cleveland Clinic. Arterioles. https://my.clevelandclinic.org/health/body/23377-arterioles. Accessed 11 Jan 2024.

[9] American society of hematology: Blood basics. https://www.hematology.org/education/patients/blood-basics (2023). Accessed 3 Dec 2023.

[10] Libretti S, Puckett Y. Physiology, Homeostasis. In: StatPearls. Treasure Island (FL): StatPearls Publishing. 2023. https://www.ncbi.nlm.nih.gov/books/NBK559138/. Accessed 3 Dec 2023.

[11] American Red Cross: What does hematocrit mean? https://www.redcrossblood.org/donate-blood/dlp/hematocrit.html (2023). Accessed 3 Dec 2023.

[12] NHS blood and transplant: What is plasma. https://www.blood.co.uk/plasma/what-is-plasma/. Accessed 3 Dec 2023.

[13] Microbiology info: Differences beetween Antigen and Antibody. https://microbiologyinfo.com/differences-between-antigen-and-antibody/ (2023). Accessed 3 Dec 2023.

which help in blood clotting, and electrolytes like sodium, potassium, bicarbonate, chloride, and calcium, which support blood pH maintenance.[14] The process of forming a blood clot to stop bleeding from a damaged blood vessel is known as blood coagulation or blood clotting. There are three stages involved in blood clotting. During the first phase, certain coagulation factors that are present in the blood or released by platelets and wounded tissue, as well as calcium ions, assist in the formation of prothrombin activator at the site of blood vessel injury. The blood protein prothrombin is changed into thrombin in the second stage by the prothrombin activator.[15] The third phase is a physiological process in the blood called the enzymatic action of thrombin on fibrinogen, which forms fibrin, a polymeric protein. Fibrin's fibrous structure forms a web of fibers that encloses blood cells and squeezes blood serum, causing clotting of the blood.[16] Plasma contains large amounts of the complex glycoprotein fibrinogen. When fibrinogen converts into fibrin, hemostasis is also boosted.[17] Hemostasis is a process or procedure utilized to stop bleeding. The creation of a platelet plug, blood clotting, and the narrowing of the bleeding blood vessel comprise the intricate process of spontaneous hemostasis.[18] The process by which blood cells are formed is called hematopoiesis.[19] The bone marrow is the spongy material found in the hollow centers of an individual's long bones.[20] Periosteum, the hard outer layer of bone, protects the bone marrow.[21] Blood cells in the bone marrow start out as stem cells, which is the first phase of all blood cells.[22] When blood cells reach maturity and are needed, a healthy bone marrow releases them into the bloodstream. Without bone marrow, our bodies are unable to produce red blood cells (RBC).[23] Bone marrow can be red and yellow. At birth, all bone marrow is red. Nearly all of the red marrow is replaced by yellow marrow by the time an individual reaches old age. However, if there is a greater demand for RBC, such

---

[14] Mathew J, Sankar P, Varacallo M. Physiology, Blood Plasma. In: StatPearls. Treasure Island (FL): StatPearls Publishing. 2023. https://pubmed.ncbi.nlm.nih.gov/30285399/. Accessed 3 Dec 2023.

[15] Hrvatska enciklopedija: Zgrušavanje krvi. https://www.enciklopedija.hr/Natuknica.aspx?ID=67187 (2023). Accessed 3 Dec 2023.

[16] Hrvatska enciklopedija: Fibrin. https://www.enciklopedija.hr/natuknica.aspx?ID=19435 (2023). Accessed 3 Dec 2023.

[17] Pieters M, Wolberg AS. Fibrinogen and fibrin: An illustrated review. Res Pract Thromb Haemost. 2019 4;3(2):161–172. https://www.ncbi.nlm.nih.gov/pmc/articles/PMC6462751/

[18] Hrvatska enciklopedija: Hemostaza. https://www.enciklopedija.hr/Natuknica.aspx?ID=24967 (2023). Accessed 3 Dec 2023.

[19] Jagannathan-Bogdan M., Zon L. I. Hematopoiesis. Development. 2013 Jun;140(12):2463–7. https://www.ncbi.nlm.nih.gov/pmc/articles/PMC3666375/.

[20] Better Health: Bone Marrow. https://www.betterhealth.vic.gov.au/health/conditionsandtreatments/bone-marrow. (2023). Accessed 4 Dec 2023.

[21] CLL society. What is bone marrow. https://cllsociety.org/2016/09/what-is-bone-marrow/ Accessed 4 Jan 2024.

[22] John Hopkins medicine. Facts about blood. https://www.hopkinsmedicine.org/health/wellness-and-prevention/facts-about-blood Accessed 10 Jan 2024.

[23] Better Health: Bone Marrow, 2023.

1.1 The Circulatory System

as in blood loss situations, the yellow marrow may turn red again.[24] Important elements of blood like RBC, white blood cells, and platelets are produced in the red bone marrow. The ends of long bones, including the ribs, spine, shoulder blades, and skull, contain red bone marrow. Cartilage, fat cells, and bones are all produced by the yellow bone marrow.[25] It is called yellow blood marrow because of its high concentration in fat cells. It can be found in the medullary cavity in the shaft of long bones, and a layer of red bone marrow surrounds it. It also aids in the storage of fats in cells named adipocytes. This helps preserve the right environment and provides the necessary nourishment for the bones to function.[26]

Erythrocytes carry oxygen that keeps all body cells alive, and in normal conditions, they live for about 120 days. Unlike other cells, RBC do not have a nucleus.[27] The normal number of erythrocytes in adult men is 4.7–6.1 and in women, 4.2–5.4 million cells/mcL.[28] An iron-rich protein found in RBC is called hemoglobin. It is what makes blood red, and a normal level of hemoglobin in adults is around 120 g/L to 180 g/L.[29] Significantly important are the body's hemoglobin and hematocrit levels. Oxygen is transported to the body's tissues with hemoglobin, a protein present in RBC. The hematocrit measures the volume of RBC in relation to the volume of whole blood, which includes both RBC and plasma.[30] Normal results of hematocrit are 40.7–50.3% for men and 36.1–44.3% for women.[31]

Leukocytes protect us against disease and illness. They are stored in lymph tissues and blood. Because certain types of white blood cells only live for 1–3 days, our bone marrow produces them continuously.[32] The normal number of leukocytes

---

[24] Medscape. Bone marrow anatomy. https://emedicine.medscape.com/article/1968326-overview?form=fpf#a2 Accessed 10 Jan 2024.

[25] Bansal hospital. What are yellow bone marrow and red bone marrow? What is their difference? https://bansalhospital.com/yellow-bone-marrow-vs-red-bone-marrow/ Accessed 10 Jan 2024and Redne

[26] Moffitt cancer center. What is bone marrow? https://www.moffitt.org/treatments/blood-bone-marrow-transplant/what-is-bone-marrow/ Accessed 10 Jan 2024. and

[27] Udruga darivatelja krvi: Eritrociti koji život znače. http://uddk.hr/jeste-li-znali/eritrociti-koji-%c5%beivot-zna%c4%8de (2023). Accessed 3 Dec 2023.

[28] Mount Sinai: RBC count. https://www.mountsinai.org/health-library/tests/rbc-count (2023). Accessed 4 Dec 2023.

[29] Canadian Blood Services: What you need to know about hemoglobin, anemia, iron and hemochromatosis. https://www.blood.ca/en/blood/am-i-eligible-donate-blood/abcs-eligibility/what-you-need-to-know-about-hemoglobin-hemochromatosis-iron-anemia#hemoglobin (2023). Accessed 4 Dec 2023.

[30] Billett HH. Hemoglobin and Hematocrit. In: Walker HK, Hall WD, Hurst JW, editors. Clinical Methods: The History, Physical, and Laboratory Examinations. third edition. Boston: Butterworths; 1990. Chap. 151. https://www.ncbi.nlm.nih.gov/books/NBK259/. Accessed 3 Dec 2023.

[31] Mount Sinai: Hematocrit. https://www.mountsinai.org/health-library/tests/hematocrit (2023). Accessed 4 Dec 2023.

[32] Stanford medicine: children's health. https://www.stanfordchildrens.org/en/topic/default?id=what-are-white-blood-cells-160-35 (2023). Accessed 3 Dec 2023.

in the blood of adults is around 4.5–11.0 × 10^9/L.[33] Granulocytes are a subset of white blood cells with tiny granules. There are proteins in this granule. Granulocytes come in three distinct varieties: neutrophils, eosinophils, and basophils.[34] Agranulocytes are made up of monocytes and lymphocytes. Although they do not have particular granules, they do have azurophilic granules.[35] Azurophilic granules contain peptides that provide strong antimicrobial activity through both oxidative and non-oxidative pathways.[36]

Small blood cells called platelets serve a variety of physiological functions, the most well-studied of which is thrombosis activation. They are essential for sustaining enough blood volume in patients with vascular injury because of their clotting activity and activation of the coagulation cascade.[37] Platelets essentially form a blood clot and aid in stopping bleeding. They migrate to the site of a blood vessel injury and form clumps.[38] Platelets have a limited lifespan; they are eliminated from the bloodstream after about 10 days.[39] Platelets are also anucleated.[40] The normal number of platelets in the blood of adults is around 150–400 × 10^9/L.[41]

Our body and its cardiovascular system enable us to carry out our daily activities. It is also important to maintain a healthy lifestyle so that our internal processes can provide us with a good quality of life.

---

[33] Mount Sinai: WBC count. https://www.mountsinai.org/health-library/tests/wbc-count (2023). Accessed 4 Dec 2023.

[34] Medlineplus: Granulocyte. https://medlineplus.gov/ency/article/003440.htm. Accessed 3 Dec 2023.

[35] Tigner A, Ibrahim SA, Murray IV. Histology, White Blood Cell. In: StatPearls [Internet]. Treasure Island (FL): StatPearls Publishing; 2023. https://www.ncbi.nlm.nih.gov/books/NBK563148/. Accessed 3 Dec 2023.

[36] Koenig J. M., Bliss J. M., Mariscalco M. M, Section XX: Developmental Immunobiology,126 - Normal and Abnormal Neutrophil Physiology in the Newborn. In: Polin R. A., Abman S. H., Rowitch D. H., Benitz W. E., Fox W. W, editors.; Fetal and Neonatal Physiology (Fifth Edition), New York. Elsevier; 2017, p. 1216–1229. https://www.sciencedirect.com/science/article/abs/pii/B9780323352147001268 Accessed 10 Jan 2024.

[37] Fountain JH, Lappin SL. Physiology, Platelet. In: StatPearls [Internet]. Treasure Island (FL): StatPearls Publishing; 2023 Jan-. https://www.ncbi.nlm.nih.gov/books/NBK470328/

[38] Canadian Cancer Society: The blood and bone marrow. https://cancer.ca/en/cancer-information/what-is-cancer/blood-and-bone-marrow. (2023) Accessed 3 Dec 2023.

[39] LeBrasseur N. Platelets' preset lifespan. J Cell Biol. 2007;23;177(2):186. https://www.ncbi.nlm.nih.gov/pmc/articles/PMC2064146/

[40] Williams O, Sergent SR. Histology, Platelets. In: StatPearls [Internet]. Treasure Island (FL): StatPearls Publishing; 2023 Jan-. https://www.ncbi.nlm.nih.gov/books/NBK557800/

[41] Mount Sinai: Platelet count. https://www.mountsinai.org/health-library/tests/platelet-count (2023). Accessed 4 Dec 2023.

References

1. American Society of Hematology: Blood basics. https://www.hematology.org/education/patients/blood-basics (2023). Accessed 3 Dec 2023.
2. American Red Cross: what does hematocrit mean? https://www.redcrossblood.org/donate-blood/dlp/hematocrit.html (2023). Accessed 3 Dec 2023.
3. Billett HH. Hemoglobin and hematocrit. In: Walker HK, Hall WD, Hurst JW, editors. Clinical methods: the history, physical, and laboratory examinations. 3rd ed. Boston: Butterworths; 1990. Chapter 151. https://www.ncbi.nlm.nih.gov/books/NBK259/ Accessed 3 Dec 2023.
4. Better health: bone marrow. https://www.betterhealth.vic.gov.au/health/conditionsandtreatments/bone-marrow. 2023. Accessed 4 Dec 2023.
5. Bansal Hospital. What are yellow bone marrow and red bone marrow? What is their difference? https://bansalhospital.com/yellow-bone-marrow-vs-red-bone-marrow/ Accessed 10 Jan 2024.
6. Cleveland Clinic: circulatory sytem. https://my.clevelandclinic.org/health/body/21775-circulatory-system (2023). Accessed 3 Dec 2023.
7. Cleveland Clinic. Arterioles. https://my.clevelandclinic.org/health/body/23377-arterioles. Accessed 11 Jan 2024.
8. Canadian Cancer Society: the blood and bone marrow. https://cancer.ca/en/cancer-information/what-is-cancer/blood-and-bone-marrow. 2023. Accessed 3 Dec 2023.
9. Canadian Blood Services: What you need to know about hemoglobin, anemia, iron and hemochromatosis. https://www.blood.ca/en/blood/am-i-eligible-donate-blood/abcs-eligibility/what-you-need-to-know-about-hemoglobin-hemochromatosis-iron-anemia#hemoglobin. 2023. Accessed 4 Dec 2023.
10. CLL society. What is bone marrow. https://cllsociety.org/2016/09/what-is-bone-marrow/. Accessed 10 Jan 2024.
11. Fountain JH, Lappin SL. Physiology, platelet. In: StatPearls [internet]. Treasure Island, FL: StatPearls Publishing; 2023. https://www.ncbi.nlm.nih.gov/books/NBK470328/. Accessed 3 Dec 2023.
12. Hrvatska enciklopedija: Zgrušavanje krvi. https://www.enciklopedija.hr/Natuknica.aspx?ID=67187 (2023). Accessed 3 Dec 2023.
13. Hrvatskaenciklopedija:Fibrin. https://www.enciklopedija.hr/natuknica.aspx?ID=19435. Accessed 3 Dec 2023.
14. Hrvatska enciklopedija: Hemostaza. https://www.enciklopedija.hr/Natuknica.aspx?ID=24967. 2023. Accessed 3 Dec 2023.
15. InformedHealth.org, Cologne, Germany: Institute for Quality and Efficiency in Health Care (IQWiG); 2006. How does the blood circulatory system work? https://www.ncbi.nlm.nih.gov/books/NBK279250/. 2010. Accessed 3 Dec 2023.
16. Jagannathan-Bogdan M, Zon LI. Hematopoiesis. Development. 2013;140(12):2463–7. https://www.ncbi.nlm.nih.gov/pmc/articles/PMC3666375/
17. John Hopkins medicine. Facts about blood. https://www.hopkinsmedicine.org/health/wellness-and-prevention/facts-about-blood Accessed 10 Jan 2024.
18. Koenig JM, Bliss JM, Mariscalco MM. Section XX: developmental Immunobiology,126 - Normal and abnormal neutrophil physiology in the newborn. In: Polin RA, Abman SH, Rowitch DH, Benitz WE, Fox WW, editors. Fetal and neonatal physiology. 5th ed. New York: Elsevier; 2017. p. 1216–29. https://www.sciencedirect.com/science/article/abs/pii/B9780323352147001268 Accessed 10 Jan 2024.
19. LeBrasseur N. Platelets' preset lifespan. J Cell Biol. 2007;177(2):186. https://www.ncbi.nlm.nih.gov/pmc/articles/PMC2064146/
20. Libretti S, Puckett Y. Physiology, homeostasis. In: StatPearls. Treasure Island, FL: StatPearls Publishing; 2023. https://www.ncbi.nlm.nih.gov/books/NBK559138/ Accessed 3 Dec 2023.
21. Medlineplus:Granulocyte. https://medlineplus.gov/ency/article/003440.htm. Accessed 3 Dec 2023.

22. Mathew J, Sankar P, Varacallo M. Physiology, blood plasma. In: StatPearls. Treasure Island, FL: StatPearls Publishing; 2023. https://pubmed.ncbi.nlm.nih.gov/30285399/ Accessed 3 Dec 2023.
23. Microbiology info: differences beetween antigen and antibody. https://microbiologyinfo.com/differences-between-antigen-and-antibody/. 2023. Accessed 3 Dec 2023.
24. Mount Sinai. WBC count. https://www.mountsinai.org/health-library/tests/wbc-count. 2023. Accessed 4 Dec 2023.
25. Mount Sinai. RBC count. https://www.mountsinai.org/health-library/tests/rbc-count (2023). Accessed 4 Dec 2023.
26. Mount Sinai. Platelet count. https://www.mountsinai.org/health-library/tests/platelet-count. 2023. Accessed 4 Dec 2023.
27. Mount Sinai. Hematocrit. https://www.mountsinai.org/health-library/tests/hematocrit (2023). Accessed 4 Dec 2023.
28. Medscape. Bone marrow anatomy. https://emedicine.medscape.com/article/1968326-overview?form=fpf#a2 Accessed 10 Jan 2024.
29. Moffitt Cancer Center. What is bone marrow? https://www.moffitt.org/treatments/blood-bone-marrow-transplant/what-is-bone-marrow/. Accessed 10 Jan 2024.
30. National Cancer Institute, seer training modules: classification and structure of blood vessels. https://training.seer.cancer.gov/anatomy/cardiovascular/blood/classification.html (2003). Accessed 3 Dec 2023.
31. NHS blood and transplant: what is plasma. https://www.blood.co.uk/plasma/what-is-plasma/ Accessed 3 Dec 2023.
32. Pieters M, Wolberg AS. Fibrinogen and fibrin: an illustrated review. Res Pract Thromb Haemost. 2019;3(2):161–72. https://www.ncbi.nlm.nih.gov/pmc/articles/PMC6462751/
33. Bay Medical Center, Northwell health: Red Bone Marrow Vs. Yellow Bone Marrow. https://www.pbmchealth.org/news-events/blog/red-bone-marrow-vs-yellow-bone-marrow. 2023. Accessed 4 Dec 2023.
34. Stanford medicine: children's health. https://www.stanfordchildrens.org/en/topic/default?id=what-are-white-blood-cells-160-35(2023). Accessed 3 Dec 2023.
35. Tucker WD, Arora Y, Mahajan K. Anatomy, blood vessels. In: StatPearls. Treasure Island, FL: StatPearls Publishing; 2023. https://www.ncbi.nlm.nih.gov/books/NBK470401/. Accessed 3 Dec 2023.
36. Tigner A, Ibrahim SA, Murray IV. Histology, white blood cell. In: StatPearls [internet]. Treasure Island (FL): StatPearls Publishing; 2023. https://www.ncbi.nlm.nih.gov/books/NBK563148/. Accessed 3 Dec 2023.
37. USA Vein Clinics: Understanding vein valves: importance and function. https://www.usaveinclinics.com/blog/what-are-vein-valves/. 2023. Accessed 3 Dec 2023.
38. Udruga darivatelja krvi: Eritrociti koji život znače. http://uddk.hr/jeste-li-znali/eritrociti-koji-%c5%beivot-zna%c4%8de (2023). Accessed 3 Dec 2023.
39. Vascular Society: circulatory system. https://www.vascularsociety.org.uk//patients/vascular_health/the_circulatory_system.aspx (2023). Accessed 3 Dec 2023.
40. Williams O, Sergent SR. Histology, platelets. In: StatPearls [internet]. Treasure Island, FL: StatPearls Publishing; 2023. https://www.ncbi.nlm.nih.gov/books/NBK557800/.

Image Source

Brands OM, Van Gieson HC. The circulatory system. An academic physiology and hygiene. Boston: B. H. Sanborn & Co; 1903. Retrieved from the Library of Congress, public domain. www.loc.gov/item/03014869/. Accessed 7 Dec 2023

The View and Study of Blood through History and its Impact on Blood Donation and Transfusion Medicine

Contents

2.1 The View on Blood in Ancient Times.. 9
2.2 Scientific Debates and Discoveries... 10
2.3 The Discovery of Different Cells and Platelets in the Human Body...................... 14
References.. 15

2.1 The View on Blood in Ancient Times

Since ancient times, stories of blood transmission have been found in many written traditions of all peoples. Fairy tales, stories, poems, Egyptian papyri, plates from ancient Nineveh, written in cuneiform, the Bible, etc. tell about it.[1] Nonetheless, these all are mythical tales. Many philosophers and doctors described blood in different forms. The Chinese book *The Yellow Emperor's Classic of Internal Medicine* has several pages, for the first time scientifically written, about blood. There are different opinions about when the book was written, but it was probably written between the periods of 260 before Christ (BC) and 220 years after our Lord (AD).[2] In the book, the court doctor Qi Bo, among other things, explains to Huang Di, the Yellow Emperor: *"The heart is responsible for blood flow. When the heart is attacked*

---

[1] Gjukić N. O transfuziji krvi. Liječnički vjesnik: glasilo Hrvatskoga liječničkog zbora. 1929; 51(6), p. 253–290. http://library.foi.hr/lib/casopis.php?%20sqlx=S01101&H=&E=&broj=192900006%20&sqlid=1&U=gjuki%E6.

[2] Wang B. The Su Wen of the Huangdi Neijing (Inner Classic of the Yellow Emperor), China: Publisher not identified]; 1115 to 1234, p. 1–67. https://www.loc.gov/item/2021666312. Accessed 3 Apr 2020.

© The Author(s), under exclusive license to Springer Nature Switzerland AG 2024
Z. Kvržić, *History of Blood Donation and Transfusion Medicine*, https://doi.org/10.1007/978-3-031-68715-0_2

by heat, the blood flows upward."[3] Publius Ovidius Naso (March 20, 43 BC–17/18 AD), a Roman poet, mentions in his book *Metamorphoses* the mythological verses of the sorceress and priestess Medea, which testify that in ancient times people wondered about the greater importance of blood for life*: "Un-sheath your blades, and let out the old blood, so that I can fill the empty veins with new!"* [4] The ancient Greeks had, in general, great knowledge of different subjects and a scientific explanation of blood. For example, they knew that blood was important for our lives and that without blood in the body, there was no life. They also knew about venous and arterial blood.[5]

Everything mentioned proves that blood was important in everyday life in ancient times, just as it is today. The early modern period (AD 1450–AD 1750) marked the beginning when people began to think about blood transfusion as an idea, and slowly, through different periods, they began with the first experiments. First with blood transfusions from animal to animal, then from animal to human, and then from human to human. The first successful blood transfusion from animal to animal was in 1665 by Richard Lower; the first from animal to human blood transfusion was in 1667 by Jean Baptiste Denys; and the first from human to human blood transfusion was in 1818 by James Blundell.

The first blood transfusion textbook was published in Bologna in 1668 and was titled "*Relazione dell'esperienze fatti Inghilerra, Francia ed Italia intorno alla celebre e famosa trasfusione del sangue per tutto maggio 1668.*" (Report of the experiences made in England, France, and Italy around the celebrated and famous blood transfusion throughout May 1668.) The report was a collection of tracts and journals from 1667 that were published in Paris and London, along with additional notes on experiments conducted by Magnani in Rome.[6]

2.2 Scientific Debates and Discoveries

Blood transfusion was discussed in the sixteenth century by Hieronymus Cardanus. Hieronymus Cardanus, also known as Girolamo Cardano (1501–1576), an Italian polymath in 1558 wrote [41, p. 141]: "*There are those who hope to be able to*

---

[3] Maoshing Ni. The Yellow Emperor's Classic of Medicine, USA: Shambhala; 1995. https:/books.google.si/. Accessed 3 Apr 2020. P. 163.
[4] Ovid.P.N. Metamorphoses (Kline) 7, the Ovid Collection, USA: Univ. of Virginia E-Text Center; 2020 https://ovid.lib.virginia.edu/trans/Metamorph7.htm. Accessed 3 Apr 2020.
[5] Meletis, J., & Konstantopoulos, K. (2010). The beliefs, myths, and reality surrounding the word hema (blood) from homer to the present. Anemia. 2010, p. 1–7. https://www.ncbi.nlm.nih.gov/pmc/articles/PMC3065807/ Accessed 4 Apr 2020.
[6] Brewer H.F., Ellis R., Greaves R. I. N., Keynes G., Mills F. W., Bodley Scott R., Till A., Whitby L. Blood transfusion. Bristol: John Wright & sons LTD. London: Simpkin Marshall (1941). LTD.;1949. Preface.

2.2 Scientific Debates and Discoveries

exchange blood with another young man of good character with a double fistula, others with a single fistula."[7]

Magnus Pegelius, also known as Magnus Pegel (1547–1619), a German doctor and mathematician, is sometimes credited as being the first to describe the possibility of blood transfusion. The date of his work is from the year 1604, but the work of Cardanus, which suggests the possibility of transferring blood from one human to another, is much older and dates from the year 1558.

Magnus Pegelius does not, in fact, explain the blood transfusion procedure, as some sources claim [41, p. 111–115].[8] His words are ambiguous; he does mention the change of some kind, but not in a specific way. Some sources have interpreted this as Pegelius referring to blood transfer of any kind.

One of the earliest claims in favor of Pegelius's ambiguous words may be found in *"Transactions of the Medical Society of the State of Pennsylvania, Fourth Series, Part I (1865)"* [42, p. 387–393].[9]

As a matter of fact, the German chemist and doctor Andreas Libavius (c. 1550–1616) in 1615 described blood transfusion in detail: *"Given, one has before oneself a strong, healthy, youth rich in spirited blood and a powerless, weak, cachectic old man scarcely capable of breathing. If now the doctor wishes to practice the rejuvenating art on the latter, he should make silver tubes which fit into each other: open then the artery of the healthy person and introduce one of the tubes into it and fasten it to the artery; thereupon he opens also the artery of the ill person and fastens the other, female tube into it. These two tubes one fits into the other and notes herewith that the warm and spirited arterial blood of the healthy person flows into the ill person and imparts to him the fountain of life and drives away all faintness."*[10]

In 1616, at the College of Physicians in England, English doctor William Harvey (April 1, 1578 to June 3, 1657) described in detail the systemic blood circulation (Image 2.1) and the role of the heart in circulation: *"It is plain from the structure of the heart that the blood is passed continuously through the lungs to the aorta as by the two clacks of a water bellows to raise water. It is shown by the application of a ligature that the passage of the blood is from the arteries into the veins. Whence it follows that the movement of the blood is constantly in a circle, and is brought about by the beat of the heart. It is a question therefore whether this is for the sake of nourishment or rather for the preservation of the blood and the limbs by the*

---

[7] Girolamo C. De rerum varietate, libri XVII. Avignon: M. Vincentius; 1558, p. 441 https://archive.org/details/dererumvarietate00card/page/440/mode/2up Accessed 7 Dec 2023.

[8] Magnus P. Thesaurus Rerum, Selectarum, Magnarum, Dignarum, Utilium, Suavium, Pro generis humani salute oblatus. Rostock; 1604, p. 111–116. https://www.zvdd.de/dms/load/met/?PPN=PPN816124795 Accessed 7 Dec 2023.

[9] The Society. Transactions of the Medical Society of the State of Pennsylvania, Fourth Series, Part I. Collins, Printer, 705 Jayne street; 1865, p. 387–393 https:/books.google.si/ Accessed 7 Dec 2023.

[10] Maluf, N. S. R. History of Blood Transfusion. Journal of the History of Medicine and Allied Sciences. 1954;9(1), p. 59–107. https://pubmed.ncbi.nlm.nih.gov/13118144/.

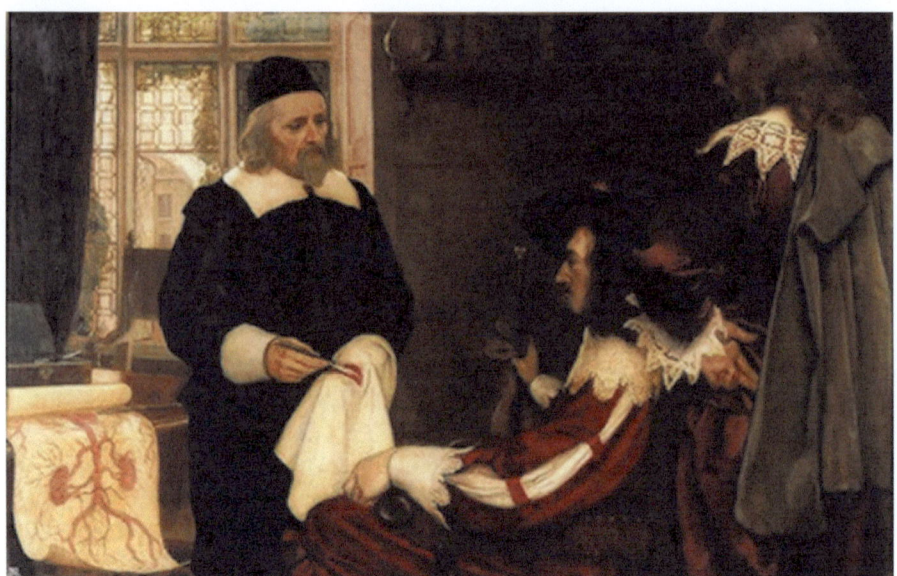

Image 2.1 William Harvey demonstrating his theory of circulation of blood before Charles I. (Source: William Harvey demonstrating his theory of circulation of blood before Charles I. Oil painting by Ernest Board. Available at: Wellcome Collection, public domain. https://wellcomecollection.org/works/skj2d74p/image?id=jwpexqb8 Accessed 7 Dec 2023)

communication of heat, the blood cooled by warming the limbs being in turn warmed by the heart."[11]

Throughout history, in addition to William Harvey and the Chinese, several doctors and philosophers from the fifth BC to the seventeenth century AD, such as *Hippocrates, Aristotle, Erysistratus, Galen, Ibn Al Nafis, Miguel Servetus, Andreas Vesalius, Realdus Columbus, Girolamo Fabrici d'Acquapendente, Marcelo Malpighi, Andrea Cesalpino,* and *Jacques Dubois,* have discussed and written on the systemic and pulmonary circulation.[12, 13] In general, some authors defend the aforementioned experts as the first to describe systemic blood circulation; some described it more accurately than others, while others explained that the most accurate description was given by William Harvey. However, the fact is that it was only after William Harvey published a detailed work on blood circulation in the book *"Exercitatio Anatomica de Motu Cordis et Sanguinis in Animalibus"* (*An Anatomical*

---

[11] Power, D.A. William Harvey. London: T Fisher Unwin; 1897, p. 62–67. https://archive.org/details/williamharvey00powerich/page/66/mode/2up?ref=ol&view=theater Accessed 15 Aug 2020.

[12] Akmal M, Zulkifle M, Ansari A. Ibn nafis—a forgotten genius in the discovery of pulmonary blood circulation. Heart Views. 2010; 11(1), p. 26–30. https://www.ncbi.nlm.nih.gov/pmc/articles/PMC2964710/.

[13] Aird WC. Discovery of the cardiovascular system: from Galen to William Harvey. J Thromb Haemost. 2011; 9(1), p. 118–29. https://pubmed.ncbi.nlm.nih.gov/21781247/.

Study of the Movement of Heart and Blood in Animals) in 1628, which was published in Frankfurt, that doctors slowly began to show interest in the realization of the idea of blood transfusion.

Giovanni Colle (1558–1630), professor of medicine at Padua in 1628, wrote about the idea of blood transfusion*:* "*Someone will rise up again, and it will be a futile attempt, while through fewer and better we can achieve what we wished for, as if some blood issuing from the vein of a healthy young man, permeates through a tube hot in the veins of the old man, drawing in breath the young man and the old man, and inhaling them so that the young man's blood is drawn in by the old man, that his blood should not come out. This dwarf's blood can restore moisture and temperance, as Aristotle taught. If an old man had the eyes of a young man, would he not see as a young man? Would he not feel and reason as a youth if he possessed the heart and brain of a youth, then even if he obtained the blood of a youth? to live as a young man.*"[14]

Robert Desgabets (1610–1678), a French Cartesian philosopher and Benedictine prior, was an early proponent of blood transfusion. He defended and described it in *"Desgabets' Discourse on the Communication or Blood Transfusion of Blood."* Desgabets presented his study in Paris in 1658.[15] He referred to blood transfusion as communication, and by that, he meant that "*communication is an effective passage of blood from a healthy man or some other animal into the veins of a weak or sick man.*" He stated that for blood transfusion, the vein of a person should be open and that a small tube should be inserted into the opening of the vein. He also described a machine for blood transfusion with two small silver tubes:[16] "*The machine that I imagine for this operation is simple and consists only of two small silver tubes, one whose end is open like a trumpet for its gentle application against the vessels that must give the blood; and the other is of a thickness proper to the insertion into the opening of the vein. The other two ends of the tubes communicate together by means of a small leather pouch of the thickness of a walnut* etc." Furthermore, Desgabets concurred that blood should be maintained warm, transfused gradually, and kept free of air. He additionally stated that the patient should not be exposed to excessive or insufficient amounts of fresh blood.[17]

Another interesting fact is that Johann Daniel Major (1634–1693), a physician in Germany in 1664, advocated for blood transfusion and intravenously administered medication.[18] Francesco Folli, a physician from Florence in 1680, based on William

---

[14] Alessandro S. Origine E vicende della transfusione del sangue. Bologna cooperativa tipografica azzoguidi-XI; 1933, p. 69–70.

[15] Easton, P., Robert Desgabets on the Physics and Metaphysics of Blood Transfusion. In: Dobre, M., Nyden, T. (eds) Cartesian Empiricisms. Studies in History and Philosophy of Science; vol 31. Springer, Dordrecht; 2013, p. 185–193.

[16] B. Noel. Les débuts expérimentaux de la transfusion sanguine, Transfusion. 1960, 3(3), p. 287–292. https://www.sciencedirect.com/science/article/abs/pii/S0372124860800367.

[17] Easton, 2013, p. 185–193.

[18] Maluf, 1954, p. 60.

Harvey's thesis, developed the theory that blood transfusions could potentially treat illnesses and revitalize the elderly.[19]

2.3 The Discovery of Different Cells and Platelets in the Human Body

The discoveries of several cells and platelets helped experts understand what size and structure the discovered cells had, and it helped them understand their functions.

Antoine Philips Van Leeuwenhoek (October 24, 1632 to August 26, 1723) was a Dutch microbiologist and microscopist first described RBC in the seventeenth century; it took more than 160 years for William Addison (1803–1881), a British physician, and Gabrielle Andral (November 6, 1797 to February 13, 1876), a French pathologist and a professor, to use improved microscopes to distinguish the much less common white blood cells (WBCs). Although he observed the WBCs with his basic monocular microscopes, Leeuwenhoek did not classify them as a distinct group. Paul Ehrlich (March 14, 1854 to August 20, 1915) was a German physician and scientist, and others then characterized the fundamental categories of WBC in terms of their morphology, with the majority of them being given one or more functions throughout the late nineteenth and early twentieth centuries. Although Astrid Fagraeus (May 30, 1913 to February 24, 1997), a Swedish immunologist, demonstrated in 1948 that immunoglobulins are produced by plasma cells, the relationship between lymphocytes and plasma cells was not confirmed until 1973.[20] William Hewson (November 4, 1739 to May 1, 1774), a surgeon, anatomist, and physiologist from Britain known as the "*father of hematology*" in the 1770s, contributed to our understanding of RBC, the lymphatic system, the thymus, and the spleen in addition to identifying fibrinogen.[21] Throughout the nineteenth century, Rudolph Virchow (October 13, 1821 to September 5, 1902) was, among others, a German pathologist, scientist, and doctor who produced a lot of discoveries. He discovered via observation that only specific cells or cell types can get ill, not an entire body. One of Virchow's many discoveries was the discovery of cells in connective tissue and bone, as well as the description of compounds like myelin. Leukemia was initially identified by him. He was the first to describe the pulmonary thromboembolism mechanism. He provided evidence that venous thrombi can be the source of blood clots in the pulmonary artery. Virchow recognized the connection between human and animal diseases and created the term "*zoonosis*" to denote this relation-

---

[19] Keynes G. The history of blood transfusion, section I. In: Brewer H.F., Ellis R., Greaves R. I. N., Keynes G., Mills F. W., Bodley Scott R., Till A., Whitby L. Blood transfusion. Bristol: John Wright & sons LTD. London: Simpkin Marshall (1941). LTD.;1949, p. 4–7.

[20] Doherty, P., The Red and white: ancient history, Nat. Rev. Immunol., 2016. 16,77: 1. https://www.nature.com/articles/nri.2016.1#citeas.

[21] Doyle, D., William Hewson (1739–74): the father of haematology. British Journal of Haematology. 2006; 133(4), p. 375–381. https://onlinelibrary.wiley.com/doi/full/10.1111/j.1365-2141.2006.06037.x.

ship between infectious diseases affecting both human and animal health.[22] Italian pathologist Giulio Bizzozero (March 20, 1846 to April 8, 1901) made the discovery of platelets in 1882. In the circulating blood of living creatures as well as in blood that had been drawn from blood vessels, he viewed them under a microscope.[23] In the late 1920s, Max Wintrobe (October 27, 1901 to December 9, 1986), an Austrian-born American physician, defined normal blood levels. He improved the hematocrit as a quantitative indicator of red cells and was the first to classify anemias[24] according to their size, including microcytic, normocytic, and macrocytic.[25] In 1959, Max Ferdinand Perutz (May 19, 1914 to February 2002), a molecular biologist, and his colleague, another structural biologist, John Kendrew, discovered the structure of hemoglobin and a related oxygen-carrying protein found in muscles, myoglobin.[26]

The presented cases demonstrate that people always knew that blood was important. Ideas and beliefs about blood changed as medicine advanced, leading to the realization that not only was blood transfusion possible but that it could also benefit humanity. Experts from the past needed to understand how the body functioned, not just for their everyday lives but also for medicine. Experts wanted to understand how they could help their patients with their health problems and how to treat their diseases so that they would get healthy. A lot of times, experts lived in periods where modern technology, as we know it today, was not available. For those reasons, they had to constantly develop new methods, approaches, and techniques for treating patients. Understanding how systemic circulation functions, as well as blood itself, was just one of many important things for doctors to understand. This all encouraged experts to experiment with blood transfusions.

References

1. Alessandro S, Origine E vicende della blood transfusione del sangue. Bologna cooperativa tipografica azzoguidi –XI.; 1933. p. 69–70.
2. Akmal M, Zulkifle M, Ansari A. Ibn nafis—a forgotten genius in the discovery of pulmonary blood circulation. Heart Views. 2010;11(1):26–30. https://www.ncbi.nlm.nih.gov/pmc/articles/PMC2964710/
3. Aird WC. Discovery of the cardiovascular system: from Galen to William Harvey. J Thromb Haemost. 2011;9(1):118–29. https://pubmed.ncbi.nlm.nih.gov/21781247/

---

[22] Schultz M., Rudolph Virchow, Emerg. Infect. Dis., 2008; 14 (9): 1480—1841. https://www.ncbi.nlm.nih.gov/pmc/articles/PMC2603088/.

[23] Ribatti D, Crivellato E. Giulio Bizzozero and the discovery of platelets, Leuk Res., 2007; 31(10): 1339–41. https://pubmed.ncbi.nlm.nih.gov/17383722/.

[24] Anaemia is Anemia is a condition that occurs when your blood produces fewer healthy RBC than is typical.

[25] NEJM Resident 360. History of Hematology. https://resident360.nejm.org/content-items/history-of-hematology (2020). Accessed 23 May 2020.

[26] Steensma D.P., Shampo M. A., Kyle R. A. Max Perutz and the structure of hemoglobin. Mayo Clin Proc., 2015; 90(8), p. 89. https://pubmed.ncbi.nlm.nih.gov/26250737/. Accessed 23 May 2020.

4. Noel B. Les débuts expérimentaux de la blood transfusion sanguine. Blood Transfus. 1960;3(3):287–92. https://www.sciencedirect.com/science/article/abs/pii/S0372124860800367
5. Brewer HF, Ellis R, Greaves RIN, Keynes G, Mills FW, Bodley SR, Till A, Whitby L. Blood transfusion. Bristol: John Wright & sons LTD. London: Simpkin Marshall (1941). LTD. Preface; 1949.
6. Keynes G. The history of blood transfusion, section 1. In: Brewer HF, Ellis R, Greaves RIN, Keynes G, Mills FW, Bodley Scott R, Till A, Whitby L, editors. Blood transfusion. Bristol: John Wright & sons LTD. London: Simpkin Marshall (1941). LTD.; 1949. p. 4–7.
7. Doherty P. The red and white: ancient history. Nat Rev Immunol. 2016;16(77):1. https://www.nature.com/articles/nri.2016.1#citeas
8. Doyle D. William Hewson (1739–74): the father of haematology. Br J Haematol. 2006;133(4):375–81. https://doi.org/10.1111/j.1365-2141.2006.06037.x.
9. Easton P. Robert Desgabets on the physics and metaphysics of blood transfusion. In: Dobre M, Nyden T, editors. Cartesian empiricisms. Studies in history and philosophy of science, vol. 31. Dordrecht: Springer; 2013. p. 185–93.
10. Girolamo C. De rerum varietate, libri XVII. Avignon: M. Vincentius; 1558. p. 441. https://archive.org/details/dererumvarietate00card/page/440/mode/2up. Accessed 7 Dec 2023
11. Gjukić NO. transfuziji krvi. Liječnički vjesnik: glasilo Hrvatskoga liječničkog zbora. 1929;51(6):253–90. Liječnički vjesnik : glasilo Hrvatskoga liječničkog zbora. - (foi.hr)
12. Maluf NSR. History of blood transfusion. J Hist Med Allied Sci. 1954;9(1):59–107. https://pubmed.ncbi.nlm.nih.gov/13118144/
13. Ni M. The Yellow Emperor's classic of medicine, USA: Shambhala; 1995, p. 163. https://books.google.si/, Accessed 3 Apr 2020.
14. Meletis J, Konstantopoulos K. The beliefs, myths, and reality surrounding the word hema (blood) from homer to the present. Anemia. 2010, 2010:1–7. https://www.ncbi.nlm.nih.gov/pmc/articles/PMC3065807/. Accessed 4 Apr 2020
15. Magnus P, Rerum T, Selectarum M, Dignarum U. Suavium, Pro generis humani salute oblatus. Rostock. 1604:111–6. https://www.zvdd.de/dms/load/met/?PPN=PPN816124795. Accessed 7 Dec 2023
16. NEJM Resident 360. History of hematology. https://resident360.nejm.org/content-items/history-of-hematology (2020). Accessed 23 May 2020.
17. Ovid.P.N. Metamorphoses (Kline) 7, the Ovid collection, USA: Univ. of Virginia E-Text Center; 2020 https://ovid.lib.virginia.edu/trans/Metamorph7.htm Accessed 3 Apr 2020.
18. The Society. Transactions of the Medical Society of the State of Pennsylvania, Fourth Series, Part I. Collins, Printer, 705 Jayne street; 1865. P. 387–393 https:/books.google.si/ Accessed 7 Dec 2023.
19. Power DA. William Harvey. London: T Fisher Unwin; 1897. https://archive.org/details/williamharvey00powerich/page/66/mode/2up?ref=ol&view=theater. Accessed 15 Aug 2020
20. Ribatti D, Crivellato E. Giulio Bizzozero and the discovery of platelets. Leuk Res. 2007;31(10):1339–41. https://pubmed.ncbi.nlm.nih.gov/17383722/
21. Steensma DP, Shampo MA, Kyle RA. Max Perutz and the structure of hemoglobin. Mayo Clin Proc. 2015;90(8):–89. Available at: https://pubmed.ncbi.nlm.nih.gov/26250737/ Accessed 23 May 2020
22. Schultz M. Rudolph Virchow. Emerg Infect Dis. 2008;14(9):1480–841. https://www.ncbi.nlm.nih.gov/pmc/articles/PMC2603088/
23. Wang B. The Su Wen of the Huangdi Neijing (Inner Classic of the Yellow Emperor), China: Publisher not identified]; 1115 to 1234. https://www.loc.gov/item/2021666312. Accessed 3 Apr 2020.

Image Source

William Harvey demonstrating his theory of circulation of blood before Charles I. Oil painting by Ernest Board. Available at: Wellcome Collection, public domain. https://wellcomecollection.org/works/skj2d74p/image?id=jwpexqb8. Accessed 7 Dec 2023.

The Curious Case of Pope Innocent VIII

3

Contents

3.1 The Origin of the Story and Later Impact... 19
3.2 Conclusion... 23
References.. 23

3.1   The Origin of the Story and Later Impact

Pope Innocent VIII (1432–1492) was born in Genoa, Italy, as Giovanni Battista Cybo, or Cibo. He was, among others, Cardinal of Santa Cecilia in the Trastevere Rione and Bishop of Molfettha; he then became head of the Catholic Church and ruled the Papal States from September 8, 1484, until his death on July 7, 1492. He assumed the name Innocent VIII as a newly elected pontiff.[1] He was seriously ill several times between 1484 and 1492. The pontiff was also falsely pronounced dead a couple of times. Every time it appeared that the pontiff was dead, he surprised everyone with his recovery. His health rapidly deteriorated from March to July of 1492. His medical issues recurred and worsened due to abdominal pains, feverish attacks, and inflammation of an old sore on his leg. In the last 5 days of his life, he suffered and died in agony. Following his death, the republican and Roman Senate secretary, Infessura Stephanus (c. 1436–1500), spread the rumor of the pontiff's alleged blood therapy. One of the reasons why Infessura could have spread the

---

[1] Pastor L. F. V. The history of the popes from the close of the Middle Ages: drawn from the secret archives of the Vatican and other original sources, volume V. London: Kegan Paul, Trench, Trübner and CO; 1901, p. 238–320. https://ia600203.us.archive.org/12/items/historyofthepope05pastuoft/historyofthepope05pastuoft.pdf Accessed 7 Apr 2020.

© The Author(s), under exclusive license to Springer Nature
Switzerland AG 2024
Z. Kvržić, *History of Blood Donation and Transfusion Medicine*,
https://doi.org/10.1007/978-3-031-68715-0_3

rumor can be found in the fact that, immediately after Innocent VIII was elected as pope, he had pledged his word to the magistrates to bestow all civic offices and benefits on Roman citizens only. The pontiff failed to keep his promise due to various political reasons, such as rewarding his important electors and their adherents. Failed promises enraged Infessura, leading him to compose a series of caustic epigrams against the pontiff.[2] Also, Infessura was an ardent Republican who looked at the papal government from Rome with unfriendly eyes. Besides Pope Innocent VIII, he sharply criticized Pope Sixtus IV.[3] Infessura, in his book *Diario della città di Roma*, wrote that a Jewish doctor took blood from the veins of three young boys, each of whom was 10 years old, with the promise of giving each boy a ducat. He wanted to cure the pontiff with their blood, but soon after the bloodletting, they died. The Jewish doctor fled, and the pontiff was not cured.[4, 5] What is also interesting is that the people who were present at that time, for example, chroniclers, ambassadors, and colleagues of the pope, did not mention anything about the Pope receiving any kind of blood therapy.[6] It must be pointed out that some sources claim as a fact or as a suggestion that the pontiff drank blood, but it is clear that Infessura does not mention how the blood was actually administered to the pontiff.

"*The New Catholic Dictionary*" from 1929 rejects Infessura as a reliable chronicler because of the preposterous and malevolent rumors in his book.[7] An early mention of the death of Pope Innocent VIII is mentioned in a book *Volume XXII. Commentariorum Urbanorum Libri* by the author, the historian Raffaello Maffei (1451–1522), known among others as Raphael de Volterra or Volaterranus. Maffei mentions the Pope's death but does not mention anything about a blood therapy that was supposedly performed on Pope Innocent VIII as a healing method to prolong life.[8] However, in the eighteenth century, it was possible to trace the first claim about the Pope's alleged blood therapy.

In 1754, Italian historian and oratorian Odorico Raynaldo (1595–January 22, 1671) wrote that the pontiff was treated with a preparation of blood, with no mention of how the blood was administered.[9] The story about the pontiff receiving a blood transfusion was written in the nineteenth century by the Swiss historian Jean

---

[2] Lbid.

[3] Mandell C. A history of the papacy during the period of reformation. England: Longmans, Green and CO; 1887. P. 284. https://books.google.si Accessed 7 Apr 2020.

[4] Morselli E. La trasfusione del sangue. Loescher; 1876, p. 12. https://books.google.si/ Accessed 7 Apr 2020.

[5] Infessura S. Diario della città di Roma di Stefano Infessura scribasenato. Nuova edizione a cura di Oreste Tommasini. Roma Forzani e c; 1890, p. 275–276. https://archive.org/details/diariodellacitt01infeuoft/page/276/mode/2up?q=sanatus Accessed 10 Dec 2023.

[6] G.A. Lindeboom. The Story of a Blood Transfusion to a Pope. Journal of the History of Medicine and Allied Sciences. 1954; 9(4), p. 459. https://pubmed.ncbi.nlm.nih.gov/13212030/.

[7] The New Catholic Dictionary. The Universal knowledge foundation, New York; 1929, p. 509. https://archive.org/details/TheNewCatholicDictionary_201906 Accessed 7 Apr 2020.

[8] Lindeboom, 1954, p. 459.

[9] Hebbel E. Hoff and Roger Guillemin. "The first experiments on transfusion in France." Journal of the History of Medicine and Allied Sciences. 1963; 18 (2), p. 103–124.

Charles Léonard de Sismondi (May 9, 1773–June 25, 1842). In his version, the three boys were subjected to the device, which was to make their blood transfuse to the pontiff and his blood enter their veins. The boys allegedly died of an air embolism.[10]

Sismondi knew about blood transfusions since the first from animal to human was performed in the late seventeenth century. However, there was no device capable of performing a blood transfusion in 1492. Sismondi's motives for mentioning blood transfusions are not known. It remains unclear if someone told him the story as a fact and believed it to be true or if he fabricated the whole thing. However, it is clear that Infessura's story influenced Sismondi's version because of the similarities between them.

In 1927, Holmes à Court wrote that the Jewish doctor's name who took the blood from the children was Abraham Myers. In the Middle Ages, barber-surgeon guilds had absolute rights for bloodletting, not doctors.[11] Barber-surgeons performed bloodletting by executing miniature, sharp cuts in the skin and allowing the patient's blood to flow into a bowl. Sometimes healers would use leeches to draw out the blood.[12]

The surname of this doctor is also sometimes written as Mayr. He was a real person. Abraham di Mayr de Balmes of Lecce was a doctor whom Pope Innocent VIII granted the privilege to graduate in medicine in Naples and to practice on all patients without regard for their religion in 1492. He died in 1523 in Venice and was also respected by the Catholic community. He was the doctor of Cardinal Grimani. In the Middle Ages, Jewish doctors were educated at the same universities as their colleagues of other religions.[13]

It could be that the author Holmes à Court chose the Jewish doctor Abraham di Mayr de Balmes as a result of Pope Innocent VIII's help in becoming a doctor. He was, of course, not a personal doctor of Pope Innocent VIII. It could also be possible that Infessura mentioned that the doctor was Jewish as a result of Pope Innocent VIII showing favor to Jewish doctors, perhaps because Infessura despised them. The assumption that Infessura had something against the Jews comes from the fact that he specifically pointed out that the supposed doctor was a Jew.

Throughout history, for example, in the Middle Ages, Jews were falsely accused of blood libel. In those cases, they were accused of murdering Christians and using

---

[10] Sismondi J. C. L., Histoire des républiques italiennes du moyen âge, vol. 6. Société typographique belge, 1839, p. 215. https://www.google.si/books/edition/Histoire_des_r%C3%A9publiques_italiennes_du/1DdBAAAAcAAJ?hl=sl&gbpv=0 Accessed 7 April 2020.

[11] Gottlieb A.M. History of the First Blood Transfusion but a Fable Agreed Upon: The Transfusion of Blood to a pope, Transfusion Medicine Reviews, 1991, 5(3), p. 228–235. https://pubmed.ncbi.nlm.nih.gov/1821180/.

[12] Toney A. Medieval medicine and disease. San Diego, CA: ReferencePoint Press, Inc.; 2015. p. 23. https://archive.org/details/medievalmedicine0000allm/page/22/mode/2up?q=bloodletting Accessed 9 Dec 2023.

[13] Friedenwald H. Jewish physicians in italy: their relation to the papal and italian states, Publications of the American Jewish Historical Society, 28; 1922, p. 133–211. https://www.jstor.org/stable/pdf/43059382.pdf. Accessed 7 Apr 2020.

their blood in their rituals.[14] Early Christians were also accused of blood libel by the Romans.[15]

It is worth noting that Jewish and Christian doctors did not promote blood intake therapy to their patients because the Jewish dietary regulations, Kashrut, and the biblical prohibition on drinking blood strictly prohibited blood intake. People in the Middle Ages were very religious and afraid of God's wrath if they disobeyed the holy rules. There are sources that mention drinking blood in different rituals across the world and in different periods of time. However, reading such claims must be done with caution because the whole population of the past did not drink blood on an everyday basis. Consuming blood on a daily basis may result in an iron overload in the body as well as the spread of pathogens that may cause various illnesses.

In the present time, there is another doctor who is accused of allowing or performing the controversial blood therapy on Pope Innocent VIII. He goes by the name of Giacomo di San Genesio. There are different versions that claim that di San Genesio was a doctor who, by chance, was in Rome when the pontiff was dying, or that he was his Jewish doctor who allowed the blood therapy and afterward quickly fled. These are all completely fictional stories.

Several doctors served Pope Innocent VIII. They were Ludovico Podocataro, the bishop of Carpaccio, who later became cardinal; the ecclesiastic and later cardinal Ferdinando Ponzetti; Benedetto Porcocinti; Pietro Macerata; and Giacomo di San Genesio.[16] Regarding their religion, they were all Catholics. So the story about the pontiff having an official Jewish doctor is absolutely not true.

Giacomo di San Genesio was the most famous and skilled of the five. His real name was "*Giacomo (Jacopo) di Agnolo Solleciti da San Ginesio.*" He was born in the town of San Ginesio, near the city of Macerata, in the region of Marche. His nickname was "*il Sanginesio.*" Jacopo was the Latin translation of his name, Giacomo, and his real surname was Solleciti. All the sources who wrote about his biography agree that he was born in 1415, but the year of his death ranges from

---

[14] Dundes A., The Blood Libel Legend: A Casebook in Anti-Semitic Folklore, University of Wisconsin Press.; 1991. p. 32.

[15] Luijk R. V., Children of Lucifer: The Origins of Modern Religious Satanism. New York: Oxford University Press; 2016. p. 26.

[16] Marini G. L. Degli Archiatri Pontifici, volume 1. Roma: nella stamperia Pagliarini; 1784, p. 218–233.

1482 to 1495. Some wrote that he died in San Ginesio, others in Ancona, and still others in Rome.[17, 18, 19, 20, 21, 22, 23]

The year and place of his death are debatable. He could not have possibly died in 1482 or 1484, as some claim. Interestingly, some sources agree that he died before Pope Innocent VIII, while others claim the year of his death to be 1495. He could not have died before Pope Innocent VIII because he treated him until he died. Whatever the year and location of his death, he successfully treated the pontiff a couple of times with his knowledge. Nevertheless, if he was alive or dead at the time the pontiff was dying, it is clear that despite the pontiff having five doctors, their knowledge and experience could not have helped them save his life. There were also no compelling reasons why they should have sought advice at that time, particularly from the less experienced doctor, Abraham di Mayr.

3.2 Conclusion

There is no real evidence that could support the stories, from the pontiff's death to the present, that the pontiff received any kind of blood therapy. The official report about his death does not mention anything about this, and there were no eyewitnesses to support these alleged claims. A great injustice is being done to Pope Innocent VIII because of the fabricated stories. There are numerous online sources where people can read and comment on the fabricated stories about this case. A lot of the commentaries on Pope Innocent VIII and the Catholic Church are very disrespectful. More than 500 years have passed since the death of Pope Innocent VIII, and this case proves how a rumor can echo through time and do unnecessary damage to someone's reputation. The question remains: how long will this case continue to be presented as a truth despite the fact that it never happened?

References

1. Colucci G. Antichità picene, X; 1791, XXIV–XXXI.
2. Colucci G. Antichità picene, XXIII; 1795, 228–233.
3. Claudi GM, Catri L. Dizionario biografico dei marchigiani ad vocem; 2002, 463.

---

[17] Panelli G., Memorie degli uomini illustri e chiari in medicina del Piceno o sia della Marca di Ancona, vol. 2; 1758, p. 65–66.

[18] Marini,1784, p. 206–216.

[19] Colucci G., Antichità picene, vol. X; 1791, p. XXIV–XXXI.

[20] Colucci G., Antichità picene, vol. XXIII; 1795, p. 228–233.

[21] Gentili G. A., 'Jacopo da Sanginesio Archijatro di Sisto IV e Innocenzo VIII,' in "Rivista di storia delle scienze mediche e naturali", gennaio-aprile n. 1; 1952, p. 50–77.

[22] Claudi G. M., Catri L., Dizionario biografico dei marchigiani ad vocem; 2002, p. 463.

[23] Staffeti di L., *Il libro de' ricordi della famiglia Cybo,* pubblicato con introduzione, appendice di documenti inediti, note illustrative e indice analitico di Luigi Staffetti, "Atti della Società ligure di storia patria, 38; 1910, p. 225.

4. Dundes A. The blood libel legend: a casebook in anti-semitic folklore. University of Wisconsin Press; 1991. p. 32.
5. Friedenwald H. Jewish physicians in Italy: their relation to the papal and italian states. Publications of the American Jewish Historical Society. 1922;28:133–211. https://www.jstor.org/stable/pdf/43059382.pdf. Accessed 7 Apr 2020
6. Luijk RV. Children of Lucifer: the origins of modern religious Satanism. New York: Oxford University Press; 2016. p. 26.
7. Lindeboom GA. The story of a blood transfusionto a pope. J Hist Med Allied Sci. 1954;9(4):459. https://pubmed.ncbi.nlm.nih.gov/13212030/
8. Gottlieb AM. History of the first blood transfusionbut a fable agreed upon: the blood transfusion of blood to a pope. Blood Transfus Med Rev. 1991;5(3):228–35. https://pubmed.ncbi.nlm.nih.gov/1821180/
9. Gentili GA. Jacopo da Sanginesio Archijatro di Sisto IV e Innocenzo VIII. In "Rivista di storia delle scienze mediche e naturali", gennaio-aprile n. 1; 1952, p. 50–77.
10. Hoff HE, Guillemin R. The first experiments on blood transfusion in France. J Hist Med Allied Sci. 1963;18(2):103–24.
11. Infessura S. Diario della città di Roma di Stefano Infessura scribasenato. Nuova edizione a cura di Oreste Tommasini. Roma Forzani e c. 1890:275–6. https://archive.org/details/diariodellacitt01infeuoft/page/276/mode/2up?q=sanatus. Accessed 10 Dec 2023
12. Mandell C. A history of the papacy during the period of reformation. England: Longmans, Green and CO; 1887. p. 284. https://books.google.si Accessed 7 Apr 2020
13. Morselli E. La trasfusione del sangue. Loescher. 1876:12. https://books.google.si/. Accessed 7 Apr 2020
14. Marini GL. Degli Archiatri Pontifici, volume 1. Roma: nella stamperia Pagliarini; 1784. p. 218–33.
15. Pastor LFV. The history of the popes from the close of the middle ages: drawn from the secret archives of the Vatican and other original sources, volume V. London: Kegan Paul, Trench, Trübner and CO; 1901. p. 238–320. https://ia600203.us.archive.org/12/items/historyofthepope05pastuoft/historyofthepope05pastuoft.pdf Accessed 7 Apr 2020
16. Panelli G. Memorie degli uomini illustri e chiari in medicina del Piceno o sia della Marca di Ancona. 2; 1758, 65–66.
17. Sismondi JCL. Histoire des républiques italiennes du moyen âge, vol. 6. Société typographique belge, 1839, p. 215. https://www.google.si/books/edition/Histoire_des_r%C3%A9publiques_italiennes_du/1DdBAAAAcAAJ?hl=sl&gbpv=0. Accessed 7 April 2020.
18. Staffeti di L. Il libro de' ricordi della famiglia Cybo, pubblicato con introduzione, appendice di documenti inediti, note illustrative e indice analitico di Luigi Staffetti, "Atti della Società ligure di storia patria, 38; 1910, 225.
19. The New Catholic Dictionary. The universal knowledge foundation. New York; 1929. p. 509. https://archive.org/details/TheNewCatholicDictionary_201906. Accessed 7 Apr 2020
20. Toney A. Medieval medicine and disease. San Diego, CA: ReferencePoint Press, Inc.; 2015. p. 23. https://archive.org/details/medievalmedicine0000allm/page/22/mode/2up?q=bloodletting. Accessed 9 Dec 2023

Animal Blood Donors for Human Patients

Contents

4.1 Early Experiments.. 25
4.2 Jean Denys Xenotransfusion.. 26
References... 29

4.1 Early Experiments

As described in the following cases, early experiments were carried out from one animal to another. Francis Potter in 1652 advocated blood transfusion for curing different diseases. He tried to perform a blood transfusion on the hen, but he could not find its vein.[1] A German horseman named Georg von Wahrendorff administered the first injections into the bloodstream in 1642 by injecting wine into the veins of his hunting dogs using tiny fowl bones. It is claimed that he used a variety of medications to treat sick dogs in this way. Christopher Wren (1632–1723), just 24 years old, made a vivacious dog drunk in Oxford in 1656 by injecting wine and beer directly into its veins. In 1663, the physician Timothy Clarke demonstrated injecting different medications into the veins of living animals.[2]

The first successful blood transfusion performed among animals is credited to English doctor Richard Lower (ca. 1631–January 17, 1691), who performed the first blood transfusion of this kind from artery to vein.

---

[1] Surgenor D., The red blood cell, New York and London: Academic press inc. 1974, p. 25. Available at: https://www.google.si/books/edition/The_Red_Blood_Cell/wDAxXpY4TCsC?hl=sl&gbpv=1. Accessed 16 Aug 2020.

[2] Maluf, 1954, p. 60.

In February 1665, Lower drew blood from an exposed jugular vein of a medium-sized dog with a cannula. The dog was severely weakened, and Lower bound the larger dog along with the smaller dog and allowed its blood to flow from the cervical artery into the smaller dog. This rushing in of blood soon transfused too much, as evidenced by the returning restlessness of the engorged dog. The artery of the blood donor was ligated, and blood was again withdrawn from the recipient. This withdrawal was repeated with another large dog until neither blood nor life remained. In the meantime, blood was being drawn away and turned loose from the small dog, equaling, in the amount that Lower would judge, the weight of its body. Nevertheless, its jugular was again joined, and its chains were unfastened. The animal immediately leaped down from the table and, apparently forgetful of its injuries, fawned upon its master. It then cleansed itself of blood, rolled in the grass, and apparently was no more inconvenienced than if it had been thrown into a flowing stream. Lower presented his case in December 1666 in the Transactions of the Philosophical Society.[3] For this reason, some sources incorrectly mention that Lower performed his first blood transfusion in 1666, when in fact he actually performed it in 1665.

4.2   Jean Denys Xenotransfusion

In the second half of the seventeenth century, experts mainly used lamb and calf blood to perform xenotransfusions. The first case of blood xenotransfusions from an animal to a human was carried out by the French doctor and Professor of philosophy and mathematics Jean-Baptiste Denys (ca.1635–1704) and the surgeon Paul Emmerez in 1667. Denys was convinced that animal blood is inherently purer than human blood because unhealthy lifestyles such as eating unhealthy and drinking are not common in animals and because healthy animal blood can cure a person of various diseases. He was convinced that if people could drink milk from animals and eat their meat, they could also receive their blood. Denys and Emmerez transfused lamb's blood to a 15- or 16-year-old youth suffering from a severe form of violent fever (Image 4.1). In the hope of reducing the fever, the doctors bled him twenty times, as a result of which he was further weakened. With the help of surgeon Emmerez, Denys decided to perform the xenotransfusions based on the young man's greater blood loss as a result of the blood leak. At 5 a.m., the patient's vein was punctured and the blood flowed into the container. They noted that the blood was "*thick and black*." They then transfused 3 ounces of lamb blood (about 90 mL) from the lamb's carotid artery into the patient's vein. During the blood transfusion, the patient reported feeling intense heat moving up his arm, which was a classic example of a hemolytic transfusion reaction.[4] After the procedure, it was reported that the young man was functioning normally, that he ate his meal without

---

[3] Hollingsworth M. W., Blood Transfusion by Richard Lower in 1665. Annals of medical history. 1928; 10(3), p. 213–225. https://www.ncbi.nlm.nih.gov/pmc/articles/PMC7940049/

[4] Haemolytic transfusion reaction is the breakdown of RBC.

4.2 Jean Denys Xenotransfusion

Image
4.1 Xenotransfusion from lamb to man. (Source: Xenotransfusion from lamb to man. Available at: Wellcome Collection https://wellcome.org/. Published under CC BY 4.0 DEED. Accessed 20 April 2020)

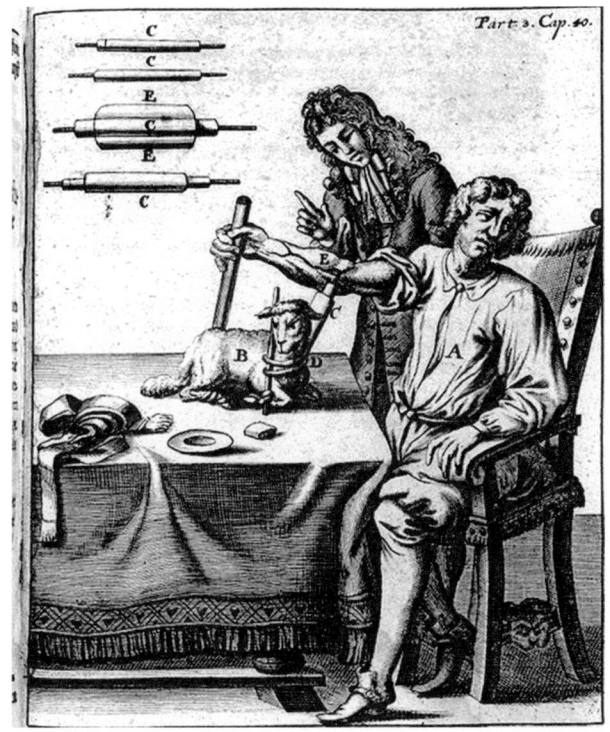

hindrance, and that he was calm and happy. A few hours later, he had a minor nosebleed.[5, 6]

It is repeatedly stated that Jean Baptiste Denys, with the aid of surgeon Paul Emmerez, performed the first blood transfusion from an animal to a human on June 15, 1667, in Paris. However, Denys met with his 15-year-old patient on June 15, 1667, and observed him while eating dinner and later breakfast. The blood transfusion took place at 5 o'clock in the morning. That means that it was performed on June 16 or even 17.[7]

Fortunately, compared to other cases of xenotransfusions, the young man survived because of the smaller amount of transfused blood. In cases where patients received more animal blood, blood transfusion reactions were more intense, leading to death.

In one of Denyse's xenotransfusions in 1668, his patient died, and he found himself in court. He was found not guilty, but on April 17, 1668, the Chatalet court

---

[5] Farr AD. The first human blood transfusion. Med Hist. 1980; 24(2) p. 143–62. Available at: https://www.ncbi.nlm.nih.gov/pmc/articles/PMC1082701/. Accessed 17 Apr 2020.

[6] Roux, F.A, Saï, P, Deschamps, J.Y.Xenotransfusions, past and present, Xenotransplantation the official journal of the international xenotransplantation association.2007;14(3), p. 208–216. Available at: https://pubmed.ncbi.nlm.nih.gov/17489860/. Accessed 17 Apr 2020.

[7] Farr 1980, page 152.

legally adopted a decision on a partial ban on blood transfusions: "*Blood transfusions on humans will not be performed without the prior consent of the doctors of the Paris Medical Faculty.*" Doctors at the Paris Medical School opposed blood transfusions, and in the seventeenth century, they no longer approved any. The judgment of the Paris parliament confirmed the decision on January 10, 1670.[8]

Not long after the French legal ban, English doctors also distanced themselves from the practice of blood transfusion, but they did not ban it by law. In some literature, it is mistakenly mentioned that the English banned the practice of blood transfusions. Xenotransfusions in other countries were still performed.

Denyse, in his letter of May 15, 1668, wrote to Henry Oldenburg: "*You obliged me significantly by having assured me, in your last letter of April 29, that the London Magistrates have never had the thought of issuing any orders to prohibit the practice of blood transfusion but that, on the contrary, your doctors continue to research its benefits with great success.*"[9]

In 1679, the German author Georg Abraham Mercklin published the book *Tractatio medica curiosa de ortu et occasu blood transfusionis sanguinis*, in which he recommended caution when carrying out blood transfusions. In the book, he relies on the arguments of the Bible and the alleged position of the Pope on blood transfusion. Many authors later incorrectly expanded this information to include the fact that Pope Innocent XI himself banned blood transfusions in 1679. However, historians have never found any proof that this statement was true. The Catholic Church has always been very careful, and no Pope in history has ever banned blood transfusions. Jacques Ruffié (1921–2004), a French hematologist, geneticist, and anthropologist, and Jean-Charles Sournia (1917–2000), a surgeon, stated in 1996 that this was confirmed in their book *La blood transfusion sanguine* in 1993 by the Vatican Archives Service.[10] There is also a story that the Pope issued an edict in 1875, but Dr. Cyrus Cressey Sturgis (1891–1966) also did a lot of investigation and found no evidence that this alleged story is true.[11]

In 1876, the physiologist Pierre Cyprien Oré reported on 154 human blood transfusions with blood from lambs, sheep, and calves and claimed 64 cures, some improvements, but 26 deaths. In 1872, the Italian Giuseppe Albini carried out two blood transfusions of sheep blood for a woman. Other blood transfusions of blood from sheep or calves were also reported by Franz Gesellius from Vilnius (1873), Oscar Hasse in Germany (1874), Henry Gradle in Chicago (1874), Emil Ponfick

---

[8] Ore, C.P. Etudes historiques, physiologiques et cliniques sur la transfusion du sang- 2è éd. (second ed.). France: Paris: JB Baillière; 1876,p. 42–44. Available at: https://archive.org/details/BIUSante_43169/page/42/mode/2up. Accessed 17 Apr 2020.

[9] Denis J. B. Lettre écrite à M. Oldenburg...par Jean Denis,... touchant les différents qui sont arrivez à l'occasion de la transfusion du sang, 1668, p. 1. Bibliothèque nationale de France, département Sciences et techniques, 4-TE13–13. https://gallica.bnf.fr/ark:/12148/bpt6k5788995z/f3.image.r=transfusion?lang=EN

[10] Ruffié J., Sournia J. C. La transfusion sanguine, Fayard Paris,1996, p. 50–51.

[11] Sturgis C. C. The history of blood transfusion, Bull Med Libr Assoc. 1942; 30(2), p. 105–12. Available at: https://www.ncbi.nlm.nih.gov/pmc/articles/PMC193993/. Accessed 20 Apr 2020.

(1874) in Germany, and Leonard Landois (1875) in Germany.[12] However, Emil Ponfick and Leonard Landois warned about the potentially harmful effects of xenotransfusions from 1874 onward.[13] Searching for cases of xenotransfusions in the 1890s in newspapers, there was one case found in Paris in 1891 that reported blood transfusion of goat blood to humans for treating tuberculosis.[14] In 1896, there was a report published about the case of the use of defibrinated sheep's blood for blood transfusion.[15] In 1922, in Paris, there was a report of using the blood of horses and sheep mixed with citrate for blood transfusion into humans.[16] In 1944, there was a report from the USA regarding a clinical trial of the use of bovine blood for human blood transfusions.[17] In 1955, there was an unsuccessful complete blood transfusion of bovine red cells to a patient.[18]

Many had high hopes that xenotransfusion was the future, but as experience has shown, these sorts of blood transfusions are not long-term beneficial for patients. They were mostly disappointing, with a few successful cases. Those who advocated xenotransfusion were largely convinced that the blood of animals was healthier than that of humans because of their food and lifestyle. The discovery of blood groups in 1900 further established the importance of human blood for treating human patients with blood transfusions.

References

1. Anon. A new system for the cure of tuberculosis. Deseret evening news. [volume] (Great Salt Lake City [Utah]), May 15, 1891, Page 5, Image 5. The Library of Congress, Chronicling America. https://www.loc.gov/. Accessed 17 Dec 2023.
2. Anon. Novel Blood transfusion. Pall Mall Gazette—Tuesday 17 October 1922, p. 4. https://britishnewspaperarchive.co.uk/ Accessed 17 Dec 2023.
3. Anon. Cattle blood transfusions for humans. Halifax Evening Courier—Saturday 15 January 1944, p. 4. https://britishnewspaperarchive.co.uk/. Accessed 17 Dec 2023.
4. Bateman WA. The use of defibrinated sheep's blood for blood transfusion. Br Med J. 1827;1896(1):17. https://pubmed.ncbi.nlm.nih.gov/20755930/

---

[12] Dunea G. Xenotransfusion: blood from animals to humans. 2023. https://hekint.org/2022/03/04/xenotransfusion-blood-from-animals-to-humans/. Accessed 17 Dec 2023.

[13] Roux 2007, p. 208.

[14] Anon. A new system for the cure of tuberculosis. Deseret evening news. [volume] (Great Salt Lake City [Utah]), May 15, 1891, Page 5, Image 5. The Library of Congress, Chronicling America. https://www.loc.gov/. Accessed 17 Dec 2023.

[15] Bateman WA. The Use of Defibrinated Sheep's Blood for Transfusion. Br Med J. 1896;1(1827), p.17. https://pubmed.ncbi.nlm.nih.gov/20755930/

[16] Anon. Novel Transfusion. Pall Mall Gazette - Tuesday 17 October 1922, p. 4. https://britishnewspaperarchive.co.uk/. Accessed 17 Dec 2023.

[17] Anon. Cattle blood transfusions for humans. Halifax Evening Courier - Saturday 15 January 1944, p. 4. https://britishnewspaperarchive.co.uk/. Accessed 17 Dec 2023.

[18] Wiener A. S., Unger LJ, Cohen L, Feldman J. Type-specific cold auto-antibodies as a cause of acquired hemolytic anemia and hemolytic transfusion reactions: biologic test with bovine red cells. Ann Intern Med. 1956;44(2), p. 221–40. https://pubmed.ncbi.nlm.nih.gov/13292836/

5. Dunea G. Xenotransfusion: blood from animals to humans. https://hekint.org/2022/03/04/xenotransfusion-blood-from-animals-to-humans/. Accessed 17 Dec 2023.
6. Denis JB. Lettre écrite à M. Oldenburg...par Jean Denis... touchant les différents qui sont arrivez à l'occasion de la transfusion du sang, 1668, p. 1. Bibliothèque nationale de France, département Sciences et techniques, 4-TE13–13. https://gallica.bnf.fr/ark:/12148/bpt6k5788995z/f3.image.r=transfusion?lang=EN
7. Farr AD. The first human blood transfusion. Med Hist. 1980;24(2):143–62. https://www.ncbi.nlm.nih.gov/pmc/articles/PMC1082701/. Accessed 17 Apr 2020
8. Hollingsworth MW. Blood transfusionby Richard Lower in 1665. Ann Med Hist. 1928;10(3):213–25. https://www.ncbi.nlm.nih.gov/pmc/articles/PMC7940049/
9. Ore CP. Etudes historiques, physiologiques et cliniques sur la blood transfusion du sang- 2è éd. 2nd ed. France: Paris: JB Baillière; 1876. p. 42–4. https://archive.org/details/BIUSante_43169/page/42/mode/2up Accessed 17 Apr 2020
10. Roux FA, Saï P, Deschamps JY. Xenotransfusions, past and present, Xenotransplantation the official journal of the international xenotransplantation association. 2007;14(3):208–16. https://pubmed.ncbi.nlm.nih.gov/17489860/. Accessed 17 Apr 2020
11. Ruffié J, Sournia JC. La blood transfusion sanguine, Fayard Paris, 1996, p. 50–51.
12. Sturgis CC. The history of blood transfusion. Bull Med Libr Assoc. 1942;30(2):105–12. https://www.ncbi.nlm.nih.gov/pmc/articles/PMC193993/. Accessed 20 Apr 2020
13. Surgenor D. The red blood cell, New York and. London: Academic press; 1974. p. 25. https://www.google.si/books/edition/The_Red_Blood_Cell/wDAxXpY4TCsC?hl=sl&gbpv=1. Accessed 16 Aug 2020
14. Wiener AS, Unger LJ, Cohen L, Feldman J. Type-specific cold auto-antibodies as a cause of acquired hemolytic anemia and hemolytic blood transfusion reactions: biologic test with bovine red cells. Ann Intern Med. 1956;44(2):221–40. https://pubmed.ncbi.nlm.nih.gov/13292836/

Image Source

Xenotransfusion form lamb to man. Available at: Wellcome Collection https://wellcome.org/. Published under CC BY 4.0 DEED. Accessed 20 April 2020.

The First Human to Human Blood Transfusion in 1818

Contents

5.1 James Blundell and His Fascination with Blood Transfusion Medicine.................... 31
5.2 The Impellor and the Gravitator.. 35
5.3 Influence of James Blundell on Blood Transfusion Medicine............................. 37
References.. 38

5.1 James Blundell and His Fascination with Blood Transfusion Medicine

Dr. James Blundell (Image 5.1) was born in London. He obtained his general education from the reverend Thomas Thomason, and when he reached the usual age, he started studying medicine at the United Borough hospitals, under the direct supervision of his uncle Dr. Haighton (c. 1755–March 23, 1823), the renowned obstetrician and physiologist. Afterwards, he traveled to Edinburgh, where on June 24, 1813, he received his Doctor of Medicine degree. In his work (*D.M.I. de Sensu, quo Melos sentitur*), he attempted to establish the independence of the senses of hearing and music while also demonstrating their interdependence. Returning to London, Dr. Blundell started lecturing on midwifery in 1814 alongside Dr. Haighton, and he commenced a course in physiology a few years later. He succeeded Dr. Haighton's position as lecturer at Guy's Hospital, where he oversaw the largest midwifery class in London for many years. In 1836, he stopped lecturing. On June 25, 1818, Dr. Blundell was admitted as a Licentiate of the College of Physicians, and on August

Image 5.1 James Blundell. (Source: James Blundell. Wellcome Collection https://wellcome.org/. Published under CC BY 4.0 International. Accessed 20 Dec 2023)

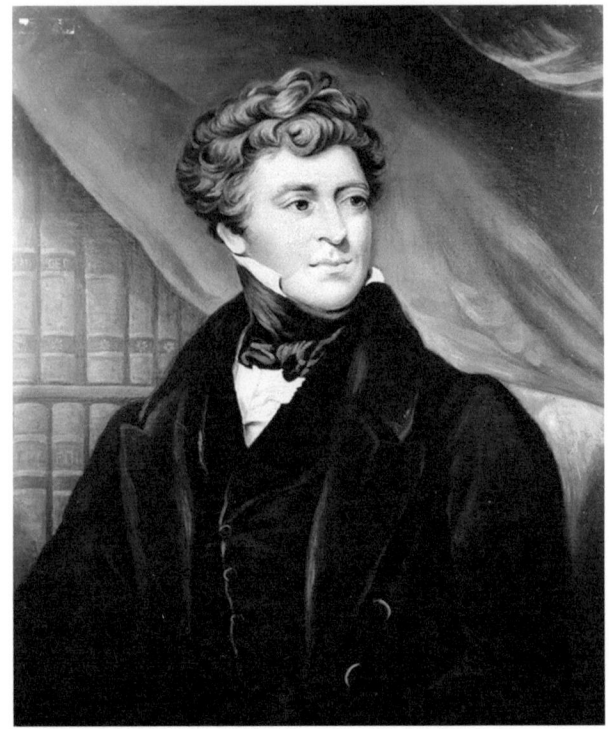

6, 1838, he was made a Fellow.[1] In 1847, Dr. Blundell stopped working as a physician.[2]

In the year 1816, a Scottish physician, John Henry Leacock (1793–1828), reported systematic experiments on cats and dogs and concluded that blood donor and patient of blood transfusion must be of the same species, and he also recommended the blood transfusion of human blood for human patients.[3] This was an important and strong statement for the safety of patients.

Experts continued to employ animal blood transfusions in the nineteenth century. Direct injection of the lamb's blood into human veins was advised at that time by

---

[1] Munk W. The roll of the Royal College of Physicians of London, comprising biographical sketches of all the eminent physicians whose names are recorded in the Annals. James Blundell p. 180. 2nd ed. London: The College, pall Mall East; 1878, p. 180. https://archive.org/details/rollofroyalcolle03royaiala/page/n3/mode/2up?q=blundell Accessed 19 Dec 2023.

[2] Ellis H. James Blundell, pioneer of blood transfusion, British Journal of Hospital Medicine.2007; 68 (8), p. 447–447. https://www.magonlinelibrary.com/doi/abs/10.12968/hmed.2007.68.8.24500.

[3] Schmidt PJ. Leacock AG. Forgotten transfusion history: John Leacock of Barbados, BMJ. 2002; 325(7378), p. 1485–1487. https://www.ncbi.nlm.nih.gov/pmc/articles/PMC139049/. Accessed 20 Apr 2020.

Oré, Gesellius, Hasse, and Albini; the potential risks of this procedure have been highlighted by Landois, Panum, Ponfick, Albertoni, Beel, and Kuster.[4]

Blundell noted that for his first notions on blood transfusion, he was wholly indebted to Dr. Leacock from Barbados. In comparison, Blundell transfused in his early experiments venous blood instead of arterial blood; he used human blood instead of lamb blood and performed his blood transfusions with a syringe, not a tube as Leacock did. Blundell also observed the work of Dr. Goodridge. Blundell's experiments involved the blood transfusion of blood from the arteries of one dog to the veins of another using the syringe; blood transfusion by the syringe from the arteries to the veins of the same animal; experiments in which the blood was exposed for a short time in the cup; experiments in which the dog was drained of its own and supplied with human blood; experiments using venous blood instead of arterial blood; experiments on the injection of air into the veins; and experiments on the time required for the coagulation of canine blood.[5, 6] Blundell also advocated the idea that the blood donor and patient must be of the same species. It was based on the awareness that in cases of extensive bleeding, such as postpartum, it would be dangerous to transfuse animal blood instead of human blood because of the incompatibility of blood between the two species. In 1825, James Blundell advised that men should be used as blood donors, claiming that men's blood flows more freely than women's blood and that men faint less when donating blood.[7] The author Moulin stated that in the nineteenth century, women were rarely blood donors, due to the belief at the time that women's blood was less abundant and vital.[8] Today, women are also successful blood donors, despite in general having less blood volume in their bodies than men due to their weight and height and lower levels of hemoglobin and iron.

James Blundell was also a visionary. He had foreseen that blood transfusions in the future would be beneficial for mankind.[9] The first officially documented blood transfusion with human blood was on December 22, 1818. It was performed by Dr. James Blundell, who used a syringe to transfuse 12 ounces (about 355 mL) of human blood into a male patient who was vomiting and weak from cirrhosis of the

---

[4] Dujardin-Beaumetz G. The blood from a therapeutic standpoint. In: Brodie W., Mulheron J. J., Lyons A. B., editors. Therapeutic Gazette, Volume 7, Detroit, Michigan: G. S. Davis, medical publisher. 1883, p. 401. Available at: https://books.google.si/ Accessed 20 Apr 2020.

[5] Blundell J. Researches physiological and pathological: instituted principally with a view to the improvement of medical and surgical practice. Operation of transfusion. E. Cox and son. 1825, p. 90–91. https://wellcomecollection.org/works/d5vdhnnb. Accessed 2 May 2020.

[6] Blundell J. Experiments on the Transfusion of Blood by the Syringe, Med Chir Trans.1818; 9(1) p. 56–92. https://www.ncbi.nlm.nih.gov/pmc/articles/PMC2128869/. Accessed 2 May 2020.

[7] Blundell, 1825, p. 97–125.

[8] Moulin A.M. Le dernier langage de la médecine: Histoire de l'immunologie de Pasteur au Sida. 1re éd. ed. Paris: Presses universities de France. 1991, p. 154.

[9] Pettigrew T. J. Medical portrait gallery: biographical memoirs of the most celebrated physicians, surgeons, etc., who have contributed to the advancement of medical science: James Blundell. London: Fisher, son & co.,1838–1840, p. 5. https://wellcomecollection.org/works/a5zsh3e9. Accessed 20 Dec 2023.

pylorus (gastric carcinoma). After the blood transfusion, the patient felt better but unfortunately died 56 hours later. The first failed case gave him additional impetus to deal with blood transfusions. In August 1825, he performed his first successful blood transfusion of human blood, assisted by his colleague Dr. Charles Waller. The blood donor was the husband of the patient. Together, they transfused four ounces (about 118 mL) of blood to a patient with postpartum hemorrhage. Despite the successful blood transfusion, they wondered if the small transfused amount of blood managed to save the patient. They both later agreed that the patient's blood transfusion helped to improve her health. In October 1825, Dr. Blundell and Dr. Edward Doubleday (1810–1849) successfully transfused 14 ounces (about 414 mL) of blood to a dying patient named Cocklin, who was bleeding from her uterus after giving birth. Her husband was the blood donor. After the blood transfusion, patient Cocklin said she *"felt strong as a bull."* Between 1818 and 1829, Dr. Blundell and his colleagues performed ten blood transfusions, with the fact that two of the patients were already dead before the blood transfusion, and the third was dying of cancer. So out of ten cases of blood transfusions, five out of eight were successful. His successful blood transfusions were in cases of *uterine hemorrhage, postpartum bleeding, hemorrhage following placental delivery, hemorrhage following leg amputation*, and *uterine hemorrhage*. All unsuccessful cases of blood transfusion were in a dying man from gastric carcinoma, placental hemorrhage, where the young woman was dead for 5–6 minutes with severe hemorrhage during childbirth, a woman with severe hemorrhage during childbirth, a woman ill with puerperal fever, and a young man already dead for 3–4 minutes of hemorrhage due to the burst of an artery. Blundell explained that blood does not lose its vital agents when passing through the instrument. He explained that blood must be transfused slowly and developed methods for determining the amount of blood. With his work, in addition to other experts in this field, he significantly influenced the development of today's blood transfusion medicine.[10, 11, 12, 13, 14, 15, 16]

---

[10] Jones H.W, Mackmull G., The influence of James Blundell on the development of blood transfusion, Annals of Medical history. 1928;10(3,) p. 242–248. https://www.ncbi.nlm.nih.gov/pmc/articles/PMC7940050/.

[11] Blundell, 1818, p. 56–92.

[12] Blundell J. Some account of a case of obstinate vomiting, in which an attempt was made to prolong life by the Injection of blood into the veins, Medico Chirurgical Transactions. 1819, 10(2), p. 296–311. https://pubmed.ncbi.nlm.nih.gov/20895389/.

[13] Doubleday, E. Case of uterine hemorrhage, successfully treated by the operation of Transfusion, The London medical and physical journal.1826; 54(328), p. 380–386. https://www.ncbi.nlm.nih.gov/pmc/articles/PMC5646564/.

[14] Waller, C. Case of uterine hemorrhage, in Which the operation of transfusion was successfully performed, The London medical and physical journal. 1825; 54 (320), p. 273–277. https://pubmed.ncbi.nlm.nih.gov/30494818/.

[15] Waller, C. Case of uterine hemorrhage, in Which the operation of transfusion was successfully performed, The London medical and physical journal. 1825; 54 (320), p. 273–277. https://pubmed.ncbi.nlm.nih.gov/30494818/.

[16] Blundell J. Observations on transfusion of blood, The Lancet. 1829; 12(302), p. 321–324. https://www.thelancet.com/journals/lancet/article/PIIS0140-6736(02)92543-2/fulltext.

5.2 The Impellor and the Gravitator

Dr. Blundell, in his experiments with human-to-human blood transfusion, first used a cannula for blood transfusion from artery to vein; he then later collected the blood in a vessel and injected it with a syringe into the patient's vein (Image 5.2); and finally, he constructed two instruments for blood transfusion called "*Impellor*" and the "*Gravitator*" for the blood transfusion of venous blood.[17] The Impellor (Image 5.3) was a complicated instrument, but this was done to prevent the admission of the smallest quantity of air that could potentially cause a fatal outcome. The Impellor consisted of an outer compartment that formed a water bath surrounding an inner cup for receipt of the blood donor's blood. The water bath was filled with what Blundell described as "*milk-warm*" water (35.5 °C), and before use, air was displaced from the tubing and cannula by pumping warm water through the apparatus. For the operation, the blood donor was seated in a chair, to which the Impellor was clamped.[18] The Impellor was fixed to give it stability and accommodation the blood donor, while blood was flowing from his vein into the funnel-shaped part. Two opposing spring-loaded valves under the funnel allowed the action of the pump on one side to force the blood forward along the tube toward the cannula, which was inserted into the patient's vein.[19] The object of the Gravitator (Image 5.4) was to give help to this last extremity by transmitting the blood in a regulated stream from one individual to another with as little exposure as may be to air, cold, and inanimate surfaces. The operation was performed with venesection on the person who emitted the blood with the insertion of a small tube into the vein, usually laid open in bleeding. A syringe, scalpel, lancet, and silver probe were connected to the apparatus.[20] The main technical difficulties were clumping and breakdown of transfused blood cells and infection and clotting of the blood in the Impellor.[21, 22] To summarize the methods of these two instruments, it can be explained that the impellor, after the blood was collected into a warm clamp, "impelled" the blood into the recipient via a fixed syringe. The Gravitator delivered to the recipient the collected blood by means of gravity through a long vertical cannula.[23]

---

[17] Mcloughlin G, The British contribution to blood transfusion in the nineteenth century, British Journal of Anesthesia. 1959; 31(11), p. 503–516. https://academic.oup.com/bja/article/31/11/503/256941.

[18] Ibid., p. 504–508.

[19] Keynes, 1949, p. 22.

[20] Blundell, 1829, p. 321.

[21] Bird G.W.G. The history of blood transfusion, Injury 1971; 3 (1), p. 40–44. https://www.sciencedirect.com/science/article/abs/pii/S0020138371801389.

[22] Bird, 1971, p. 40–44.

[23] Rossi E. C., Simon T. L. Chap. 1 - Transfusion in the new millennium. In: Simon TL, McCullough J., Snyder E. L., Solheim BG, Strauss RG., editors. Rossi's Principles of Transfusion Medicine, fifth Edition. USA: Wiley Blackwell. 2016, p. 1–14. https://www.blackwellpublishing.com/content/BPL_Images/Content_store/Sample_chapter/9781405175883/9781405175883_4_001.pdf. Accessed 2 Mar 2024.

Image 5.2 Blood transfusion apparatus, designed by James Blundell, made by Savigny & Co.; Anon. n.d. (Source: Blood-blood transfusion apparatus, designed by James Blundell, made by Savigny & Co.; Anon., n.d. Wellcome Collection https://wellcome.org/. Published under CC BY 4.0 DEED. Accessed 12 Jan 2024)

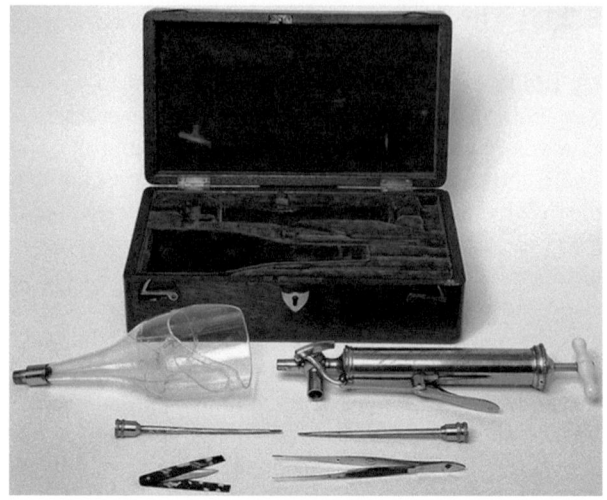

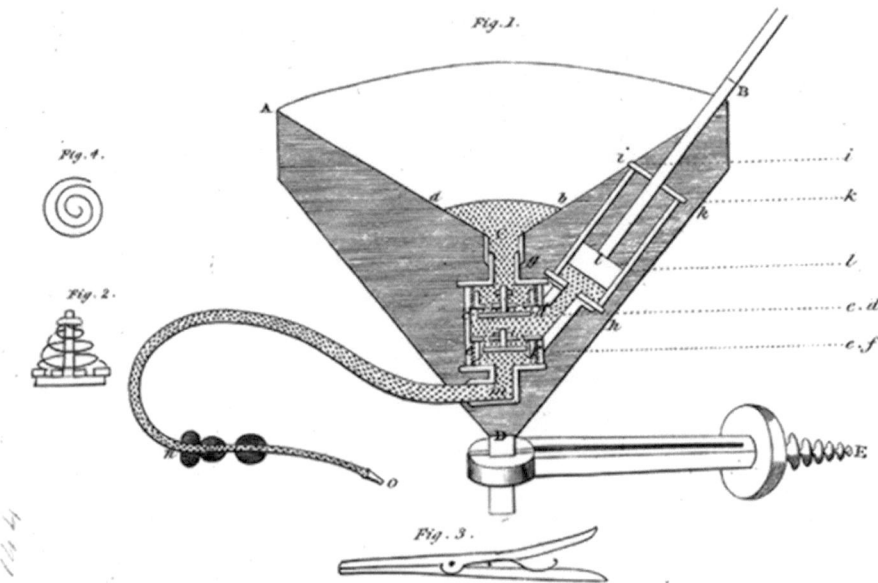

Image 5.3 James Blundell's Impellor. (Source: James Blundell Impellor. Wellcome Collection https://wellcome.org/. Public domain. Accessed 20 Dec 2023)

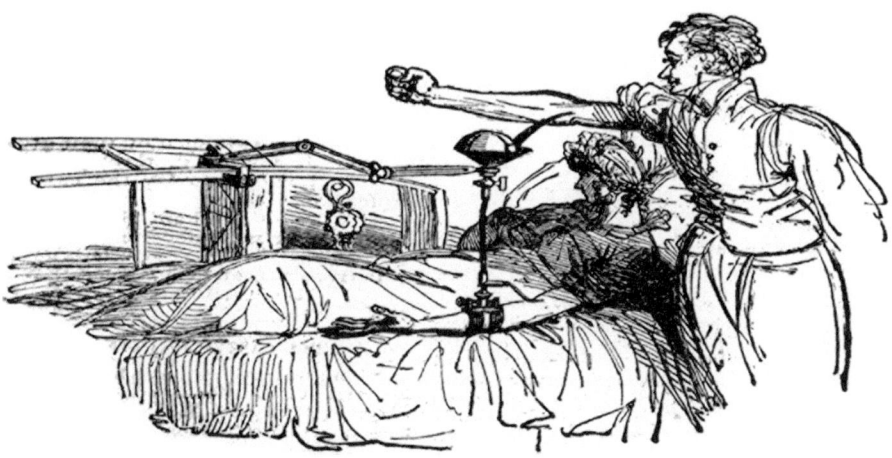

Image 5.4 Blood transfusion method of Blundell with the Impellor and Gravitator. (Source: Blood transfusion method of Blundell with the Gravitator. Wellcome Collection https://wellcome.org/. Published under CC BY 4.0 DEED. Accessed 2 May 2020)

5.3 Influence of James Blundell on Blood Transfusion Medicine

Dr. Blundell was undoubtedly the pioneer of his time. He was very enthusiastic and talented, and he successfully revived blood transfusions, set an example, and gave hope to many other experts. His clinical experiences with severe hemorrhage led him to turn to blood transfusion as an important and beneficial treatment. Important decisions for using blood transfusion in practice were also based on experiments carried out by Leacock. It did not take Blundell long to start experimenting with human-to-human blood transfusions. He certainly had many trials but with successful outcomes. He also invented two apparatuses that were highly useful. One of the most important realizations of Blundell, whom he also knew as Leacock, was that the blood transfusion must be used only on the same species. He understood that healthy blood donors with a higher volume of blood were needed in order to reduce unwanted reactions that could have occurred to the blood donor, like fainting. He systematically presented blood transfusion both in a theoretical and practical way and realized its importance. According to some versions, Blundell administered the first human autotransfusion and was aware of hemophilia A. These two assertions are untrue. Other colleagues occasionally sought his advice regarding blood transfusions, and some of them also used his creative devices.

References

1. Blundell J. Researches physiological and pathological: instituted principally with a view to the improvement of medical and surgical practice. Operation of blood transfusion. E. Cox and son. 1825, p. 90–91. https://wellcomecollection.org/works/d5vdhnnb Accessed 2 May 2020.
2. Blundell J. Experiments on the blood transfusion of blood by the syringe. Med Chir Trans. 1818;9(1):56–92. https://www.ncbi.nlm.nih.gov/pmc/articles/PMC2128869/. Accessed 2 May 2020
3. Blundell J. Some account of a case of obstinate vomiting, in which an attempt was made to prolong life by the injection of blood into the veins. Med Chir Trans. 1819;10(29):296–311. https://pubmed.ncbi.nlm.nih.gov/20895389/
4. Blundell J. Observations on blood transfusion of blood. Lancet. 1829;12(302):321–4. https://www.thelancet.com/journals/lancet/article/PIIS0140-6736(02)92543-2/fulltext
5. Bird GWG. The history of blood transfusion. Injury. 1971;3(1):40–4. https://www.sciencedirect.com/science/article/abs/pii/S0020138371801389
6. Dujardin-Beaumetz G. The blood from a therapeutic standpoint. In: Brodie W, Mulheron JJ, Lyons AB, editors. Therapeutic gazette, vol. 7. Detroit, Michigan: G. S. Davis, medical publisher; 1883. p. 401. https://books.google.si/. Accessed 20 Apr 2020.
7. Doubleday E. Case of uterine hemorrhage, successfully treated by the operation of blood transfusion. Lond Med Phys J. 1826;54(328):380–6. https://www.ncbi.nlm.nih.gov/pmc/articles/PMC5646564/
8. Ellis H. James Blundell, pioneer of blood transfusion. Br J Hosp Med. 2007;68(8):447. https://www.magonlinelibrary.com/doi/abs/10.12968/hmed.2007.68.8.24500
9. Jones HW, Mackmull G. The influence of James Blundell on the development of blood transfusion. Ann Med Hist. 1928;10(3):242–8. https://www.ncbi.nlm.nih.gov/pmc/articles/PMC7940050/
10. Munk W. The roll of the Royal College of Physicians of London, comprising biographical sketches of all the eminent physicians whose names are recorded in the Annals. James Blundell. 2nd ed. London: The College, pall Mall East; 1878. p. 180. https://archive.org/details/rollofroyalcolle03royaiala/page/n3/mode/2up?q=blundell. Accessed 19 Dec 2023
11. Mcloughlin G. The British contribution to blood transfusionin the nineteenth century. Br J Anesth. 1959;31(11):503–16. https://academic.oup.com/bja/article/31/11/503/256941
12. Moulin AM. Le dernier langage de la médecine: Histoire de l'immunologie de Pasteur au Sida. 1re éd. Paris: Presses universites de France; 1991. p. 154.
13. Schmidt PJ, Leacock AG. Forgotten blood transfusion history: John Leacock of Barbados. BMJ. 2002;325(7378):1485–7. https://www.ncbi.nlm.nih.gov/pmc/articles/PMC139049/. Accessed 20 Apr 2020
14. Pettigrew TJ. Medical portrait gallery: biographical memoirs of the most celebrated physicians, surgeons, etc., who have contributed to the advancement of medical science: James Blundell. London: Fisher, Son & Co.; 1838. p. 5. –1840 https://wellcomecollection.org/works/a5zsh3e9. Accessed 20 Dec 2023
15. Rossi EC, Simon TL. Chapter 1 - transfusion in the new millennium. In: Simon TL, McCullough J, Snyder EL, Solheim BG, Strauss RG, editors. Rossi's principles of transfusion medicine. 5th ed. USA: Wiley Blackwell; 2016. p. 1–14. https://www.blackwellpublishing.com/content/BPL_Images/Content_store/Sample_chapter/9781405175883/9781405175883_4_001.pdf Accessed 2 March 2024.
16. Waller C. Case of uterine hemorrhage, in, which the operation of blood transfusion was successfully performed. Lond Med Phys J. 1825;54(320):273–7. https://pubmed.ncbi.nlm.nih.gov/30494818/

Image Sources

Blundell J. Wellcome Collection https://wellcome.org/. Published under CC BY 4.0 International. Accessed 20 Dec 2023.

Blood-blood transfusion apparatus, designed by James Blundell, made by Savigny & Co.; anon., n.d. Wellcome Collection https://wellcome.org/. Published under CC BY 4.0 DEED. Accessed 12 Jan 2024.

James Blundell's Impellor. Wellcome Collection https://wellcome.org/. Public domain. Accessed 20 Dec 2023.

Blood transfusion method of Blundell with Impellor and the Gravitator. Wellcome Collection https://wellcome.org/. Published under CC BY 4.0 DEED. Accessed 2 May 2020.

Interesting Cases of Blood Transfusion in the Nineteenth Century

6

Contents

6.1	Blood Transfusion Medicine in the Nineteenth Century.	41
6.2	Nurse Tender in Ireland Gives Blood to Save a Woman.	48
6.3	Women as a Blood Donor for Patients with Hemophilia.	48
6.4	A Blood Transfusion for a Boy with Hemophilia.	49
6.5	Blood Donation for Sister.	50
6.6	Early Case of a Successful Autotransfusion During an Operation in Europe.	50
6.7	Blood Transfusions in the USA.	52
	6.7.1 Early Case of Autotransfusion in USA.	53
References.		54

6.1 Blood Transfusion Medicine in the Nineteenth Century

In the nineteenth century, blood was donated by healthy volunteer neighbors of patients, assistants of doctors, and spouses of patients who unselfishly donated their blood to the endangered patients. Blood transfusions were also performed in the nineteenth century for a variety of medical conditions, including hemophilia, an inherited disease caused by a lack of certain blood clotting factors 8 and 9. Blood transfusion was also used for severe injuries such as amputations, work or war injuries, uterine hemorrhage, cholera, and more. In the nineteenth century, blood from animals, such as calves and lambs, was used for blood transfusions in addition to human blood. The described cases are a testimony to how doctors cured health conditions with blood transfusions using human blood, with remarkable results in many cases. Some of them were the first reported cases at the time.

© The Author(s), under exclusive license to Springer Nature
Switzerland AG 2024
Z. Kvržić, *History of Blood Donation and Transfusion Medicine*,
https://doi.org/10.1007/978-3-031-68715-0_6

Swiss doctor Joseph Antoine Roussel (1837–1901) was one of the biggest proponents of blood transfusions in the nineteenth century.[1] Dr. Roussel obtained in his native town the diploma of bachelor and master of arts, did his medical studies in Paris, and, after cruises in Labrador and Newfoundland as a marine surgeon, he became a doctor in Paris in 1863 with the presentation of a *Thesis on the rheumatism of the marrow envelopes*. Then he settled in Geneva, practicing in the city in winter and in summer in the Geneva countryside, in Troinex, where he ran a small clinic. In 1880, Roussel again settled in Paris. He wrote several publications on blood transfusion.[2] In 1864, he invented his blood transfusion device for direct hand-to-hand blood transfusion known as *Transfuser* (Image 6.1). In 1865 with Transfuser he made his first successful transfusion in a case of puerperal hemorrhage. In 1867 the design and the description of the Transfuser were inserted in the Gazette des Hôpitaux and the Archives de Médecine of Paris.[3] His device, which employed a lancet connected by rubber tubes to a manual pump to collect venous blood, was acknowledged as the best one for transfusing entire venous human blood at the 1873 Vienna World's Fair.[4] In 1888, he founded a journal *La Medecine hypodermique*, which lasted for 10 years. In his book on blood transfusion from 1877, Roussel wrote that after reviewing the literature from various authors, he found that blood transfusion from blood donors between 1818 and 1875 was carried out in 190 cases. Of the 80 cases of dying women due to childbirth hemorrhages, 30 were due to war wounds or surgical wounds; 50 were due to blood diseases and anemia problems; 20 were due to typhus,[5] cholera,[6] rabies,[7] syphilis,[8] and dangerous fevers[9]; and 10 were due to blood poisoning due to asphyxia[10] or scurvy.[11,12] Surgeon Austin Meldon, in his article from 1890, wrote that blood transfusions were carried out in large numbers from 1818 to 1874. He reported 737 blood transfusions, of which 302

---

[1] Roussel J. Transfusion of human blood, England: J & A Churchill; 1877, p. 25–26. https://books.google.si. Accessed 27 March 2023.

[2] Oliver J. Le Dr. Roussel, La Croix-Rouge suisse. 1952; 61, p. 9–12. https://www.e-periodica.ch/digbib/view?pid=acf-002:1952:61::231#13.

[3] Roussel, 1877, 25–26.

[4] Sergeeva MS, Panova E. L. Blood transfusions for the wounded: promising method of battlefield surgery or utopia of the mid-1870s? History of Medicine 7.2021; 2, p. 133–139. https://historymedjournal.com/wp-content/uploads/volume7/number2/en/2.Sergeeva.pdf.

[5] Typhus, also known as typhus fever, is a group of infectious diseases that are caused by specific types of bacterial infection.

[6] Cholera is an infection of the small intestine by some strains of the bacterium *Vibrio cholerae*.

[7] Rabies is a viral disease caused by lyssaviruses, including the rabies virus and Australian bat lyssavirus.

[8] Syphilis is a sexually transmitted infection caused by the bacterium *Treponema pallidum* subspecies *pallidum*.

[9] Fever, also known as pyrexia, is characterized by a temperature that is higher than normal due to an elevation in the body's temperature set point.

[10] Asphyxia is the cessation of breathing.

[11] Roussel, 1877, 37–38.

[12] Scurvy is a disease due to a vitamin C deficiency.

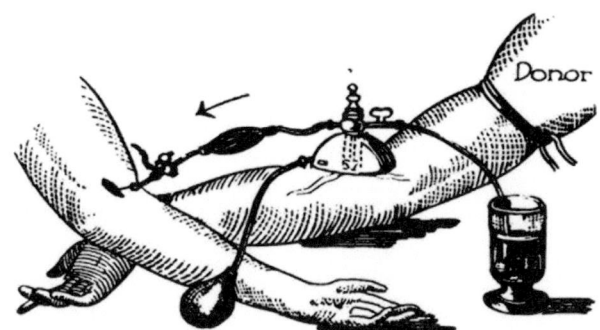

Fig. 19.—J. Roussel (1867). Instrument devised for transfusion of unmodified blood with rubber bulb for suction and pressure and suction chamber over donor's vein for collection of blood.

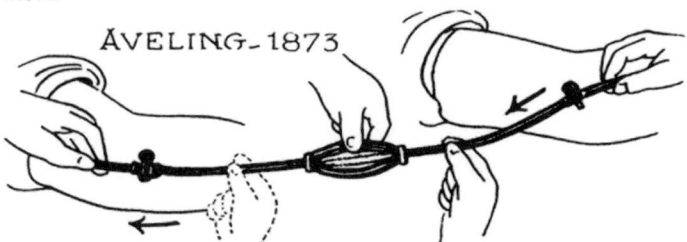

Fig. 20.—Aveling. Apparatus for transfusion of blood with rubber bulb for aspiration and ejection of blood.

Image 6.1 Roussel (1867) and Aveling's (1873) blood transfusion apparatus. (Source: Roussel (1867) and Aveling's (1873) blood transfusion apparatus. Source: Chapter I history. In: Kilduffe, R. A., DeBakey, M. E. The blood bank and the technique and therapeutics of blood transfusions. Mosby, St. Louis, 1942, p. 33. Permission for usage of the image was granted by the copyright holder, Elsevier, on January 23, 2024. https://babel.hathitrust.org/cgi/pt?id=uc1.$b595310&seq=1. Accessed 24 Jan 2024)

(41%) were successful.[13] Experts in the nineteenth century used the injection of defibrinated blood,[14] indirect blood transfusions with different apparatuses, and direct blood transfusions uniting two circulations by a simple closed and direct channel. This was used with instruments tubes of ivory, glass, silver, and caoutchouc for blood transfusion of arterial human blood taken from a brachial artery. They also practiced direct venous to venous blood transfusion. The instrument for the direct arterial xenotransfusion was a 6 inches long tube made of natural caoutchouc that was put inside the carotid or femoral artery of a lamb, which was 4–5 months old. The blood of animals was also used in direct vein-to-vein blood transfusion. Roussel had several good opinions on described methods of blood transfusion. He advocated that the blood for blood transfusion should be of the same species. He explained that the blood should continue to be vital and unaltered in its

---

[13] Meldon, A., Transfusion of blood and intravenous injection of milk and saline fluid, Trans. RAM Ireland.1891;9(1), p. 214–222. https://link.springer.com/article/10.1007/BF03170599.

[14] Defibrinated blood is whole blood from which fibrin, which is one of the clotting factors, has been removed during the blood clotting process.

most intimate composition not having been subjected to contact with air or any other modifying materials, and it should have lost neither its motion nor its temperature nor its gases nor its density. The quantity of the blood to be transfused and the rapidity of its flow should be subject to the discretion of the expert operator. The operation should be conducted without danger to either subject. Roussel believed that a good operator should have a direct and uninterrupted channel, but it should not be attached to a cannula at the afferent extremity or made of a substance that degrades blood when it comes into touch with it.[15]

Dr. Roussel had a great understanding of blood and blood transfusions. He also performed a lot of blood transfusions, invented his own apparatus, and saved many lives. The nineteenth century was a period where blood transfusions expanded in all fields of medicine for the treatment of patients, with new successful discoveries and approaches. This period introduced many great and ambitious experts in Europe to early blood transfusion medicine.

In the nineteenth century, there were a couple of instruments for blood transfusion. Ineffective tests were conducted by Professor Maisonneuve of Paris using a gray caoutchouc ball with valves contained in ivory and glass tubes and silver cannulas. Professor Neudörder of Vienna, Küster of Berlin, and James Hobson Aveling of London used cannulas made of copper or silver and hollow spheres made of sulphuretted India rubber (Image 6.1). The same flaws existed in these devices. They were made of substances that, when they came in touch with blood, they deteriorated it. Some thinkers have attempted to demonstrate that if a certain amount of air was introduced into the veins, it would not necessarily be fatal, reasoning from the fact that one can never be certain that no air bubbles are contained in them, even if they were filled with water prior to the procedure. Their primary flaw was that the glass, metal, or plastic cannulas or trocars used to create their afferent extremities were inserted into and tied to the vein that supplied the blood. This procedure required a delicate and painful surgery for the blood donor, which was typically followed by phlebitis.[16] The severity of the phlebitis depended on the amount of manipulation the vein had undergone. If the surgeon had been justified in taking a few ounces of blood from one man to save the life of another, it was only under the condition that he took every care to avoid injuring the patient. Additionally, from the perspective of the operator, this cannula had the inherent flaw of having a too-small diameter. Blood could exit through this narrow channel, but slowly, and it took far too long to fill the instrument's ball. As a result, the blood stagnated and coagulated against the tube's walls, obstructing the passage, which caused the blood transfusion to stop in the first few jets.[17] Higginson revived the syringe technique in 1837, and Waller enhanced it in 1838 with the use of a funnel, a two-ounce syringe, and a

---

[15] Roussel, J. 1877, p. 27–39.
[16] Phlebitis is inflammation of the veins.
[17] Roussel, J. 1877, p. 35–36.

two-way tap linking the blood donor and the patient. The syringe technique was, however, first used by Blundell in 1818.[18]

Blood transfusion was a procedure that was only carried out as a last option in the nineteenth century. Both the patient and the blood donor frequently feared phlebitis. Even when human blood was utilized, reactions were frequent, and occasionally fatalities happened. There were numerous technical issues, especially problems with blood coagulating.[19] The blood transfusion device's tubes were obstructed by the blood clot that formed as the blood coagulated. Because of the creation of clots, it is likely that some of the patients who got animal blood transfusions in the past would not have survived if there had not been a technical issue. It is quite likely that the patients would have received enough blood to kill them.[20] However, some improvements have been made in addressing these latter issues. Blood that had been defibrinated and that had been rendered incoagulable by the inclusion of caustic soda[21] were the subjects of Prevost and Dumas' experiments.[22] The use of defibrinated blood was first proposed by Prevost in 1821, but it did not gain much popularity until Sir Thomas Smith in 1873 described his apparatus.[23] Dieffenbach devised these tests in 1826 after discovering that fibrin[24] embedded in water or serum could not revive patients with a severe hemorrhage. Bischoff went further in 1835 and demonstrated that while defibrinated blood from the same species was well tolerated and successful in reviving animals after a debilitating hemorrhage when injected into these animals, whole blood from animals of another species was poisonous. He came to the conclusion that fibrin is poisonous and suggested that only blood that has been defibrinated should be transfused. Larsen performed the first real blood transfusion of defibrinated blood in 1847.[25] The English doctors tried to perfect their methods. They avoided the method of their German surgeon colleagues by injecting defibrinated blood, which was filtered, cooled, or rewarmed. They also gave up using animal blood and sought blood donation from a suitable, healthy man.[26] Blood was stirred up with beads or by *shaking and whipping* in the 1800s. For instance, Sir Thomas Smith, in 1873, at St. Bartholomew Hospital in London, used this method. Blood lysis or hemolysis[27] that followed raised suspicions. In

---

[18] Inwood M. J., The evolution of modern blood transfusion apparatus, Western University, UWOMJ. 1966; (37)1, p. 3–7. https://ir.lib.uwo.ca/uwomj/218.

[19] Zimmerman LM, Howell KM, History of Blood Transfusion, Ann Med Hist. 1932; 4(5), p. 415–433. https://pubmed.ncbi.nlm.nih.gov/33944186/.

[20] Keynes, 1949, p. 27.

[21] Caustic, known as sodium hydroxide, is an extremely strong base, used in the manufacture of hard soaps.

[22] Zimmerman LM, Howell KM, 1932, p. 415–433.

[23] Inwood, 1966, p. 4.

[24] Fibrin is a fibrous protein that forms the scaffold of a blood clot in the blood-clotting process and is one of the so-called clotting factors.

[25] Zimmerman LM, Howell KM, 1932, p. 423.

[26] Roussel, J. 1877, p. 24.

[27] Hemolysis is the breakdown of RBC and the release of hemoglobin from them.

1868, British obstetrician John Braxton Hicks described chemical methods or blood additives to prevent blood from clotting during blood transfusion.[28] In 1869, Dr. Hicks reported on a series of blood transfusions performed with the use of phosphate of sodium, stating that it was an effective anticoagulant.[29] He was influenced by Dr. Pavy, who experimented with different solutions and recommended to Hicks the use of phosphate of sodium, which he considered to be the safest salt to employ. Dr. Hicks' patients who required blood transfusions all died, and not even phosphate of sodium helped. In different sources, it is stated that Hicks experimented with phosphate of sodium in 1868 or 1869. But the truth is, his first case with this method was actually in the morning of December 23, 1863.[30] It was also confirmed that the phosphate sodium was harmful and dangerous.[31] John Berry Haycraft, a British professor of physiology, discovered the anticoagulant characteristics of hirudin[32] in 1884, and Leonard Landois, professor of physiology at the University of Greifswald in Germany, proposed using it during blood transfusion in 1892. It was eventually discovered that using hirudin was harmful.[33]

The Germans were performing blood transfusions, which were mostly deterred by the coagulation that unimpaired blood produces in bad apparatus. Consequently, the majority of German operators made experiments on and practiced with trifling success the injection of defibrinated blood. The only Germans who have performed the real blood transfusion were *Klott, Schroegler, Bickersteth, Schneemann, Meyer, Seyferth*, and *O. Heyfelder*. In France the experts for blood transfusion were *Clement, Savy, Olivier, Abèle, Danyaux, Roux, Nélaton, Marmonnier, G. Devay, Desgranges, B. Maisonneuve, Michaux, Courcy, Gentil, Blondeau, Oré, Raynaud, Lande, Béhier, Brouardel*, and *Roussel*. From 1820 to 1830, the following English operators stood out: *Blundell, Doubleday, Urvins, Waller, Brigham, Jewell, Boyle, Baxton Brown, Howell, Daviss, Savvy Pointer*, and *Douglas Fox*. From 1830 to 1840: *Blundell, Ingleby, Bird, Healey, Fraser, Ashwell, Banner, Tweedy, Collins*, and *Samuel Lane*. From 1840 to 1850: *May, Brown, Greaves*, and *Waller*. Between 1850 and 1860: *Blundell, Brigham, Higginson, Simpson, Wheatkrop, Lever*, and *Bryant*. Between 1860 and 1870: *Higginson, Braxton Hicks, Greenhalgh, Thorne, Currey*, and *Playfair*. Between 1870 and 1876: *Lister, Aveling, Barnes, Thomas*,

---

[28] Roets M, Sturgess DJ, Wyssusek K, van Zundert AA., Intraoperative cell salvage: A technology built upon the failures, fads and fashions of blood transfusion, Anaesthesia and Intensive Care.2019;47(3), p. 17–30. https://journals.sagepub.com/doi/10.1177/0310057X19860161#b ibr3-0310057X19860161.

[29] Keynes, 1949, p. 27.

[30] Braxton Hicks J. Cases of transfusion with some remarks on a new method of performing the operation. Guy's hospital reports. London Churchill & Sons New Burlington Street 1869; 14(3). https://www.google.si/books/edition/Guy_s_hospital_reports/Ky1TAAAAcAAJ?hl=sl&gbpv=1 &dq=guys+hospital&printsec=frontcover. Accessed 6 Jan 2024.

[31] Wiener A. S. Chapter IV: history of blood transfusion. In: Blood groups and transfusion. Charles C. Thomas publisher; 1948, p. 58.

[32] Hirudin is a naturally occurring peptide in the salivary glands of blood-sucking leeches.

[33] Roets M, Sturgess DJ, Wyssusek K, van Zundert AA., 2019, p. 17–30.

Ringland, Wagstaffe, and numerous others.[34] Several of the cases that were discussed were ground-breaking in the blood transfusion profession and had astounding outcomes. Nevertheless, despite the expansion of blood transfusion medicine in the nineteenth century, experts instead also used saline and milk for blood substitution because they believed that with these infusions, there would not be the same technical problems as with blood. But they soon realized that this was not enough, nor was it good for the substitution of blood.

Doctor Thomas Aitchison Latta (1796–1833), from Scotland, was the first to use saline as a means of treatment. He used saline in 1832 to treat patients with cholera in Great Britain.[35] Dissatisfaction with blood transfusions led to a brief use of milk as a substitute for blood.[36] Dr. Edward Hodder performed this procedure in Toronto, Canada, in 1850 on three patients suffering from cholera. Milk was boiled, and up to 14 ounces (414 mL) of milk was injected, and two patients survived.[37] After this, there was a brief period when other doctors were inspired to use an injection of milk instead of a blood transfusion. Milk cannot be successfully used instead of a blood transfusion. The reason why patients survived was probably due to not-so-life-threatening situations.

Milk was used from cows, goats, and women. The side effects were as minor as an intense headache, fever, and tachycardia[38] and the patient also died. In the USA, this method was used from 1873 to 1880.[39] According to the available literature, the use of saline as a substitute for blood transfusion was first mentioned in 1881, when the German surgeon Albert Landerer used an infusion of saline solution for a patient with acute anemia instead of blood on July 10, 1881.[40] As medicine advanced, so did the challenges for professionals. They began to realize that the procedures themselves—blood transfusion, surgery, childbirth, etc.—were not sufficiently successful for the survival of the patients. They noticed that after successful procedures, the patients had many infections, blood poisoning, and the like due to the poor hygienic conditions in which the treatments took place. The solution was found in eliminating the causes of infections by preparing the room, materials, and patient without infection.

Only after 1865, when Louis Pasteur (December 27, 1822 to September 28, 1895), a French chemist and microbiologist, discovered that bacterial and fungal

---

[34] Roussel, J. 1877, page 23–26.

[35] MacGillivray N., Dr. Latta of Leith: Pioneer in the treatment of cholera by intravenous saline infusion, The journal of the Royal College of Physicians of Edinburgh. 2006; 36(1), p. 80–85. https://pubmed.ncbi.nlm.nih.gov/17146955/.

[36] Oberman, H.A., Early History of Blood Substitutes: Transfusion of Milk, Transfusion. 1969;9 (2), p. 74–77. https://onlinelibrary.wiley.com/doi/abs/10.1111/j.1537-2995.1969.tb04920.x

[37] Jennings C. E. The intravenous injection of milk. The British medical journal. 1885;1(1275), p. 1147–1149. https://www.ncbi.nlm.nih.gov/pmc/articles/PMC2256321/.

[38] Tachycardia means fast heartbeat.

[39] Oberman 1969, p- 74—76.

[40] Landerer, A. Ueber Transfusion und Infusion. Archiv f. pathol. Anat. 1886; 105, 351–372. https://link.springer.com/article/10.1007/BF01940368.

contaminations cause putrefaction, were instrument sterilization and aseptic work methods gradually introduced. In 1867, the English surgeon Dr. Joseph Lister (April 5, 1827 to February 10, 1912) started antiseptic surgery with carbolic acid to prevent infections.[41, 42]

6.2 Nurse Tender in Ireland Gives Blood to Save a Woman

In Ireland the first blood transfusion is attributed to an Irish surgeon Robert McDonnell (March 15, 1828 to May 6, 1889), who performed it in April 1865.[43] But I have found an even older case of blood transfusion that was performed in Ireland in 1827.

Doctor Pebbles of Dominick Street, who was a member of the Royal College of Surgeons and was in Ireland, assisted by some other medical gentlemen, performed a blood transfusion in Wellesley Fever Hospital. He transfused 296 mL of blood from a nurse's arm into a woman who was paralyzed from uterine hemorrhage. It was marked as the first blood transfusion in Ireland with salutary effects.[44]

6.3 Women as a Blood Donor for Patients with Hemophilia

A Philadelphia doctor named John Conrad Otto (March 15, 1774 to June 26, 1844) published *An account of a hemorrhagic disposition prevailing in some families* in 1803; it contains the first description of hemophilia in contemporary times. He had a thorough understanding of the defining characteristics of hemophilia, including the genetic propensity for men to bleed. Yet, Friedrich Hopff from the University of Zurich used the term "hemophilia" for the first time in an essay that was published in 1828. In 1937, Harvard researchers Patek and Taylor discovered a way to fix the coagulation problem by using plasma-derived material. The term for this was antihemophiliac globulin. In 1944, Argentinean researcher Alfredo Pavlovsky (November 24, 1907 to April 26, 1984) demonstrated how blood from one hemophiliac may treat the coagulation disorder of another, and vice versa. He had discovered two patients who lacked the various proteins, factor VIII and factor IX. These findings enabled a precise diagnosis and formed the cornerstone of the current

---

[41] Newsom, S.W.B., Pioneers in infection control - Joseph Lister, Journal of Hospital Infection. 2003; 55(4), p. 246–253. https://pubmed.ncbi.nlm.nih.gov/14629967/.

[42] Cannas G, Thomas X., Supportive care in patients with acute leukemia: historical perspectives, Blood Transfus.2015; 13(2), p. 205–220. https://www.ncbi.nlm.nih.gov/pmc/articles/PMC4385068/.

[43] Leyden S., Kelly R. Blood work, Instruments and Innovations, Ireland. 2019; p. 11. https://issuu.com/rcsi/docs/rcsi_heritage_collections_-_instruments_innovati. Accessed at 20 Sep 2021.

[44] Anon. Transfusion, The Berkshire Chronicle, Apr 7, 1827, p. 3. https://www.Britishnewspaperarchive.co.ukAccessed 20 Sep 2021.

treatment for this inherited hemorrhagic condition.[45] Dr. Pavlovsky discovered two types of hemophilia, A and B, in 1947.[46, 47] These findings enabled a precise diagnosis and formed the cornerstone of the current treatment for this inherited hemorrhagic condition.[48]

Hemophilia A, B, and C are the three types of hemophilia. Hemophilia type A is the most prevalent form, which is caused by factor VIII deficiency. Hemophilia B occurs due to the absence or severe deficiency of clotting factor IX; this kind of hemophilia exists. Hemophilia C is an uncommon variant of hemophilia, commonly known as "factor XI deficiency." It was originally identified in 1953 in patients with significant bleeding after dental extractions. There are also other factor deficiencies, such as factor I, II, V, VII, X, XII, and XIII.[49,50]

6.4   A Blood Transfusion for a Boy with Hemophilia

Dr. Samuel Lane (1802–1892), a lecturer on anatomy and surgery, performed a blood transfusion in 1840 on a boy who was dying from hemorrhage after a slight surgical operation. The patient was a 11-year-old boy named George Firmin. He was brought to Dr. Lane by his father to perform Dieffenbach's operation to relieve the deformity of squinting. Dr. Lane reported that nothing special occurred during the procedure, except that the boy fainted and that he lost more blood compared to other patients with the same operation. The bleeding eventually subsided, and the patient was able to go home. However, on the same evening, Dr. Lane was sent for because the bleeding from the eye repeated. Dr. Lane was able to stop the bleeding in half an hour. He was also informed that the boy started to bleed for a quarter of an hour when he returned to his home and that he was actually bleeding for 6–7 h before Dr. Lane arrived. He also found out that this was not the first time the boy had severely bled and that he was in danger. He also bled before from slight injuries (tooth extraction, cut from a finger, affection of a knee joint). For 6 days and five nights, with occasional intermissions, Dr. Lane struggled to stop the bleeding. He stopped the bleeding with intermissions by several methods: applying pressure, putting the boy in an upright position to induce faintness, applying powdered gum, a natural gum tragacanth, and beaver hair obtained from a hat, which with the blood

---

[45] Franchini M, Mannucci P. M., Past, present and future of haemophilia: a narrative review, Orphanet J Rare Dis. 2012; 7(24), p. 1–8. https://www.ncbi.nlm.nih.gov/pmc/articles/PMC3502605/.

[46] Great Lakes, hemophilia foundation. History of bleeding disorder. https://glhf.org/resources/facts-about-bleeding-disorders/history-of-bleeding-disorders/. Accessed 20 Sep 2021.

[47] Haemophilia A patients do not have clotting protein factor VIII, and patients with haemophilia B lack blood clotting factor IX.

[48] Franchini, Mannucci, 2012, p.2.

[49] Healthline. Haemophilia. https://www.healthline.com/health/hemophilia. Accessed at 20 Sep 2021.

[50] National bleeding disorders foundation. Other factor deficiencies. https://www.hemophilia.org/bleeding-disorders-a-z/types/other-factor-deficiencies. Accessed 20 Sep 2021.

formed a coagulated mass, firmly concealing the whole orbit. Unfortunately, the boy's condition deteriorated, and on the fifth day, he was almost in a state of continual syncope with spasms of muscle in both the features and limbs. He was also in danger of suffocating because the contents of his stomach were inside his mouth, but he was not able to eject them. On the sixth day, the patient's health worsened, as he was in a state of shock. As a last resort, Dr. Lane decided to perform a blood transfusion. He consulted with Dr. Blundell, with whom he fully complied with all professional instructions. The blood donor was a strong and healthy woman. Lane's colleague, Dr. Ancell, successfully opened the blood donor's vein. About 5.5 ounces (about 162 mL) of blood were successfully transfused. After 3 weeks, the boy's health was completely restored, and his eye returned to its correct position. The instrument that was used was a syringe with a pipe and funnel ready for use.[51] It is clear from the described signs that the young boy suffered from hemophilia.

6.5 Blood Donation for Sister

On December 3, 1865, Dr. Joseph Antoine Roussel was called to the home of a 19-year-old patient who had an abortion after 4 months of pregnancy. The patient had no pulse and was not breathing; the heart only had a weak contraction. Dr. Roussel decided to perform a blood transfusion. Her 30-year-old sister was a blood donor. Due to the patient's weakness, Roussel had difficulty finding her vein. The patient's sister donated 320 mL of her blood directly into the vein in order to save her sister's life. After the blood transfusion, the patient opened her eyes; her face turned red; and her heart began to beat rapidly. Her sister fainted with tears of joy and fell off her chair, pulling Dr. Roussel's blood transfusion device with her, which made Dr. Roussel stop the blood transfusion. The patient fully recovered after 18 days. She later became a mother and had several children.[52]

6.6 Early Case of a Successful Autotransfusion During an Operation in Europe

Autotransfusion is a procedure followed when the blood donor and the patient are one and the same person. In this case, usually blood is collected from the patient, and later it is transfused back to him, for example, during a surgical procedure. This type of blood transfusion is called autologous. Allogenic blood transfusions are procedures followed when a blood donor and the recipient are not the same person.[53]

---

[51] Lane, S.A., Hemorrhagic diathesis Successful transfusion of blood. The Lancet. 1840; 35(896), p. 185–188. https://www.sciencedirect.com/science/article/abs/pii/S0140673600400310.
[52] Roussel, 1877, 54–57.
[53] AABB. About Blood and Cellular Therapies. Facts About Blood. https://web.archive.org/web/20080612135452/http://www.aabb.org/Content/About_Blood/Facts_About_Blood_and_Blood_Banking/fabloodautoallo.htm. Accessed 1 April 2024.

6.6 Early Case of a Successful Autotransfusion During an Operation in Europe

One of the early cases of autotransfusion during an operation in Europe, was performed on October 21, 1885, by surgeon John Duncan at the Royal Hospital in Edinburgh, who used autotransfusion during a leg amputation.

The patient was a man who, after a serious injury on the railroad, had a crushed left leg in the lower third of the thigh, which required amputation. Dr. Lindsay Porteous from Kirkcaldy sent the patient to Dr. Duncan, despite the fact that the patient was initially not bleeding as a result of preventive measures. He loosely placed a compression bandage around the patient's limb, with instructions to tighten the bandage as needed. While going to the hospital, the patient started bleeding; the dressing was not tight enough, and the patient lost a lot of blood before he even got to the hospital. When the patient arrived at the hospital, he was pale, and his heartbeat was rapid and irregular upon detection. Alcohol, ether injection, and limb elevation had barely any noticeable effect, and Dr. Duncan came to the conclusion that it was impossible for a patient to survive surgery in such a way with the loss of a leg. He decided to give the patient his own blood back. The patient was anesthetized with chloroform and then with ether. While Dr. Duncan quickly removed the limb, his assistant caught about three ounces of the patient's blood (about 89 mL) flowing from the limb into a container containing a solution of sodium phosphate. After the arteries were sutured, it was difficult to tell for a while whether the patient was dead or alive. Dr. Duncan then injected the blood and phosphate of soda[54] mixed with distilled water in the last syringe to increase the volume injected. In total, about eight ounces (about 237 mL) of the mixture were injected into the femoral isthmus. The patient was quickly put to bed, placed before the fire, and frequently given small quantities of brandy and water. The heartbeat became quite noticeable when they got the patient into bed. Overnight, the patient's condition steadily improved, and he made a full recovery.[55]

In this particular case, different sources claim that this was the first successful autotransfusion performed in Europe. But it is necessary to take into account an even older case. It is mentioned that in 1874, a German doctor, Peters, transfused 350 cubic centimeters of defibrinated blood from a patient whose feet were both frozen. The blood was transfused into the left posterior tibial artery, and he believed that he thereby preserved a portion of the frozen part. The right foot, untransfused, suffered significant damage, and the patient survived. Some sources claim that this blood transfusion was carried out by Dr. Hueter. But in the article itself, it is written that Hueter wrote this review and Peters wrote the dissertation, in which he described the only case of blood transfusion done so far by him.[56,57] Autotransfusion gained popularity after 1914. Other special types of blood transfusion, for example, in 1942

---

[54] Phosphate of soda (a combination of soda water, phosphoric acid, and flavoring).
[55] Duncan J. On Re-Infusion of Blood in Primary and Other Amputations, Br Med J. 1886; 1(1309), p. 192–193. https://pubmed.ncbi.nlm.nih.gov/20751443/. Accessed 1 June 2020.
[56] Jarcho S., Halsted W. On refusion of blood in carbon monoxide poisoning (1883), Am J Cardiol.1961, p. 589–97. https://pubmed.ncbi.nlm.nih.gov/13789548/.
[57] Peters E. Die arterielle Transfusion and ihre Anwendung bei Erfrierung. Greifswald. 1874, p. 378–381. https://ia800708.us.archive.org/view_archive.php?archive=/22/items/crossref-pre-

were also exsanguinotransfusion, which may be defined as the simultaneous withdrawal of part of the patient's blood and its replacement by blood obtained from a healthy blood donor. This procedure was performed experimentally by Burmeister in 1916 in a case of acute mercuric chloride poisoning. Then reciprocal or exchange blood transfusion may be defined as the continuous simultaneous blood transfusion of equal quantities of blood from blood donor to patient and from patient to blood donor. Also, immunotransfusion was considered a special type of blood transfusion. In this type, a blood transfusion was performed from a previously immunized blood donor. There were two types of immunotransfusion: specific and nonspecific.[58]

6.7 Blood Transfusions in the USA

In the USA, the first mentions of blood donation begin in the nineteenth century, when in 1825, in the *Philadelphia Journal of the Medical and Physical Sciences*, the editors, at the request of James Blundell, described his successful case of blood transfusion in collaboration with Dr. Waller. They wrote that an exactly identical blood transfusion was performed in 1795 by the American doctor Philip Syng Physick, who was considered the *father of surgery* in the USA.[59]

The problem with this claim for the late eighteenth century is that, aside from this mention, there is actually no written evidence anywhere in the case mentioned to confirm that Dr. Philip Syng Physick actually performed the first blood transfusion with human blood. Dr. James Blundell therefore remains the first expert to perform a successful blood transfusion with human blood.

It is stated that blood transfusions were used on cholera patients in 1832. In a documented case of cholera in 1854 where the patient was transfused with human blood, about 296 mL of blood were donated by a blood donor who was a nurse at Charity Hospital in New Orleans. Blood was transfused into the patient with a syringe. The patient died shortly after the blood transfusion, probably due to the large amount of air in the circulation. In 1858, a case of blood transfusion was reported in New Orleans in which a young female patient who had yellow fever received blood from a survivor of the same disease. She was transfused with about 74 mL of blood, which was enough to save her life. During the winter of 1860–1861, Dr. Austin Flint Jr. transfused about 207 mL of blood to a woman patient from her husband. The blood transfusion helped the patient survive for 24 h. In Chicago, Illinois, in 1860, it was reported that Dr. Brainard performed a leg amputation on a patient, and his assistant collected blood from the patient in a heated container

---

1909-scholarly-works/10.1007%252Fbf02808070.zip&file=10.1007%252Fbf02811113.pdf. Accessed 8 Jan 2024.

[58] Kilduffe, R. A., DeBakey, M. E. Chapter IV special types of transfusion. In: The Blood Bank and the Technique and Therapeutics of Transfusions. Mosby, St. Louis, 1943, p. 130–142. https://babel.hathitrust.org/cgi/pt?id=uc1.$b595310&seq=7. Accessed 28 Jan 2024.

[59] Blundell J., Transfusion of blood. The Philadelphia Journal of the Medical and Physical Sciences. 1825;11(1), p. 205–207. https://catalog.hathitrust.org/Record/000524072

during the operation and defibrinated it. Dr. Brainard revived the same patient after a leg amputation with about 59 mL of defibrinated blood. Warfare in the nineteenth century resulted in numerous serious injuries. When limbs were shattered, amputation was necessary. Surgeons cleaned their severe wounds with naphtha and creosote[60] and sawed off their damaged limbs. The best that surgeons could do to improve the chances of survival was to operate as quickly as possible, thereby minimizing shock to the human body system. During the American Civil War, four cases of blood transfusion were recorded. The first two battlefield cases, which occurred in 1864 on the side of the Union army, were described in detail. In both cases, the soldiers were shot. In the first case, 37-year-old soldier J. Mott had the upper third of his left leg amputated due to extensive bleeding and complications. The next day, he received about 473 mL of blood by syringe from a young and healthy man. Ether was used as an anesthetic. Nine days later, he unfortunately passed away due to the repeated effects of bleeding. The transfusion was carried out by assistant surgeon B. E. Fryer. In another case, surgeon E. Bentley transfused about 59 mL of blood to a 19-year-old soldier, G.P. Cross, from the temporal artery of a strong and healthy German after having his leg amputated due to bleeding from the posterior tibial artery. The soldier survived and recovered. An opening was made into the wounded soldier's median basilica vein, and about 59 mL of blood was transfused by means of a Tiemann's syringe.[61, 62] In Europe, during the Second Italian War of Independence in 1859, the Austro-Prussian War in 1866, and the later Franco-Prussian War from 1870 to 1871, a couple of cases of blood transfusions were also reported.[63]

6.7.1 Early Case of Autotransfusion in USA

One of the early cases of autotransfusion was in the USA. It was performed by an American surgeon named William Stewart Halsted (September 23, 1852 to September 7, 1922) in 1883. The patient was poisoned by carbon dioxide.

A 57-year-old patient of medium size and good physique was found unconscious in a stateroom. A strong smell of gas was sensed in the room. The patient arrived at the hospital in an ambulance. There, the surgeon noticed that the patient could not be aroused. Respirations were superficial, the pulse was fairly strong, the temperature was not taken, and he had pale and cold skin. His lips were slate-colored, and his pupils were somewhat dilated. He was placed in a hot air bath and given whisky

---

[60] Creosote is a mixture of phenol and phenolic ethers obtained from wood and coal tar.
[61] Schmidt P.J. Transfusion in America in the eighteenth and nineteenth centuries, The New England journal of medicine. 1968;279(24), p. 1319–1320. https://pubmed.ncbi.nlm.nih.gov/4880439/.
[62] Kuhns, W.J. Historical Milestones Blood Transfusion in the Civil War. Transfusion,1965;5(1), p. 92–94. https://pubmed.ncbi.nlm.nih.gov/14255506/.
[63] Boel B. Strange Blood the Rise and Fall of Lamb Blood Transfusion in nineteenth Century Medicine and Beyond, 3. Blood on the battlefield in: Strange Blood, Bielefeld: transcript Verlag. 2020; 45–59. https://d-nb.info/1211992861/34. Accesed 1 Aug 2020.

intravenously. The patient was still in very poor condition when Dr. Halsted decided to perform a blood transfusion. The patient's both arms were flexed, the right more than the left. After 20 minutes, the right radial artery was exposed above the wrist for about 1 inch, and two ligatures were passed under it. The cannula was introduced centripetally into the artery, and it was held in place by one ligature. The other was used to occlude the vessel peripherally. Dr. Halsted then drew 512 mL of the patient's blood from his artery via cannula. He then defibrinated, strained, and kept the blood at a temperature of about 37.5 °C in a blood transfusion apparatus. After 42 min, the patient's condition was slowly improving. The patient's limbs were no longer stiff, and even though his eyes were closed, he could be made to open them. From the 512 mL of defibrinated blood, 288 mL were returned through the cannula in the artery toward the heart. After 50 min, Halsted had withdrawn 300 mL of blood as before through the cannula, defibrinated it, and mixed it with 128 mL of defibrinated blood taken from another patient. Later, he infused 192 mL of the mixed blood. He noted that the patient's color returned to his face rapidly when 80–100 mL of blood was injected. The patient gradually regained consciousness. Two days later, he was allowed to go home. On October 1, the patient reported not having any single symptom of the poisoning.[64] In this interesting case, different sources claim that this was the first successful autotransfusion in the USA. But from the evidence shown, it is not clear if the patient's own blood helped him or if this was because he received another blood transfusion mixed with another patient's blood. Perhaps the reason the patient survived was accidentally because he received a larger quantity of blood or his emergency condition was not severe, and perhaps the second patient, who served as a blood donor, had the same blood group as him.

References

1. Anon. Blood transfusion. The Berkshire Chronicle; 1827. p. 3. https://www.Britishnewspaperarchive.co.uk Accessed 20 Sep 2021
2. AABB. About blood and cellular therapies. Facts About Blood. https://web.archive.org/web/20080612135452/http://www.aabb.org/Content/About_Blood/Facts_About_Blood_and_Blood_Banking/fabloodautoallo.htm Accessed 1 April 2024.
3. Blundell J. Blood transfusion of blood. Phila J Med Phys Sci. 1825;11(1):205–7. https://catalog.hathitrust.org/Record/000524072
4. Boel B. Strange blood the rise and fall of lamb blood transfusion in 19th century medicine and beyond, 3. Blood on the battlefield in: Strange Blood, Bielefeld: transcript Verlag. 2020; 45–59. https://d-nb.info/1211992861/34. Accessed 1 Aug 2020.
5. Braxton HJ. Cases of blood transfusion with some remarks on a new method of performing the operation. Guy's hospital reports. London Churchill & Sons New Burlington Street 1869; 14(3). https://www.google.si/books/edition/Guy_s_hospital_reports/Ky1TAAAAcAAJ?hl=sl&gbpv=1&dq=guys+hospital&printsec=frontcover. Accessed 6 Jan 2024.
6. Cannas G, Thomas X. Supportive care in patients with acute leukemia: historical perspectives. Blood Transfus. 2015;13(2):205–20. https://www.ncbi.nlm.nih.gov/pmc/articles/PMC4385068/

---

[64] Jarcho S., Halsted W. On refusion of blood in carbon monoxide poisoning (1883), Am J Cardiol.1961, p. 589–97. https://pubmed.ncbi.nlm.nih.gov/13789548/.

References

7. Curling J, Goss N, Bertolini J. Production of plasma proteins for therapeutic use. Hoboken, New Jersey: John Wiley and sons Inc.; 2012. p. 3–22.
8. Duncan J. On re-infusion of blood in primary and other amputations. Br Med J. 1886;1(1309):192–3. https://pubmed.ncbi.nlm.nih.gov/20751443/. Accessed 1 June 2020
9. Peters E. Die arterielle Blood transfusion and ihre Anwendung bei Erfrierung. Greifswald. 1874, 378–381. https://ia800708.us.archive.org/view_archive.php?archive=/22/items/crossref-pre-1909-scholarly-works/10.1007%252Fbf02808070.zip&file=10.1007%252Fbf02811113.pdf Accessed 8 Jan 2024.
10. Franchini M, Mannucci PM. Past, present and future of haemophilia: a narrative review. Orphanet J Rare Dis. 2012;7(24):1–8. https://www.ncbi.nlm.nih.gov/pmc/articles/PMC3502605/
11. Great Lakes, hemophilia foundation. History of bleeding disorder. https://glhf.org/resources/facts-about-bleeding-disorders/history-of-bleeding-disorders/. Accessed 20 Sep 2021.
12. Healthline. Haemophilia. https://www.healthline.com/health/hemophilia. Accessed 20 Sep 2021.
13. Inwood MJ. The evolution of modern blood transfusion apparatus, Western University. UWOMJ. 1966;37(1):3–7. https://ir.lib.uwo.ca/uwomj/218
14. Jarcho S, Halsted W. On refusion of blood in carbon monoxide poisoning (1883). Am J Cardiol. 1961:589–97. https://pubmed.ncbi.nlm.nih.gov/13789548/
15. Jennings CE. The intravenous injection of milk. Br Med J. 1885;1(1275):1147–9. https://www.ncbi.nlm.nih.gov/pmc/articles/PMC2256321/
16. Kuhns WJ. Historical milestones blood transfusion in the civil war. Blood Transfus. 1965;5(1):92–4. https://pubmed.ncbi.nlm.nih.gov/14255506/
17. Kilduffe RA, DeBakey ME. Chapter IV special types of blood transfusion. In: The blood bank and the technique and therapeutics of blood transfusions. St. Louis: Mosby; 1942. p. 130–42. https://babel.hathitrust.org/cgi/pt?id=uc1.$b595310&seq=7 Accessed 28 Jan 2024.
18. Landerer A. Ueber blood transfusion und infusion. Archiv f Pathol Anat. 1886;105:351–72. https://link.springer.com/article/10.1007/BF01940368
19. Lane SA. Hemorrhagic diathesis successful blood transfusion of blood. Lancet. 1840;35(896):185–8. https://www.sciencedirect.com/science/article/abs/pii/S0140673600400310
20. Leyden S, Kelly R. Blood work, instruments and innovations, Ireland. 2019; p. 11. https://issuu.com/rcsi/docs/rcsi_heritage_collections_-_instruments_innovati. Accessed at 20 Sep 2021.
21. Meldon A. Blood transfusion of blood and intravenous injection of milk and saline fluid. Trans RAM Ireland. 1891;9(1):214–22. https://link.springer.com/article/10.1007/BF03170599
22. MacGillivray N. Dr. Latta of Leith: Pioneer in the treatment of cholera by intravenous saline infusion. J R Coll Physicians Edinb. 2006;36(1):80–5. https://pubmed.ncbi.nlm.nih.gov/17146955/
23. Newsom SWB. Pioneers in infection control—Joseph Lister. J Hosp Infect. 2003;55(4):246–53. https://pubmed.ncbi.nlm.nih.gov/14629967/
24. National Bleeding Disorders Foundation. Other factor deficiencies. https://www.hemophilia.org/bleeding-disorders-a-z/types/other-factor-deficiencies. Accessed 20 Sep 2021.
25. Oliver J. Le Dr. Roussel, La Croix-Rouge suisse. 1952; 61, p. 9–12. https://www.e-periodica.ch/digbib/view?pid=acf-002:1952:61::231#13.
26. Oberman HA. Early history of blood substitutes: blood transfusion of Milk. Blood Transfus. 1969;9(2):74–7. https://onlinelibrary.wiley.com/doi/abs/10.1111/j.1537-2995.1969.tb04920.x
27. Roets M, Sturgess DJ, Wyssusek K, van Zundert AA. Intraoperative cell salvage: a technology built upon the failures, fads and fashions of blood transfusion. Anaesth Intensive Care. 2019;47(3):17–30. https://journals.sagepub.com/doi/10.1177/0310057X19860161#bibr3-0310057X19860161
28. Roussel J. Blood transfusion of human blood. England: J & A Churchill; 1877. p. 25–6. https://books.google.si. Accessed 27 March 2023
29. Schmidt PJ. Blood transfusion in America in the eighteenth and nineteenth centuries. N Engl J Med. 1968;279(24):1319–20. https://pubmed.ncbi.nlm.nih.gov/4880439/

30. Sergeeva MS, Panova EL. Blood transfusions for the wounded: promising method of battlefield surgery or utopia of the mid-1870s? Hist Med. 2021;7(2):133–9. https://historymedjournal.com/wp-content/uploads/volume7/number2/en/2.Sergeeva.pdf
31. Wiener AS. Chapter IV: history of blood transfusion. In: Blood groups and blood transfusion. Charles C. Thomas Publisher; 1948. p. 58.
32. Zimmerman LM, Howell KM. History of blood transfusion. Ann Med Hist. 1932;4(5):415–33. https://pubmed.ncbi.nlm.nih.gov/33944186/

Image Source

Roussel (1867) and Aveling's (1873) blood transfusion apparatus. Chapter I history. In: Kilduffe, R. A., DeBakey, M. E. The blood bank and the technique and therapeutics of blood transfusions. Mosby, St. Louis, 1942, p. 33. Permission for usage of the image was granted by the copyright holder, Elsevier, on January 23, 2024. https://babel.hathitrust.org/cgi/pt?id=uc1.$b595310&seq=1. Accessed 24 Jan 2024.

The Discovery of Blood Groups in the Twentieth Century

7

Contents

7.1 The Discovery of Blood Groups and Later Achievements.................................. 57
    7.1.1 Some Early Observations on Hemolysis and Agglutination...................... 58
    7.1.2 The Discovery of ABO Blood Group System by Karl Landsteiner 1900–1901. 59
    7.1.3 Further Discoveries on ABO Blood Group System by Other Experts............ 60
    7.1.4 Some Interesting Facts About ABO Blood Group System........................ 61
    7.1.5 Blood Grouping.. 62
7.2 The Discovery of Rh Blood Group System.. 63
7.3 Erythroblastosis Fetalis... 64
7.4 Discovery of Other Blood Group Systems... 67
7.5 Compatibility of Blood Donors and Patients Cross-Match Testing.................... 69
7.6 Definition of Universal Blood Donor and Patient... 70
7.7 Coombs Tests... 70
7.8 Important Events in Immunohematology and Serology................................. 71
    7.8.1 Some Important Achievements in Serology in the 1950s........................ 71
    7.8.2 Some Important Achievements in Immunohematology from the 1950s to 1970s.. 71
7.9 Organ Transplantation.. 72
7.10 Hematopoietic Stem Cell Transplantation.. 73
References.. 74

7.1 The Discovery of Blood Groups and Later Achievements

Blood groups are antigenic determinants on the surface of blood cells, but the use of the term is generally restricted to antigens on RBC. A blood group system is one or more blood group antigens encoded by either a single gene or a cluster of two or

© The Author(s), under exclusive license to Springer Nature Switzerland AG 2024
Z. Kvržić, *History of Blood Donation and Transfusion Medicine*,
https://doi.org/10.1007/978-3-031-68715-0_7

more closely linked, homologous genes.[1] A person's biological parents determine their blood group. The RhD and ABO genes are inherited from the parents. A person may not have the exact same blood group as their parents due to the large number of potential combinations. A person usually has the same blood group throughout their entire life. Yet occasionally, blood groups can alter. The change is typically related to particular events, such as receiving a bone marrow transplant, developing a specific form of leukemia, or contracting an infection. Not all of these blood group alterations are long-lasting.[2]

7.1.1 Some Early Observations on Hemolysis and Agglutination

In the nineteenth century, xenotransfusions were occasionally performed with sheep's blood or with the blood of other domestic animals. Fatal reactions that occurred intrigued physiologist Leonard Landois (December 1, 1837 to November 17, 1902) and others to investigate this problem.[3] In 1869, as a medical student, Adolf Creite published a paper in which he wrote that serum proteins had the property of both dissolving and bringing about clustering of RBC, that is, lysis and agglutination.[4, 5] Landois in 1875 found that if human blood is mixed with the blood of other animals in vitro, hemolysis or agglutination of the blood cells occurs. This work, as well as Bordet's, in which he immunized animals with the serum or blood of animals of different species, led to the concept of species specificity of blood.[6, 7] Doctor Edoardo Maragliano in Genoa in the year 1892 reported that an infected person's serum may have a "globulicidal" effect on another person's RBC, causing them to hemolyze entirely.[8]

---

[1] Reid M. E. Blood Group Systems. In: Maloy S., Huges K., editors. Brenner's Encyclopedia of Genetics (Second Edition). Academic Press; 2013, p. 351–352. https://www.sciencedirect.com/science/article/abs/pii/B9780123749840001595. Accessed 12 Jan 2024.

[2] Cleveland Clinic, Blood types. https://my.clevelandclinic.org/health/articles/21213-blood-types. Accessed 9 Dec 2021.

[3] Wiener, 1948, p. 4.

[4] Hughes-Jones NC, Gardner B. Red cell agglutination: the first description by Creite (1869) and further observations made by Landois (1875) and Landsteiner (1901), Br J Haematol. 2022;119 (4), p. 889–893. https://pubmed.ncbi.nlm.nih.gov/12472564/.

[5] Agglutination is the aggregation of cellular elements into larger and smaller aggregates as a result of a reaction between a cell surface antigen or flagellum and an appropriate antibody.

[6] Wiener, 1948, p. 4.

[7] Bird 1971, p. 42.

[8] Pierce S. R., Reid M. E. Section 1: ABO: The Birth of Blood Groups: 1. Blood Groups—From Then 'Til Now. In: Bloody Brilliant! A History of Blood Groups and Blood Groupers. AABB Press, Bethesda, Maryland; 2016, p. 1.

7.1.2 The Discovery of ABO Blood Group System by Karl Landsteiner 1900–1901

Karl Landsteiner was born in Vienna on June 14, 1868. He entered the University of Vienna in 1885, and after 6 years of study, he graduated as a doctor of medicine in 1891. In 1896, he became an assistant at the Institute of Hygiene at the University of Vienna. From 1898 to 1908, he was an assistant at the Pathological Institute. In 1908, he was a prosector at the Wilhelminenspital, where he served as a pathologist from 1909 to 1919, earning the rank of professor. After World War I, he moved to Holland, where he worked as a pathologist in The Hague at the R. K. Ziekenhuis from 1919 to 1922. He was then in New York. In 1922, he became a member of the Rockefeller Institute for Medical Research, where he continued to work for more than 20 years. In 1939, he was made an emeritus member of the Institute. He completed the preparation of a new edition of his book, *The Specificity of Serological Reactions*, which was already a classic when he died on June 26, 1943, at the Rockefeller Institute Hospital. Landsteiner published about 330 papers on his investigations in chemistry, pathological anatomy, experimental pathology,[9] serology,[10] and immunology.[11] His studies of syphilis and poliomyelitis were particularly important. Probably his most far-reaching work was in immunochemistry.[12]

Landsteiner, in 1900, made the first observations on differences between the blood of normal individuals belonging to the same species in human beings. His investigations were prompted by the discovery of serological species specificity. He mixed the serum of one individual with the RBC of other individuals.[13] He predicted that possible reactions would be minor since the blood of individuals was of the same species. As he anticipated, many of his tests came back negative, and some of the reactions were weak. Nevertheless, certain red cells strongly clumped together. The agglutination was just as intense when compared to the reactions when blood from different species was mixed together. Landsteiner's observations showed that a person's own serum and red cells never reacted. It is interesting that not all of the blood samples Landsteiner tested were from healthy people; some of them were from patients.[14] In 1900, in a footnote to a paper published in the journal *Zentralblatt für Bakteriologie*, Landsteiner mentioned the agglutination that occurred between

---

[9] Pathology is a knowledge of diseases and disease processes in organisms.

[10] Serology is science of serums: to deal with serology.

[11] Immunology is knowledge of the organism's resistance to a specific infection: immunology laboratory; immunology; and virology.

[12] Stevenson L. F. Nobel prize winners in medicine and physiology, 1901–1950, New York, Schuman.1953, p. 143–147. https://archive.org/details/nobelprizewinner0000stev/page/142/mode/2up Accessed 10 Oct 2021.

[13] Wiener A. S. Chapter I: introduction. In: Blood groups and transfusion. Charles C. Thomas publisher; 1948, p. 4.

[14] Pierce, Reid, 2016, p. 1.

blood serum and blood cells from different humans.[15] On November 14, 1901, in the journal *Wiener klinische Wochenschrift*,[16] followed up with a full paper, *On the Agglutination of Normal Human Blood*, in which he was able, on the basis of the isoagglutination[17] reaction, to divide human blood into three groups: A, B, and C, which was later changed into O.[18, 19, 20]

7.1.3 Further Discoveries on ABO Blood Group System by Other Experts

In 1902, Landsteiner's associate, Adriano Sturli (1873–1964), working with Alfred von Decastello, described the fourth group, AB.[21] Landsteiner originally called group "O" as "C."[22] The name "*O*" was first used in 1911 by Emil von Dungen (November 26, 1867 to September 4, 1961), a German internist, and Ludwik Hirszfeld (August 5, 1884 to March 7, 1954), a Polish microbiologist and serologist. Blood groups A, B, AB, and O were categorized by a Czech serologist, neurologist, and psychiatrist Jan Jansky (April 3, 1873 to September 8, 1921) and an American physician in 1907 and professor of medicine William Lorenzo Moss (August 23, 1876 to August 12, 1957) in 1910.[23] Jansky and Moss differently categorized blood groups using Roman numerals, which was confusing (Fig. 7.1).

Von Dungern and Hirszfeld in 1910 proved that blood groups are inherited. In 1911, they also discovered that there were subdivisions in two of the four human blood groups. Sergei Natanovich Bernstein, in 1925, determined the exact mechanism of heredity.[24] The American Association of Immunologists therefore sponsored in 1927 a new classification suggested by Karl Landsteiner (A, B, AB, O).[25]

---

[15] Shaw, L. B., & Shaw, R. A. The Pre-Anschluss Vienna School of Medicine—The medical scientists: Karl Landsteiner (1868–1943) and Otto Loewi (1873–1961), Journal of Medical Biography. 2016; 24(3), p. 289–301. https://pubmed.ncbi.nlm.nih.gov/25052151/.

[16] Schwarz, H. P., & Dorner, F., Karl Landsteiner and his major contributions to haematology, British Journal of Haematology. 2003; 121(4), p. 556–565. https://pubmed.ncbi.nlm.nih.gov/12752096/.

[17] Isoagglutination is the clumping of the RBC by a transfusion of the blood or serum of a genetically different individual of the same species.

[18] Shaw, L. B., & Shaw, R. A. 2016, p.2.

[19] Brewer H. F. The blood groups, section IV. In: Brewer H.F., Ellis R., Greaves R. I. N., Keynes G., Mills F. W., Bodley Scott R., Till A., Whitby L. Blood transfusion. Bristol: John Wright & sons LTD. London: Simpkin Marshall (1941). LTD.;1949, p. 213.

[20] Maluf, 1954, p. 90.

[21] Grenfell Stevenson 1953, p. 146.

[22] Learoyd P. Chapter 1 Historical perspective. In: Thomas D., Thompson J., Ridler B., editors. All blood counts. Publishing Limited, Castle Hill Barns, Harley, Nr Shrewsbury; 2016, p. 18–19.

[23] Durand J. K., Willis M. S., Landsteiner K. Transfusion Medicine, Laboratory Medicine. 2010; 41(1), p. 53–55. https://academic.oup.com/labmed/article/41/1/53/2504910.

[24] Wiener A. S. 1948, p. 5.

[25] Maluf 1954, p. 90.

7.1 The Discovery of Blood Groups and Later Achievements   61

Fig. 7.1 Classification of blood groups, 1907–1927

JANSKY 1907	MOSS 1910	INTERNATIONAL 1927
I	IV	O
II	II	A
III	III	B
IV	I	AB

Today's classification system is known as the Landsteiner nomenclature, named after the person who discovered blood groups.[26] This classification eventually became internationally confirmed and used.

7.1.4 Some Interesting Facts About ABO Blood Group System

The ABO blood group system is considered the first and clinically most important system, as far as the blood transfusion of blood is concerned.[27, 28] Antibodies and antigens are all important for understanding our blood groups. A antigens are present on the blood group A's RBC, with anti-B antibodies in the plasma. The B group has B antigens on the RBC and anti-A antibodies in the plasma. The term "universal" refers to blood group O, which contains no AB antigens on the RBC, but antibodies anti-A and anti-B are present in the plasma. People with the AB blood group have both anti-A and anti-B antigens on their RBC, but their plasma does not contain any ABO antibodies. The ability to receive blood from any other blood group is made possible by this. Because of a lack of antibodies, their plasma is universal, which is why they are referred to as universal patients and universal plasma blood donors. It may be fatal to get blood from the incorrect ABO group. When a person with group A blood receives group B blood, for instance, the anti-B antibodies in that person's body will attack the group B cells.[29] A blood transfusion must not be performed if it carries an ABO antigen that the patient lacks. Blood transfusion accidents with serious outcomes, including death on some occasions, are most often caused by ABO incompatibility involving blood transfusion of the wrong ABO group blood. Fortunately, determining the ABO groups of blood donors and patients is relatively straight forward (Fig. 7.2).[30]

---

[26] Durand, Willis, 2010, p. 53–55.
[27] ISBT. Red Cell Immunogenetics and Blood Group Terminology. 001 ABO Alleles. https://www.isbtweb.org/resource/001aboalleles.html Accessed 12 Jan 2024.
[28] Issit P. D. Applied blood group serology. Durham, N. C.: Montgomery Scientific Publications; 1998, p. 175. https://archive.org/details/appliedbloodgrou0000issi_ed04/page/174/mode/2up?view=theater. Accessed 13 Jan 2024.
[29] NHS, Blood Groups. https://www.nhs.uk/conditions/blood-groups/. Accessed 8 Dec 2021.
[30] Issit, 1998, p. 175.

BLOOD GROUP	CAN BE TRANSFUSED TO THESE BLOOD GROUPS	CAN GET THE BLOOD TRANSFUSION FROM THESE BLOOD GROUPS
A+	A+, AB+	A+, A-, O+, O-
A-	A-, A+, AB+, AB-	A-, O-
B+	B+, AB+	B+, B-, O+, O-
B-	B-, B+, AB+, AB-	B-, O-
AB+	AB+	AB+, AB-, A+, A-, B+, B-, O+, O-
AB-	AB-, AB+	AB-, A-, B-, O-
O+	O+, A+, B+, AB+	O+, O-
O-	O-, O+, A+, A-, B+, B-, AB+, AB-	O-

Fig. 7.2 Blood group matching

7.1.5 Blood Grouping

Because of the presence of the expected ABO agglutinins whenever an antigen is absent, ABO typing can be performed on both cells and serum. It is of great importance that all patients and blood donors have cell and serum typing determined in order to reduce the possibility of mismatches and consequent dangers with blood transfusion (Image 7.1).[31]

Landsteiner described his own grouping technique in 1901. He said: *Equal amounts of serum and 5 percent red blood cell suspension in 0.6 percent sodium chloride were mixed and observed in a hanging drop preparation or in the test tube.* Moss in 1910 improved the tube technique, which Landsteiner had initially proposed in 1901. In 1916, a complex testing protocol was developed by Brem in which two "Platinum loopfuls" of serum were combined with one coverslip containing a 5% cell suspension. The coverslip was then placed over a microscope cavity slide and sealed with petroleum jelly.[32] By the year 1929, the most popular method was the one that Moss developed. The Moss test technique was as follows: One drop of test serum III was placed in the middle of a microscope slide, and one drop of test serum II was placed toward the end of the slide. Now, by pricking the finger or the ear of the one whose blood it was intended to test, one drop of blood was obtained, and with the help of a lancet or the end of a microscope slide, a small amount of that blood was transfused to one of the drops of test serum, and there it was mixed a little, and then, after the lancet was wiped, the same amount of blood was transfused with it or the other end of the microscope slide to another drop of test serum and mixed with it. Then the slide was easily tilted to one side and the other, but not so that the serum was spilled or the drops were mixed, and the agglutination reaction, if it occurred, would occur in a short time and at a higher temperature rather than a lower one. Agglutination occurred in the form of very small grains, which soon

---

[31] Ibid.
[32] Farr, 1979, p. 219.

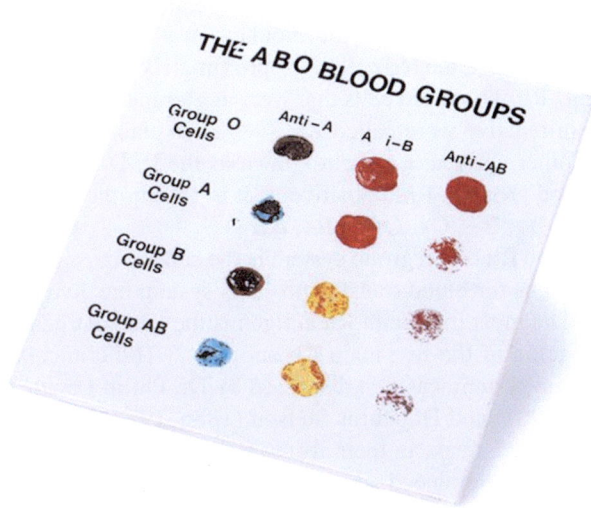

Image 7.1 Blood-grouping tile. (Source: Science Museum Group. Copy of a blood-grouping tile. 1981–476 Pt1. Science Museum Group Collection Online. Accessed 8 March 2024. Creative Commons Attribution 4.0 license. https://collection.sciencemuseumgroup.org.uk/objects/co137154/copy-of-a-blood-grouping-tile-blood-grouping-tile)

became larger and clearer, and between which there was a clear serum.[33] As an example, in 1948, there were also a variety of ways to determine blood groups. This included the tube method, the centrifuge method, and the third method, which was carried out by mixing the cell suspensions and serum directly on a glass slide.[34] Today, procedures for ABO grouping can be done by slide, tube, gel cards or cassettes (column agglutination technique, CAT), and microplate.[35] In 1949, for example, blood was taken from the blood donor by a needle prick of the ear or finger.[36] Today, we only prick the finger.

7.2 The Discovery of Rh Blood Group System

The Rhesus (Rh) blood group system was discovered in 1937 by Landsteiner and Alexander Solomon Wiener (March 16, 1907 to November 6, 1976), an American biologist and physician, but their research wasn't published until 1940 to enable the development of better anti-rhesus serum manufacturing techniques.[37, 38] Landsteiner and Weiner reported the findings of studies conducted in 1940 and 1941, where they

---

[33] Gjukić, 1929, p. 264–265.

[34] Wiener A. S. Chapter II: The four blood groups. In: Blood groups and transfusion. Charles C. Thomas publisher; 1948, p. 13–14.

[35] Goubran, H. Blood group serology. ISBT Science Series. 2009; 4 1–5. https://onlinelibrary.wiley.com/action/showCitFormats?doi=10.1111%2Fj.1751-2824.2009.01206.x. Accessed 13 Jan 2024

[36] Brewer, p. 227.

[37] Grenfell Stevenson, 1953, p. 147.

[38] Schwarz, Dorner, 2003, p. 556–565.

used RBC from rhesus monkeys (*Macaca mulatta*) to immunize rabbits and guinea pigs. The blood from the monkeys was injected into them. The antibody raised agglutinated the red cells of approximately 85% of random humans and was named anti-Rh. Those red cells that were agglutinated were said to be Rh+; those that were non-reactive were called Rh-.[39, 40] To explain more precisely, RBC sometimes has another antigen, a protein known as the RhD antigen. If this is present, a person's blood group is RhD-positive. If it is absent, the blood group is RhD-negative (A+, A−, B+, B−, O+, O−, AB+, AB−).[41]

The Rh blood group system is the second most significant blood group system in humans for blood transfusion. This system has five major antigens: D, C, E, c, and e. The most important Rh antigen is the RhD antigen, because it is the most immunogenic of the five main Rh antigens.[42] The clinical significance of the Rh blood group system was first discussed by Dr. Philip Levine (August 10, 1900 to October 18, 1987) and Dr. Rufus Stetson (1886–1977) in 1939, both from the USA.[43] They described a case in their article from 1937 of an immunized pregnant woman. The patient experienced adverse transfusion reactions (pains in legs and head), following the blood transfusion of her husband's blood after giving birth to a stillborn infant. Her serum agglutinated about 80% of ABO compatible human red blood cell samples.[44, 45] The safety of allogeneic transfusion was greatly enhanced by the discovery of the Rh blood group systems and the development of new techniques to show how IgG class antibodies, which were formerly known as blocking or incomplete antibodies, bound to RBC.[46]

7.3 Erythroblastosis Fetalis

Erythroblastosis fetalis (EF) is also called hemolytic disease of the newborn (HDN), and it is also known as hemolytic disease of the fetus and newborn (HDFN), and as alloimmune HDFN.

EF is mostly caused by Rho (D) incompatibility, which can occur when a woman with RhD-negative blood becomes pregnant with a man who has RhD-positive

---

[39] Issit, 1998, p. 315.

[40] Schwarz, Dorner, 2003, p. 556–565.

[41] NHS- Blood Groups, 2021.

[42] Goubran, 2009, p. 3.

[43] Rahorst L. The History of the Rh Blood Group & How Genomics Is Changing RhD Typing, New York blood center, NYBC Genomics laboratory. Available at: https://www.bloodgroupgenomics.org/blog-blood-experts/articles/history-rh-blood-group-how-genomics-changing-rhd-typing/. Accessed 10 Nov 2021.

[44] Levine P., Stetson R.E. An unusual case of intra-group agglutination. JAMA. 1939;113(2):126–127. https://jamanetwork.com/journals/jama/article-abstract/290521.

[45] Rahorst, 2024.

[46] Högman, C.F. Transfusion Medicine: Historical Overview. In: Smit Sibinga, C.T., Das, P.C., Cash, J.D. (eds) Transfusion Medicine: Fact and Fiction. Developments in Hematology and Immunology, vol 27. Springer, Boston, MA; 1992. p. 139–151.

7.3 Erythroblastosis Fetalis

blood and conceives a fetus with RhD-positive blood. EF can also result from fetomaternal incompatibility involving, among others, the antigen systems of Kell, Duffy, Kidd, MNSs, Lutheran, Diego, Xg, P, Ee, and Cc, among others. EF is not caused by ABO blood type incompatibilities.[47] In EF maternal immunoglobulin G (IgG) antibodies destroy the RBC of the neonate or fetus. The process when the maternal antibodies form in response to a fetal antigen is called Isoimmunization. The formation of these antibodies occurs when fetal erythrocytes cross the placenta and obtain access to maternal blood, expressing specific RBC antigens that are not present in the mother. Hemolysis, the production of bilirubin, and anemia could result from this antibody response's ability to damage fetal RBC.[48] Unless the woman has experienced prior miscarriages or abortions, firstborn babies are typically unaffected. Her immune system will become more sensitive as a result. This is due to the mother's prolonged production of antibodies. It might harm all of her later-born RhD-positive offspring.[49] Treatment of EF may involve intrauterine fetal transfusion or neonatal exchange transfusion. The prevention of EF is with RhoGAM (rhod immune globulin human) medicine.[50] Rho(D) immune globulin is a preparation of human IgG containing antibodies against the Rho(D) antigen of the red cell.[51] RhoGAM are special immune globulins made from human plasma. RhoGAM prevents RH incompatibility in mothers who are RhD-negative. If the father of the infant is RhD-positive or if his blood type is not known, the mother is given an intramuscular injection of RhoGAM during the second trimester. If the baby is RhD-positive, the mother will get a second injection within a few days after giving birth. These injections prevent the development of antibodies against RhD-positive blood. However, women with RhD-negative blood type must get injections during every pregnancy, after a miscarriage or abortion, after prenatal tests such as amniocentesis and chorionic villus biopsy or after injury to the abdomen during pregnancy.[52, 53] RhoGAM was developed by Columbia researchers John Gorman, MD, and Vincent Freda, MD, and a pharmaceutical company researcher, William Pollack, PhD, in the early 1960s. Also important contribution for this research was provided by two physicians Cyril Clarke, MD, and Ronald Finn, MD. The medicine was approved by Food and drug administration of USA (FDA) in 1968. The first patient who received RhoGAM was a pregnant woman named Marianne Cummins, who

---

[47] MSD Manual. Hemolytic disease of the fetus and neonate. https://www.msdmanuals.com/professional/gynecology-and-obstetrics/antenatal-complications/hemolytic-disease-of-the-fetus-and-neonate?query=hemolytic%20disease%20of%20the%20newborn. Accessed 27 Feb 2024.

[48] Nassar G.N., Wehbe C. Erythroblastosis Fetalis. [Updated 2023 Jun 26]. In: StatPearls [Internet]. Treasure Island (FL): StatPearls Publishing; 2024 Jan-. https://www.ncbi.nlm.nih.gov/books/NBK513292/. Accessed 27 Feb 2024.

[49] MedlinePlus. Rh incompatibility. https://medlineplus.gov/ency/article/001600.htm. Accessed 27 Feb 2024.

[50] MSD manual, 2024.

[51] Nassar, Wehbe, 2024.

[52] MedlinePlus, 2024.

[53] RhoGAM. Your baby's life story begins. https://www.rhogam.com/rhogam-science/. Accessed 27 Feb 2024.

was given RhoGAM on May 29, 1968. One year after the release of RhoGAM almost every pregnant RhD-negative woman in the USA, Canada, and most of Europe received this medication, thus saving the lives of millions of RhD-positive newborns.[54] After discovering a link between the Rh blood group system and the prevalence of erythroblastosis fetalis (EF),[55] Wiener in general came to the conclusion that the RhD incompatibility was also responsible for blood transfusion reactions, not only due to ABO incompatibility. In order to treat newborn infants with erythroblastosis fetalis, experts performed exchange blood transfusion. This blood transfusion procedure saved the lives of thousands of infants.[56, 57, 58] However, it has to be noted that this disease was recognized in the English literature before 1900 as a form of fetal hydrops. It was also known as familial icterus gravis and congenital anemia of the newborn. From 1900 to 1920, extensive studies were made on this subject, especially by the Germans. Not long after 1920, anemia, which developed unexplainably in newborn infants, was considered a new entity.[59, 60] Exchange blood transfusion was also known as exsanguination, venesection, or substitution blood transfusion. In 1921, the Canadian surgeon Lawrence Bruce Robertson developed exsanguination blood transfusion as a treatment for the toxic shock of severe burns and sepsis.[61, 62] Dr. A.P. Hart from Toronto's Hospital for Sick Children in 1925 reported about the use of exchange blood transfusion for EF. Hart convinced his colleague, Dr. J.I. MacDonald, to perform the exchange blood transfusion using a

---

[54] Columbia Medicine. RhoGAM at 50: A Drug Still Saving Lives of Newborns. https://www.columbiamedicinemagazine.org/ps-news/spring-2018/rhogam-50-drug-still-saving-lives-newborns. Accessed 27 Feb 2024.

[55] Erythroblastosis fetalis or hemolytic disease of the newborn is a blood disorder in a fetus or newborn infant. It occurs when the blood groups of a mother and baby are incompatible.

[56] Exchange transfusion is a blood *transfusion in which the patient's blood or components of it are exchanged with (replaced by)* other blood or blood products.

[57] Wiener AS, Wexler IB. The use of heparin when performing exchange blood transfusions in newborn infants. J Lab Clin Med. 1946; 31:1016–9. https://scholar.google.com/scholar?cluster=16805773366256891543&hl=sl&as_sdt=0,5. Accessed 7 Jan 2024.

[58] Bionity.com. Rhesus blood group system. https://www.bionity.com/en/encyclopedia/Rhesus_blood_group_system.html#_note-2/. Accessed 11 Nov 2021.

[59] Pochedly C. History of the exchange transfusion; its use in treatment of erythroblastosis fetalis. Bulletin of the History of Medicine. 1970; 44(5), p. 450–460. https://www.jstor.org/stable/44450798. Accessed 13 Jan 2024.

[60] Otto, Merle Lewis, "Erythroblastosis fetalis: early recognition: indications for therapy and therapy by exchange transfusion." MD Theses. 1848. 1952, p. 1–6. https://digitalcommons.unmc.edu/mdtheses/1848. Accessed 13 Jan 2024.

[61] Robertson BA. Blood transfusions in severe burns in infants and young children: a preliminary report of the treatment of the toxic shock by blood transfusion, with or without preceding exsanguination. Can Med Assoc J. 1921;11 (10), p. 744–750. https://www.ncbi.nlm.nih.gov/pmc/articles/PMC1524233/.

[62] Alistair G. S. Philip; Historical Perspectives: The Rise and Fall of Exchange Transfusion. Neoreviews July 2003; 4 (7): p. 171. https://publications.aap.org/neoreviews/article-abstract/4/7/e169/92043/Historical-PerspectivesThe-Rise-and-Fall-of?redirectedFrom=fulltext. Accessed 13 Jan 2024.

technique developed by Dr. Lawrence Bruce Robertson. Hart's 1925 article was not largely noticed, and it was not until 1946 that exchange blood transfusions began to be used as a treatment for EF. Dr. H. Wallerstein from New York was, in 1946, the first to use exchange blood transfusion for EF. In the same year, the procedure was performed using another technique by Wiener and I. B. Wexler. Both Wallerstein's and Weiner's procedures were technically challenging and fraught with serious difficulties, and soon they were superseded by a method introduced by Dr. L.K. Diamond in 1946.[63] In 1963, an intrauterine blood transfusion[64] was introduced by Albert William Liley (March 12, 1929 to June 15, 1983),[65, 66] which made it possible to successfully treat far more severely afflicted fetuses.[67]

7.4 Discovery of Other Blood Group Systems

After the discovery of the ABO and the Rh blood group systems, Kell, Duffy, Kidd, and many other blood group systems were the next important ones to be discovered.[68] The Kell blood group system was discovered in 1946. It was named after Mrs. Kelleher, a patient whose newborn child had hemolytic disease due to anti-Kell antibodies.[69] The experts who discovered it were Robin Coombs, Rob Race, and Arthur Mourant.[70] Duffy blood group system was discovered in 1950.[71] It was named after a patient named Mr. Duffy, who had multiple blood transfusions. It was found in its serum by Cutbush, Mollison, and Parkin.[72] Kidd blood group system

---

[63] Ibid. 171.

[64] The process of injecting RBC from a blood donor into the fetus is known as intrauterine transfusion.

[65] Pasman S. A., Claes L., Lewi L., Van Schoubroeck D., Debeer A., Emonds M., Geuten E., De Catte L., Devlieger R. Intrauterine transfusion for fetal anemia due to red blood cell alloimmunization: 14 years' experience in Leuven. Facts, views & vision in ObGyn. 2015; 7(2), p. 129–136. https://www.ncbi.nlm.nih.gov/pmc/articles/PMC4498170/.

[66] O'Connor K. Albert William Liley (1929–1983). https://embryo.asu.edu/pages/albert-william-liley-1929-1983. Accessed 7 Jan 2024.

[67] Bionity.com, 2021.

[68] Westhoff CM, Reid ME, Review: The Kell, Duffy, and Kidd blood group systems, Immunohematology.2004; 20(1), p. 37–49. https://pubmed.ncbi.nlm.nih.gov/15373667/.

[69] Dean L, Blood Groups and Red Cell Antigens. US: Bethesda (MD): National Center for Biotechnology Information. 2005, Chapter 8, p. 2. https://www.ncbi.nlm.nih.gov/books/NBK2267. Accessed 7 Jan 2024.

[70] Pamphilon D.H., Scott, M.L. Robin Coombs: his life and contribution to haematology and transfusion medicine. British Journal of Haematology. 2007; 137(5), p. 404 https://pubmed.ncbi.nlm.nih.gov/17488485/.

[71] Simmons, R., Gajdusek, D., Gorman, J. et al., Presence of the Duffy Blood Group Gene Fy^b demonstrated in Melanesians. 1967; Nature, 213, p. 1148–1149. https://www.nature.com/articles/2131148a0#citeas. Accessed 7 Jan 2024.

[72] Sanger, R., Race, R.R. and Jack, J., The Duffy Blood Groups of New York Negroes: The Phenotype Fy (a − b−). British Journal of Haematology. 1955; 1(4), p. 370–374. https://pubmed.ncbi.nlm.nih.gov/13269673/.

was discovered in 1951 when an unknown antibody detected in the plasma of a patient, Mrs. Kidd, caused hemolytic disease of the fetus and was born in her infant son.[73] This blood group system was discovered by the experts Allen, Diamond, and Niedziela.[74] In 1927, Landsteiner and Levine identified three more separate properties in human blood, which they designated as M, N, and P.[75] Walsh and Montgomery (1947) found, in a sample of human serum, an agglutinin that did not coincide with any known at that time. Ruth Sanger and Robert Russell Race (1947) showed that this agglutinin subdivided the three genotypes of the MN system in such a way that a connection between the new antigen, which they called S, and the MN antigens must exist. This became known as MNS blood group system.[76] LW was discovered in 1940,[77] Lutheran in 1945, and Lewis in 1946.[78] Other blood group systems were discovered in the following years. As of July 2023, there are 45 recognized blood group systems with 360 red cell antigens. Fifty genes define the genetic makeup of the 45 systems.[79] The rarest blood group discovered in 1961 is Rh null, referred to as the "golden blood."[80] The Rh null phenotype is a rare blood group characterized by the lack of expression of all Rh antigens (D, C, c, E, and e) on the red cells.[81] If a person is RhD-negative, he or she will still have some Rh proteins, but a person who is Rh-null has none of the antigens at all.[82] Fewer than 50 people in the world have a Rh null.[83] Rh null individuals (lacking all Rh antigens) have a mild clinical condition called Rh-deficiency syndrome, characterized by membrane abnormalities and some degree of hemolytic anemia.[84]

---

[73] Hamilton JR. Kidd blood group system: a review, Immunohematology. 2015; 31(1), p. 29–35. https://pubmed.ncbi.nlm.nih.gov/26308468/.

[74] Plaut G, Ikin EW, Mourant AE, Sanger R, Race RR., A new blood-group antibody, anti Jkb., Nature. 1953; 171(4349), p. 431. https://pubmed.ncbi.nlm.nih.gov/13046499/.

[75] Wiener A. S. 1948, p. 5.

[76] Sanger R., Race R. R. The mnss blood group system. American journal of human genetics.1951;3(4), p. 332–343. https://www.ncbi.nlm.nih.gov/pmc/articles/PMC1716423/.

[77] Storry J.R. Review: the LW blood group system. Immunohematology. 1992;8(4):87–93. https://pubmed.ncbi.nlm.nih.gov/15946068/.

[78] Smart, E., Armstrong, B., Blood group systems, ISBT Science Series. 2008; 3(2), p. 68–92. https://onlinelibrary.wiley.com/doi/10.1111/j.1751-2824.2008.00188.x.

[79] International society of blood transfusion (ISBT). Red Cell Immunogenetics and Blood Group Terminology. https://www.isbtweb.org/isbt-working-parties/rcibgt.html. Accessed 6 Jan 2024.

[80] Mcnab K. In a similar vein to the gods: golden blood. 2022. https://blog.sciencemuseumgroup.org.uk/golden-blood/. Accessed 2 April 2024.

[81] Qureshi A, Salman M, Moiz B. Rhnull: a rare blood group phenotype. J Pak Med Assoc. 2010;60(11),p.960–961. https://pubmed.ncbi.nlm.nih.gov/21375204/.

[82] Mcnab, 2022.

[83] Canadian Blood Services. Rarest blood type. https://www.blood.ca/en/blood/donating-blood/what-my-blood-type. Accessed 2 April 2024.

[84] Cotorruelo C. Elucidation of the molecular bases of the Rh system and its contribution to transfusion and obstetric medicine—historical and current perspective: a review. Annals of Blood, 2023, 8, p. 3. https://aob.amegroups.org/article/view/8450/html. Accessed 2 April 2024.

7.5 Compatibility of Blood Donors and Patients Cross-Match Testing

An American pathologist, microbiologist, and immunologist, Ludvig Hektoen (July 2, 1863 to July 5, 1951), proposed in 1907 that the safety of blood transfusions could be improved and thus the occurrence of adverse effects reduced by cross-matching blood samples to determine compatibility between blood donors and patients.[85] Reuben Ottenberg performed the first blood transfusion using ABO-compatible blood grouping and cross-matching of blood between the blood donor and patient in 1908 at Mount Sinai Hospital in New York.[86] In numerous sources, it is mistakenly stated that he did this in 1907.

He was the first to recognize that blood donors with blood group O are universal blood donors, which means that their blood can, in principle, be received by patients of any ABO group.[87] Franz Oehlecker (1874–1957) of Hamburg (Germany) developed a "biological test." In 1933, he published a book in which he described his test. Increasing volumes of blood from the blood donor (5 cm^3, 10 cm^3, and 20 cm^3) were injected into the patient at two-minute intervals. Any hemolytic reactions were said to occur in the first 1–2 min after the injection, and late reactions after a successful blood transfusion were not considered hemolytic.[88]

Despite Ottenberg's evidence that pre-transfusion cross-matching between blood donor erythrocytes and patient serum is important for safe blood transfusion, it took until 1913 for this method to become accepted in everyday practice.[89]

There are several reasons why this has been the case. Many doctors relied on blood group O rather than performing pre-transfusion testing. In the case of a severely injured patient, transfusion reactions could be confused with the course of the patient's condition. In the case of a smaller volume of transfused blood, transfusion reactions were also milder, bearing in mind that in certain transfusion methods, e.g., vein-to-vein, a lot of blood was spilled on the floor and that a smaller volume of blood actually entered the patient's bloodstream. Statistically speaking, transfusion reactions may also have been milder or may not have occurred if, by chance,

---

[85] Hektoen L. Iso agglutination of human corpuscles: with respect to demonstration of opsonic index and to transfusion of blood, JAMA. 1907; 48(21), p. 1739–1740. https://Jamanetwork.com/journals/jama/article-abstract/463552.

[86] Mount Sinai Hospital. 1852–2002, The Sesquicentennial. The Mount Sinai hospital, New York. 2002, p. 33. https://icahn.mssm.edu/files/ISMMS/Assets/About%20the%20School/Academic%20IT%20(AIT)/Levy%20Library/Sesquicentennial.pdf. Accessed 5 Dec 2021.

[87] Mount Sinai Hospital. Journal of the Mount Sinai hospital, New York: Mount Sinai hospital; 1942–1943, p. 201. https://archive.org/details/journalofmountsi9194moun/page/n221/mode/2up?q=Reuben. Accessed 5 Dec 2021.

[88] Farr A.D. blood group serology-the first four decades (1900–1939). Medical History. 1979; 23, p. 219–225. https://www.ncbi.nlm.nih.gov/pmc/articles/PMC1082436/pdf/medhist00099-0101.pdf. Accessed 5 Dec 2021.

[89] Ottenberg R., Kaliski D.J. Accidents in transfusion: their prevention by preliminary blood examination: based on an experience of one hundred twenty-eight transfusions. Jama. 1913;61(24):2138–2140. https://jamanetwork.com/journals/jama/article-abstract/216837.

the donor's blood was matched to that of the patient, especially if the blood donor was a family member.[90]

7.6 Definition of Universal Blood Donor and Patient

In 1912, Dr. Roger Irving Lee proved at the Massachusetts General Hospital, USA, that any patient of any blood group can receive blood group O from blood donors and that blood from all groups of blood donors can be donated to patients of blood group AB. He defined the terms "universal blood donor" (O) and "universal patient" (AB).[91]

7.7 Coombs Tests

In 1908, an Italian scientist named Carlo Moreschi (February 28, 1876—Pavia to May 24, 1921) first described what would later be known as the Coombs test.[92] Dr. Robert Royston Amos (Robin) Coombs (January 9, 1921 to January 25, 2006), a British immunologist, rediscovered this test, but at the time of its introduction, he was unaware that Moreschi was in fact the first to work out its principles. He later fully acknowledged Moreschi's work.[93] The Coombs test was introduced in 1945.[94] Antiglobulin testing, also known as the Coombs test, is an immunology laboratory procedure used to detect the presence of antibodies against circulating RBC in the body, which then induce hemolysis. Antiglobulin testing can be either direct antiglobulin testing (DAT) or indirect antiglobulin testing (IAT). The principle of DAT is to detect the presence of antibodies attached directly to the RBC. IAT is used to detect unbound antibodies to RBC, which may be present in the patient's serum.[95]

---

[90] Pierce S. R., Reid M. E. Section 1: ABO: The Birth of Blood Groups: 1. ABO grows up. In: Bloody Brilliant! A History of Blood Groups and Blood Groupers. AABB Press, Bethesda, Maryland; 2016, p. 32.

[91] Lee R.I. A Simple and rapid method for the selection of suitable blood donors for transfusion by the determination of blood groups, British medical journal. 1917; 2(2969), p. 684–685. https://www.ncbi.nlm.nih.gov/pmc/articles/PMC2349495/ Accessed 5 Dec 2021.

[92] Pamphilon, Scott, 2007, 401–408.

[93] Dunsford I., Grant J. Identification of blood group antigens, Nature. 1960; 187(4735), p. 357. https://www.nature.com/articles/187357b0#citeas.

[94] Slieman T. A., Leheste J., Chapter 1—Introduction to immunological techniques in the clinical laboratory, Methods in Microbiology, Academic Press, Volume 47 (Editors: Charles S. Pavia, Volker Gurtler) Nederland; 2020, p. 1–16. https://www.sciencedirect.com/science/article/abs/pii/S0580951720300015/ Accessed 9 Dec 2021.

[95] Theis S.R., Hashmi M.F. Coombs Test. [Updated 2022 Sep 12]. In: StatPearls [Internet]. Treasure Island (FL): StatPearls Publishing; 2023 Jan-. https://www.ncbi.nlm.nih.gov/books/NBK547707/. Accessed 13 Jan 2024.

7.8 Important Events in Immunohematology and Serology

The study of the immune system and its diseases within the body is known as immunology. Studying blood serum, or the clear liquid that separates when blood clots, is known as serology.[96] The study of red blood cell antigens and antibodies connected to blood transfusions is known as immunohematology. The antigen–antibody interaction that results in hemolysis or red blood cell agglutination is the fundamental idea behind the majority of immunohematology tests.[97] The immune system's cells are always monitoring the circulatory system, so they are never at rest. Infections would overpower the body in the absence of the immune system. Blood transfusions with it need to be done with utmost caution. When incompatible blood is transfused, the patient's immune system attacks the donor cells because they are perceived as alien intruders. Not only is the blood transfusion rendered ineffective, but shock, renal failure, circulatory collapse, and even death may result from a potentially severe immune and coagulation system activation.[98]

7.8.1 Some Important Achievements in Serology in the 1950s

- 1945—blood group serology dominates the scientific discussion;
- 1948—the birth of blood group chemistry;
- Blood transfusion services, often founded in the late 1940s, become established with the emphasis on blood donor recruitment.[99]

7.8.2 Some Important Achievements in Immunohematology from the 1950s to 1970s

- 1953—J. Dausset discovered the first leukocyte alloantibodies and subsequently identified the Mac blood group, which was the first leukocyte blood type;
- 1961—the important findings of K. Stem, R. Finn, V. Freda, J. Gorman, C. Clarke, and others were that passive transfer of IgG class Rh antibodies to a non-Rh immunized woman shortly after delivery prevented further Rh immunization;
- 1962—B and T lymphocytes were discovered, as were their roles in humoral and cellular immunity;

---

[96] Johns Hopkins medicine. Immunology and Serology. https://www.hopkinsmedicine.org/health/treatment-tests-and-therapies/immunology-and-serology. Accessed 21 March 2024.
[97] Nedelcu, E. Pre-Analytical Issues and Interferences in Transfusion Medicine Tests. Accurate Results in the Clinical Laboratory; 2013, p. 273–294. https://www.sciencedirect.com/science/article/abs/pii/B9780124157835000177. Accessed 21 March 2024.
[98] Dean L. Blood Groups and Red Cell Antigens [Internet]. Bethesda (MD): National Center for Biotechnology Information (US); Chapter 3, Blood transfusions and the immune system; 2005. https://www.ncbi.nlm.nih.gov/books/NBK2265/ Accessed 21 March 2024.
[99] Högman, 1992, p. 140–141.

- 1966—B. Bain, F. Bach, F. Kissmeyer-Nielsen, R. Payne, J. van Rood, and P. Terasaki made great contributions to the discovery of the HLA system;
- 1970—the clinical importance of the HLA system in organ and bone marrow transplantation was established, and E.D. Thomas and others demonstrated the usefulness of bone marrow transplantation in hematological aplasia and malignancies;
- 1973—G. Opelz, P. Terasaki, and others demonstrated the anti-rejection effects of blood transfusion in kidney transplantation.[100]

7.9 Organ Transplantation

Transfusion medicine has been defined as a mini-transplant of viable cells into the recipient and is a crucial part of organ transplantation. Transfusion is linked to a number of significant complications, much like organ transplantation. These include alloimmunization, infections caused by bacteria and viruses, transfusion-associated cardiac overload, organ dysfunction that may be related to the age of blood components, and acute lung injury related to transfusions. Issues with ABO-incompatible organs and passenger lymphocyte syndrome have particular significance for organ transplantation.[101] Worldwide, there is an immense need for organs, and there are long waiting periods before an organ can be transplanted. Thanks to the development of contemporary immunosuppressive medications and transplant techniques, the reliance on ABO and HLA matching has significantly declined in recent years.[102] The year 1869 saw the first skin transplant that can be independently verified. Through the use of tiny epidermis samples that had been pinched or shaved off of superficial skin layers, Swiss surgeon Jacques-Louis Reverdin successfully demonstrated epidermic grafting.[103] The first successful kidney transplant operation was performed in 1954 by Dr. Joseph Murray in Boston. Dr. Thomas Starzl performed the world's first liver transplant in Denver, Colorado, in 1963. Unfortunately, the patient died.[104] Dr. Starzl performed the first successful liver transplant in 1967,

---

[100] Ibid.

[101] Charlewood R., Kerry G. 'Transfusion medicine and organ transplantation.' in Ernesto A. Pretto, Jr., and others (eds). Oxford Textbook of Transplant Anaesthesia and Critical Care, Oxford Textbook in Anaesthesia. Oxford: academic; 2015, p. 385. https://doi.org/10.1093/med/9780199651429.003.0036. Accessed 6 Apr 2024.

[102] Sarkar R. S., Philip J., Yadav P. Transfusion medicine and solid organ transplant—Update and review of some current issues. Medical journal, Armed Forces India. 2013; 69(2), p. 162. https://www.ncbi.nlm.nih.gov/pmc/articles/PMC3862618/.

[103] Nordham K. D., Ninokawa, S. The history of organ transplantation. Proceedings (Baylor University. Medical Center). 2021; 35(1), p. 124–128. https://www.ncbi.nlm.nih.gov/pmc/articles/PMC8682823/.

[104] NHS Blood and Transplant. A history of donation, transfusion and transplantation. https://www.nhsbt.nhs.uk/who-we-are/a-history-of-donation-transfusion-and-transplantation/. Accessed 6 Apr 2024.

with the patient surviving for more than a year.[105] In 1967, the world's first heart transplant was performed in South Africa by Dr. Christian Barnard. The patient died after 18 days.[106]

7.10 Hematopoietic Stem Cell Transplantation

Blood transfusion support for hematopoietic stem cell transplantation (HSCT) is an important part of supportive care, and compatible blood should be transfused into recipients.

Blood transfusion support for hematopoietic stem cell transplantation (HSCT) is an important part of supportive care, and compatible blood should be transfused into recipients. Some of the important techniques employed are: leukocyte antigen (HLA) matching is considered first; blood products should be irradiated, with the exception of plasma; and leukocyte reduction in blood products is frequently used. Hospital transfusion committees, patient management, and local transfusion protocols should all be taken into account in order to reduce incompatibility and adverse outcomes.[107] The first human bone marrow transfusion was given to a patient with aplastic anemia in 1939.[108] In 1957, Thomas et al. reported treating acute leukemia in humans with supralethal radiation therapy and bone marrow infusion from adult and fetal cadavers. Using bone marrow cells from an HLA-matched sibling donor, Gatti and colleagues reported the first successful allogeneic transplant in an infant with severe combined immunodeficiency (SCID) in 1968. One of the first reports of HLA-matched sibling donor transplants for hematologic malignancies was reported in 1971 by Thomas and colleagues. When Thomas and associates reported the outcomes of their allogeneic transplantation for 100 consecutive acute leukemia patients in 1977, they revealed for the first time that only a small percentage of patients could be healed of this generally fatal illness. In 1979, the first unrelated donor leukemia transplant was carried out. By 1980, the use of HSCTs in cancers that were once thought to be "incurable," including chronic myelogenous leukemia, had become more common due to their therapeutic potential. Around 10,000 transplants were carried out annually for a variety of reasons worldwide by 1990.[109]

---

[105] VA U.S. Department of Veterans Affairs. Office of Research & Development. https://www.research.va.gov/research_in_action/First-successful-liver-transplant.cfm. Accessed 6 Apr 2024.

[106] NHS Blood and Transplant. A history of donation, transfusion and transplantation, 2024.

[107] Jekarl, D. W., Kim J. K., Han J. H., Lee H., Yoo J., Lim J., Kim, Y. Transfusion support in hematopoietic stem cell transplantation. Blood research. 2003; 58(S1), S1–S7. https://www.ncbi.nlm.nih.gov/pmc/articles/PMC10133853/. Accessed 6 Apr 2024.

[108] Henig, I., Zuckerman T. Hematopoietic stem cell transplantation-50 years of evolution and future perspectives. Rambam Maimonides medical journal. 2014; 5(4), e0028. https://www.ncbi.nlm.nih.gov/pmc/articles/PMC4222417/#b9-rmmj-5-4-e0028.

[109] Singh A.K., McGuirk J. P. Allogeneic Stem Cell Transplantation: A Historical and Scientific Overview. Cancer Res. 2016; 76 (22), p. 6445–6451. https://aacrjournals.org/cancerres/article/76/22/6445/613932/Allogeneic-Stem-Cell-Transplantation-A-Historical.

References

1. Philip AGS. Historical perspectives: the rise and fall of exchange blood transfusion. NeoReviews. 2003;4(7):171. https://publications.aap.org/neoreviews/article-abstract/4/7/e169/92043/Historical-PerspectivesThe-Rise-and-Fall-of?redirectedFrom=fulltext. Accessed 13 Jan 2024
2. Bionity.com. Rhesus blood group system. https://www.bionity.com/en/encyclopedia/Rhesus_blood_group_system.html#_note-2/ Accessed 11 Nov 2021.
3. Brewer HF. The blood groups, section IV. In: Brewer HF, Ellis R, Greaves RIN, Keynes G, Mills FW, Bodley Scott R, Till A, Whitby L, editors. Blood transfusion. Bristol: John Wright & sons LTD. London: Simpkin Marshall (1941). LTD.; 1949. p. 213.
4. Columbia Medicine. RhoGAM at 50: a drug still saving lives of newborns. https://www.columbiamedicinemagazine.org/ps-news/spring-2018/rhogam-50-drug-still-saving-lives-newborns. Accessed 27 Feb 2024.
5. Cleveland Clinic. Blood types. https://my.clevelandclinic.org/health/articles/21213-blood-types. Accessed 9 Dec 2021.
6. Canadian Blood Services. Rarest blood type. https://www.blood.ca/en/blood/donating-blood/what-my-blood-type. Accessed 2 April 2024.
7. Cotorruelo C. Elucidation of the molecular bases of the Rh system and its contribution to transfusion and obstetric medicine—historical and current perspective: a review. Ann Blood. 2023;8:3. https://aob.amegroups.org/article/view/8450/html. Accessed 2 April 2024
8. Charlewood R, Kerry G. Transfusion medicine and organ transplantation. In: Pretto Jr EA, et al., editors. Oxford textbook of transplant anaesthesia and critical care, Oxford Textbook in Anaesthesia. Oxford: Academic; 2015. p. 385. https://doi.org/10.1093/med/9780199651429.003.0036. Accessed 6 Apr 2024.
9. Dean L. Blood groups and red cell antigens [internet]. Bethesda (MD): National Center for Biotechnology Information (US). Chapter 3, Blood transfusions and the immune system; 2005. https://www.ncbi.nlm.nih.gov/books/NBK2265/ Accessed 21 March 2024
10. Dean L. Blood groups and red cell antigens. US. Bethesda, MD: National Center for Biotechnology Information; 2005. Chapter 8, p. 2. https://www.ncbi.nlm.nih.gov/books/NBK2267. Accessed 7 Jan 2024
11. Dunsford I, Grant J. Identification of blood group antigens. Nature. 1960;187(4735):357. https://www.nature.com/articles/187357b0#citeas
12. Durand JK, Willis MS, Landsteiner K. Blood transfusion medicine. Lab Med. 2010;41(1):53–5. https://academic.oup.com/labmed/article/41/1/53/2504910
13. Farr AD. Blood group serology-the first four decades (1900–1939). Medical history. 1979; 23, p. 219–225. https://www.ncbi.nlm.nih.gov/pmc/articles/PMC1082436/pdf/medhist00099-0101.pdf. Accessed 5 Dec 2021.
14. Goubran H. Blood group serology. ISBT Sci Ser. 2009;4:1–5. https://onlinelibrary.wiley.com/action/showCitFormats?doi=10.1111%2Fj.1751-2824.2009.01206.x. Accessed 13 Jan 2024
15. Hamilton JR. Kidd blood group system: a review. Immunohematology. 2015;31(1):29–35. https://pubmed.ncbi.nlm.nih.gov/26308468/
16. Hughes-Jones NC, Gardner B. Red cell agglutination: the first description by Creite (1869) and further observations made by Landois (1875) and Landsteiner (1901). Br J Haematol. 2022;119(4):889–93. https://pubmed.ncbi.nlm.nih.gov/12472564/
17. Hektoen L. Iso agglutination of human corpuscles: with respect to demonstration of opsonic index and to blood transfusion of blood. JAMA. 1907;48(21):1739–40.
18. Högman CF. Transfusion medicine: historical overview. In: Smit Sibinga CT, Das PC, Cash JD, editors. Transfusion medicine: fact and fiction. Developments in hematology and immunology, vol 27. Boston, MA: Springer; 1992. p. 139–51.
19. Henig I, Zuckerman T. Hematopoietic stem cell transplantation-50 years of evolution and future perspectives. Rambam Maimonides Med J. 2014;5(4):e0028. https://www.ncbi.nlm.nih.gov/pmc/articles/PMC4222417/#b9-rmmj-5-4-e0028

References

20. Jekarl DW, Kim JK, Han JH, Lee H, Yoo J, Lim J, Kim Y. Transfusion support in hematopoietic stem cell transplantation. Blood Res. 2003;58(S1):S1–7. https://www.ncbi.nlm.nih.gov/pmc/articles/PMC10133853/. Accessed 6 Apr 2024
21. Issit PD. Applied blood group serology. Durham, NC: Montgomery Scientific Publications; 1998. p. 175. https://archive.org/details/appliedbloodgrou0000issi_ed04/page/174/mode/2up?view=the. Accessed 13 Jan 2024
22. International Society of Blood Transfusion (ISBT). Red cell immunogenetics and blood group terminology. https://www.isbtweb.org/isbt-working-parties/rcibgt.html. Accessed 6 Jan 2024.
23. ISBT. Red cell immunogenetics and blood group terminology. 001 ABO Alleles. https://www.isbtweb.org/resource/001aboalleles.html. Accessed 12 Jan 2024.
24. Johns Hopkins medicine. Immunology and serology. https://www.hopkinsmedicine.org/health/treatment-tests-and-therapies/immunology-and-serology Accessed 21 March 2024.
25. Lee RI. A simple and rapid method for the selection of suitable blood donors for blood transfusion by the determination of blood groups. Br Med J. 1917;2(2969):684–5. https://www.ncbi.nlm.nih.gov/pmc/articles/PMC2349495/. Accessed 5 Dec 2021
26. Learoyd P. Chapter 1 Historical perspective. In: Thomas D, Thompson J, Ridler B, editors. All blood counts. Castle Hill Barns, Harley, Nr Shrewsbury: Publishing Limited; 2016. p. 18–9.
27. Levine P, Stetson RE. An unusual case of intra-group agglutination. JAMA. 1939;113(2):126–7. https://jamanetwork.com/journals/jama/article-abstract/290521
28. Mount Sinai Hospital. 1852–2002, The sesquicentennial. The Mount Sinai hospital, New York. 2002, p. 33.https://icahn.mssm.edu/files/ISMMS/Assets/About%20the%20School/Academic%20IT%20(AIT)/Levy%20Li brary/Sesquicentennial.pdf. Accessed 5 Dec 2021.
29. Mount Sinai Hospital. Journal of the Mount Sinai hospital, New York: Mount Sinai hospital; 1942–1943, p. 201. https://archive.org/details/journalofmountsi9194moun/page/n221/mode/2up?q=Reuben. Accessed 5 Dec 2021.
30. MSD Manual. Hemolytic disease of the fetus and neonate. https://www.msdmanuals.com/professional/gynecology-and-obstetrics/abnormalities-of-pregnancy/hemolytic-disease-of-the-fetus-and-neonate. Accessed 27 Feb 2024.
31. MedlinePlus. Rh incompatibility. https://medlineplus.gov/ency/article/001600.htm. Accessed 27 Feb 2024.
32. Mcnab K. In a similar vein to the gods: golden blood. 2022. https://blog.sciencemuseumgroup.org.uk/golden-blood/. Accessed 2 April 2024.
33. Nassar GN, Wehbe C. Erythroblastosis fetalis. [updated 2023 Jun 26]. In: StatPearls [internet]. Treasure Island, FL: StatPearls Publishing; 2024. https://www.ncbi.nlm.nih.gov/books/NBK513292/. Accessed 27 Feb 2024.
34. Nedelcu E. Pre-analytical issues and interferences in transfusion medicine tests. Accurate Results in the Clinical Laboratory; 2013, p. 273–294. https://www.sciencedirect.com/science/article/abs/pii/B9780124157835000177. Accessed 21 March 2024.
35. O'Connor K. Albert William Liley (1929–1983). https://embryo.asu.edu/pages/albert-william-liley-1929-1983. Accessed 7 Jan 2024.
36. Ottenberg R, Kaliski DJ. Accidents in transfusion: their prevention by preliminary blood examination: based on an experience of one hundred twenty-eight transfusions. JAMA. 1913;61(24):2138–40. https://jamanetwork.com/journals/jama/article-abstract/216837
37. Nordham KD, Ninokawa S. The history of organ transplantation. Proc (Baylor Univ Med Cent). 2021;35(1):124–8. https://www.ncbi.nlm.nih.gov/pmc/articles/PMC8682823/
38. NHS Blood and Transplant. The Rh system. https://www.blood.co.uk/why-give-blood/demand-for-different-blood-types/the-rh-system/. Accessed Dec 31 2023.
39. NHS Blood and Transplant. A history of donation, transfusion and transplantation. https://www.nhsbt.nhs.uk/who-we-are/a-history-of-donation-transfusion-and-transplantation/. Accessed 6 Apr 2024.
40. Pamphilon DH, Scott ML. Robin coombs: his life and contribution to haematology and blood transfusion medicine. Br J Haematol. 2007;137(5):404. https://pubmed.ncbi.nlm.nih.gov/17488485/

41. Plaut G, Ikin EW, Mourant AE, Sanger R, Race RR. A new blood-group antibody, anti Jkb. Nature. 1953;171(4349):431. https://pubmed.ncbi.nlm.nih.gov/13046499/
42. Pasman SA, Claes L, Lewi L, Van Schoubroeck D, Debeer A, Emonds M, Geuten E, De Catte L, Devlieger R. Intrauterine blood transfusion for fetal anemia due to red blood cell alloimmunization: 14 years' experience in Leuven. Facts Views Vis Obgyn. 2015;7(2):129–36. https://www.ncbi.nlm.nih.gov/pmc/articles/PMC4498170/
43. Pierce SR, Reid ME. Section 1: ABO: the birth of blood groups: 1. Blood groups—from then till now. In: Bloody brilliant! A history of blood groups and blood groupers. Bethesda, Maryland: AABB Press; 2016. p. 1.
44. Pierce SR, Reid ME. Section 1: ABO: the birth of blood groups: 1. ABO grows up. In: Bloody brilliant! A history of blood groups and blood groupers. Bethesda, Maryland: AABB Press; 2016. p. 32.
45. Pochedly C. History of the exchange blood transfusion; its use in treatment of erythroblastosis fetalis. Bull Hist Med. 1970;44(5):450–60. https://www.jstor.org/stable/44450798. Accessed 13 Jan 2024
46. Qureshi A, Salman M, Moiz B. Rhnull: a rare blood group phenotype. J Pak Med Assoc. 2010;60(11):960–1. https://pubmed.ncbi.nlm.nih.gov/21375204/
47. Robertson BA. Blood transfusions in severe burns in infants and young children: a preliminary report of the treatment of the toxic shock by blood transfusion, with or without preceding exsanguination. Can Med Assoc J. 1921;11(10):744–50. https://www.ncbi.nlm.nih.gov/pmc/articles/PMC1524233/
48. Rahorst L. The history of the Rh blood group & how genomics is changing RhD typing, New York blood center, NYBC Genomics laboratory. https://www.bloodgroupgenomics.org/blog-blood-experts/articles/history-rh-blood-group-how-genomics-changing-rhd-typing/. Accessed 10 Nov 2021.
49. Reid ME. Blood group systems. In: Maloy S, Huges K, editors. Brenner's encyclopedia of genetics. 2nd ed. Academic Press; 2013. p. 351–2. https://www.sciencedirect.com/science/article/abs/pii/B9780123749840001595 Accessed 12 Jan 2024.
50. RhoGam. Your baby's life story begins. https://www.rhogam.com/rhogam-science/. Accessed 27 Feb 2024.
51. Sanger R, Race RR, Jack J. The Duffy blood groups of New York negroes: the phenotype Fy (a−b−). Br J Haematol. 1955;1(4):370–4. https://pubmed.ncbi.nlm.nih.gov/13269673/
52. Sanger R, Race RR. The MNSs blood group system. Am J Hum Genet. 1951;3(4):332–43. https://www.ncbi.nlm.nih.gov/pmc/articles/PMC1716423/
53. Slieman TA, Leheste J. Chapter 1—Introduction to immunological techniques in the clinical laboratory, Methods in Microbiology, Academic Press, Volume 47 (Editors: Charles S. Pavia, Volker Gurtler) Nederland; 2020, p. 1–16. https://www.sciencedirect.com/science/article/abs/pii/S0580951720300015/. Accessed 9 Dec 2021.
54. Stevenson LF. Nobel prize winners in medicine and physiology, 1901–1950. New York: Schuman; 1953. p. 143–7. https://archive.org/details/nobelprizewinner0000stev/page/142/mode/2up Accessed 10 Oct 2021
55. Storry JR. Review: the LW blood group system. Immunohematology. 1992;8(4):87–93. https://pubmed.ncbi.nlm.nih.gov/15946068/
56. Shaw LB, Shaw RA. The pre-Anschluss Vienna School of Medicine—the medical scientists: Karl Landsteiner (1868–1943) and Otto Loewi (1873–1961). J Med Biogr. 2016;24(3):289–301. https://pubmed.ncbi.nlm.nih.gov/25052151/
57. Schwarz HP, Dorner F. Karl Landsteiner and his major contributions to haematology. Br J Haematol. 2003;121(4):556–65. https://pubmed.ncbi.nlm.nih.gov/12752096/
58. Simmons R, Gajdusek D, Gorman J, et al. Presence of the Duffy blood group gene Fy^b demonstrated in Melanesians. Nature. 1967;213:1148–9. https://www.nature.com/articles/2131148a0#citeas
59. Smart E, Armstrong B. Blood group systems. ISBT Sci Ser. 2008;3(2):68–92. https://doi.org/10.1111/j.1751-2824.2008.00188.x.

60. Sarkar RS, Philip J, Yadav P. Transfusion medicine and solid organ transplant—update and review of some current issues. Med J Armed Forces India. 2013;69(2):162. https://www.ncbi.nlm.nih.gov/pmc/articles/PMC3862618/
61. Singh AK, McGuirk JP. Allogeneic stem cell transplantation: a historical and scientific overview. Cancer Res. 2016;76(22):6445–51. https://aacrjournals.org/cancerres/article/76/22/6445/613932/Allogeneic-Stem-Cell-Transplantation-A-Historical
62. Otto ML. Erythroblastosis fetalis: early recognition: indications for therapy and therapy by exchange blood transfusion. MD Theses. 1848. 1952, p. 1–6. https://digitalcommons.unmc.edu/mdtheses/1848 Accessed 13 Jan 2024.
63. Theis SR, Hashmi MF. Coombs test. [updated 2022 Sep 12]. In: StatPearls [internet]. Treasure Island, FL: StatPearls Publishing; 2023. https://www.ncbi.nlm.nih.gov/books/NBK547707/. Accessed 13 Jan 2024.
64. VA U.S. Department of Veterans Affairs. Office of Research & Development. https://www.research.va.gov/research_in_action/First-successful-liver-transplant.cfm. Accessed 6 Apr 2024.
65. Westhoff CM, Reid ME. Review: the Kell, Duffy, and Kidd blood group systems. Immunohematology. 2004;20(1):37–49. https://pubmed.ncbi.nlm.nih.gov/15373667/
66. Wiener AS, Wexler IB. The use of heparin when performing exchange blood transfusions in newborn infants. J Lab Clin Med. 1946;31:1016–9. https://scholar.google.com/scholar?cluster=16805773366256891543&hl=sl&as_sdt=0,5. Accessed 7 Jan 2024
67. Wiener AS. Chapter I: introduction. In: Blood groups and blood transfusion. Charles C. Thomas Publisher; 1948. p. 4.
68. Wiener AS. Chapter II: the four blood groups. In: Blood groups and blood transfusion. Charles C. Thomas Publisher; 1948. p. 13–4.

Image Source

Science Museum Group. Copy of a blood-grouping tile. 1981–476 Pt1. Science Museum Group Collection Online. Accessed 8 March 2024. Creative Commons Attribution 4.0 license. https://collection.sciencemuseumgroup.org.uk/objects/co137154/copy-of-a-blood-grouping-tile-blood-grouping-tile.

New Developments During World War I

8

Contents

8.1	Arteriovenous Anastomosis.	79
8.2	Anastomosis with Paraffin Wax Methods.	81
8.3	Syringe Methods During the War.	87
8.4	Introduction of Sodium Citrate as an Anticoagulant.	89
8.5	Interesting Cases of Blood Donation during World War I.	100
	8.5.1 Blood Transfusion on the Battlefield.	100
	8.5.2 Remarkable Operation.	100
	8.5.3 A Courageous Wife.	101
	8.5.4 Heroic Soldier.	101
	8.5.5 Blood Transfusion for a Wounded Captain.	101
References.		102

8.1 Arteriovenous Anastomosis

Although the discovery of blood groups led to an increased interest in blood transfusion, the problem with blood clotting during the procedure was still a major problem. Direct methods of blood transfusion from vein to vein or artery to vein were still the main methods of blood transfusion.[1] Direct blood transfusion was the only method used until 1913.[2] Problems with clotting occurred during different stages of blood transfusion: before it was stopped, during the blood transfusion, if the blood

---

[1] Keynes, p. 34.
[2] LeBlanc, H.J., "To what extent did blood transfusion systems and technologies modernize during World War II?" Young Historians Conference. 2016; 10, p. 1–6. https://pdxscholar.library.pdx.edu/younghistorians/2016/oralpres/10/. Accessed 11 Dec 2021.

© The Author(s), under exclusive license to Springer Nature
Switzerland AG 2024
Z. Kvržić, *History of Blood Donation and Transfusion Medicine*,
https://doi.org/10.1007/978-3-031-68715-0_8

was transfused too rapidly and in great quantity, or if the patient had received enough blood.[3] Arteriovenous anastomosis was a method of preventing blood clotting during a direct blood transfusion.[4, 5] Direct anastomosis of blood vessels or sewing blood vessels together was elaborated by J. B. Murphy in Chicago (1897). Murphy united the arteries by invagination and suture. However, this was too challenging to be used in general practice for blood transfusions. Erwin Payr of Gratz (1900) used a magnesium tube.[6, 7, 8] French surgeon and biologist Dr. Alexis Carrel (June 28, 1873 to November 5, 1944) pioneered his technique of blood vessel anastomosis in 1902. But the surgeon Dr. George Washington Crile (November 11, 1864 to January 7, 1943) modified Carrel's anastomosis technique to administer a faster blood transfusion and was the one who performed the first direct blood transfusion by anastomosis of human blood on December 5, 1905, at St. Alexis Hospital in Cleveland, Ohio. Unfortunately, the patient did not survive. His first successful blood transfusion by anastomosis was performed at St. Alexis Hospital on August 6, 1906.[9, 10] Dr. Carrel performed his anastomosis technique on a patient for the first time in 1908.[11] Blood transfusion itself lasted only a few minutes, but the entire operation of the direct blood transfusion with anastomosis lasted, on average, over 2 h. It could have also lasted more than 3 hours.[12, 13] Although anastomosis for blood transfusion in today's world is no longer in use, different surgical anastomosis techniques for different cases are still used in modern medicine. The procedure was performed with an end-to-end anastomosis between an artery of the blood donor and a vein of the patient. The radial artery at the wrist was the best choice for this procedure, as well as the median basilic vein or the median cephalic vein at the

---

[3] Horsley Riddell V., Blood transfusion, London: Oxford University Press, London: Humphrey Milford; 1939, p. 192. https://www.woodlibrarymuseum.org/rare-book/riddell-vh-blood-transfusion-1939/. Accessed 12 Nov 2021.

[4] Nathoo N., Lautzenheiser F. K. & Barnett G. H. The first direct human blood transfusion, Operative Neurosurgery. 2009; 64(3), p. 20–27. https://pubmed.ncbi.nlm.nih.gov/19240569/.

[5] Curling, Goss, Bertolini, 2012, p. 3–4.

[6] Till A. The technique of blood transfusion, section VI. In: Brewer H.F., Ellis R., Greaves R. I. N., Keynes G., Mills F. W., Bodley Scott R., Till A., Whitby L. Blood transfusion. Bristol: John Wright & sons LTD. London: Simpkin Marshall (1941). LTD.;1949, p. 420.

[7] Carrel, A. Results of the transplantation of blood vessels, organs and limbs. Journal of the American Medical Association, 1908, 51.20: 1662–1667. https://jamanetwork.com/journals/jama/article-abstract/428456.

[8] Kilduffe, R. A., DeBakey, M. E. Chapter I, history. In: The Blood Bank and the Technique and Therapeutics of Transfusions. Mosby, St. Louis, 1943, p. 28. https://babel.hathitrust.org/cgi/pt?id=uc1.$b595310&seq=7. Accessed 28 Jan 2024.

[9] Nathoo, N., Lautzenheiser, F. K., & Barnett, G. H, 2009, p. 20–27.

[10] Curling, Goss, Bertolini, 2012, p. 3–4.

[11] Chandler JG, Chin TL, Wohlauer MV. Direct blood transfusions, J. Vasc Surg.2012; 56(4),p. 1173–1177. https://www.ncbi.nlm.nih.gov/pmc/articles/PMC4065715/.

[12] Lewisohn R. Twenty years' experience with the citrate method of blood transfusion. Annals of surgery. 1937; 105(4), p. 602–609. https://www.ncbi.nlm.nih.gov/pmc/articles/PMC1390374/.

[13] Nathoo N., Lautzenheiser F. K. & Barnett G. H, 2009, p. 23.

elbow, because of their accessibility. The alterations made by Sauerbruch (1915) and others involved drawing the end of the radial artery through a slit in the vein's wall and into the lumen. This was less difficult to perform than anastomosis; nonetheless, the artery's obstruction due to the body's spontaneous inversion of its coats at the cut end proved challenging. This was likely to occur before much blood had passed.[14]

8.2 Anastomosis with Paraffin Wax Methods

Freund (1886) and Bordet and Gengou (1901), with their experiments, showed that the coagulation of blood was delayed if the blood was kept in vaseline and paraffin-coated containers. Brewer and Leggett (1909) used paraffin-coated glass tubes to connect the artery and vein.[15, 16, 17] Curtis and David (Image 8.1) in 1911 invented a paraffin-coated glass tube apparatus with two outlets on one end for the blood donor and patient and connected on the other end to a syringe.[18] A. R. Kimpton and J. Howard Brown (Image 8.2) in 1913 used a unique glass tube whose interior was totally covered with paraffin wax. It was feasible to draw 200 cc of blood from a blood donor's artery and then transfer the contents into the vein of the patient

---

[14] Keynes, 1949, p. 34.

[15] Till A., 1949, p. 420.

[16] Inwood, 1966, p. 5.

[17] Cramer W., Pringle H. On the coagulation of blood. Experimental Physiology, 6. 1913, p. 8. https://physoc.onlinelibrary.wiley.com/action/showCitFormats?doi=10.1113%2Fexpphysiol.1913.sp000127.

[18] Kilduffe, R. A., DeBakey, M. E. Chapter XV, methods and technique of transfusion. In: The Blood Bank and the Technique and Therapeutics of Transfusions. Mosby, St. Louis, 1943, p. 399. https://babel.hathitrust.org/cgi/pt?id=uc1.$b595310&seq=1. Accessed 27 Jan 2024.

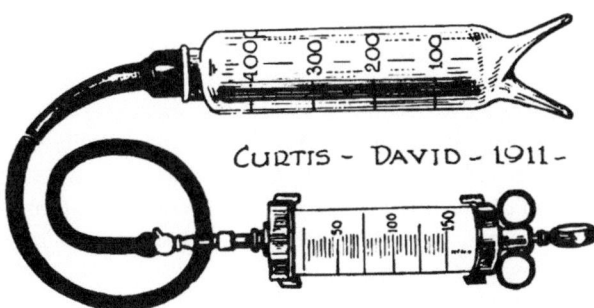

Image 8.1 Curtis and David Syringe for Blood Transfusion (1911). (Source: Curtis and David syringe for blood transfusion (1911). Chapter 15 methods and technique of blood transfusion. In: Kilduffe, R. A., DeBakey, M. E. The blood bank and the technique and therapeutics of blood transfusions. Mosby, St. Louis, 1942, p. 400. Permission for usage of the image was granted by the copyright holder, Elsevier, on January 23, 2024. https://babel.hathitrust.org/cgi/pt?id=uc1.$b595310&seq=1. Accessed 28 Jan 2024)

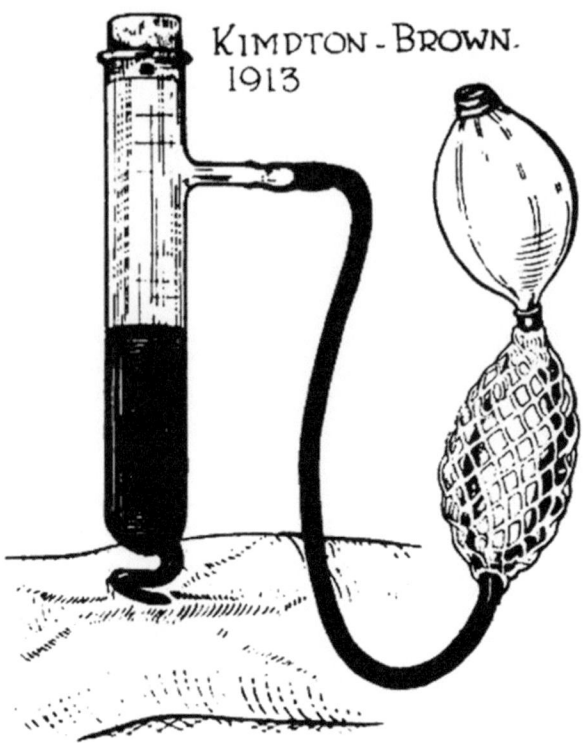

Image 8.2 Kimpton and Brown's tube for blood transfusion (1913). (Source: Kimpton and Brown's tube for blood transfusion (1913). Chapter 15 methods and technique of blood transfusion. In: Kilduffe, R. A., DeBakey, M. E. The blood bank and the technique and therapeutics of blood transfusions. Mosby, St. Louis, 1942, p. 400. Permission for usage of the image was granted by the copyright holder, Elsevier, on January 23, 2024. https://babel.hathitrust.org/cgi/pt?id=uc1.$b595310&seq=1. Accessed 28 Jan 2024)

without the occurrence of clotting. The blood donor did not always need to be present for the procedure, which solved the issue of managing blood donors when there were severe hemorrhages, etc. Satterlee and Hooker enhanced this device in 1914.[19]

Some minor adjustments to this device were also made by Nelson Mortimer Percy (1875–1958) in 1915 from Chicago (Image 8.3), Jeanbrau (1923) of France, and Dogliotti (1932) of Turin. The main changes were the addition of a suction tip to facilitate collection and a needle to the lower cannula-like extremity of the tube to prevent cutting down on the vein.[20]

---

[19] Inwood, 1966, p. 5.
[20] Horsley Riddell, 1939, p. 196.

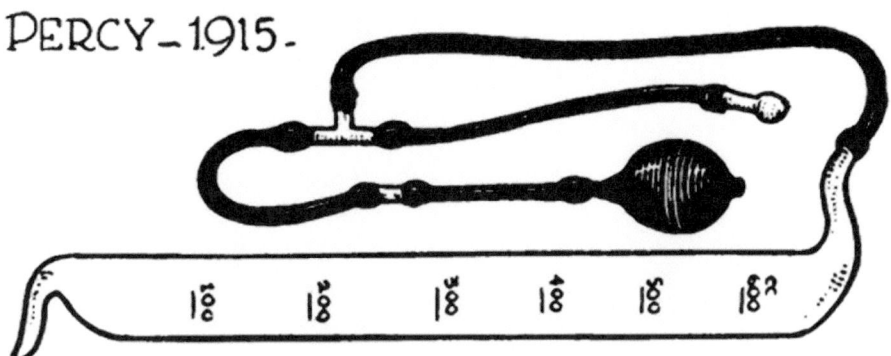

Image 8.3 Percy blood transfusion tube (1915). (Source: Percy blood transfusion tube (1915). Chapter 15 methods and technique of blood transfusion. In: Kilduffe, R. A., DeBakey, M. E. The blood bank and the technique and therapeutics of blood transfusions. Mosby, St. Louis, 1942, p. 401. Permission for usage of the image was granted by the copyright holder, Elsevier, on January 23, 2024. https://babel.hathitrust.org/cgi/pt?id=uc1.$b595310&seq=1. Accessed 28 Jan 2024)

Bernheim in 1915 used paraffin-lined tubes to connect the blood vessels of the blood donor and the patient.[21] Bernheim cannula for direct artery-to-vein blood transfusion was still being performed, at least in 1925 (Image 8.4).[22]

In cases where both the patient and the blood donor were in the same room, they both had cannulas placed into their veins. Subsequently, a sterile paraffin-lined container was filled with blood obtained via suction from the blood donor. The patient's vein was then attached to the container, which had been detached from the blood donor's cannula, and pressure was applied to drive the blood into the vein. Before clotting started, a 250-mL flask of blood needed to be drawn and injected, which took around 8 min. It was an inconvenient process that needed several individuals to complete. Both the patient's and the blood donor's veins were typically tied after the surgery. It was assumed that citrated blood was contraindicated for the surgery.[23] Colonel Andrew Fullerton reported using a thin rubber tube with a silver cannula in 1917. Before the blood transfusion, the apparatus was first coated on the inside with a thin layer of paraffin wax in order to prevent clotting in the tube itself, and the cannulas were inserted into the blood donor's artery and the vein of the patient.[24] With cannula anastomosis, various cannulas were devised by which the artery of the blood donor was connected with the vein of the patient. In essence, this was comparable to vessel anastomosis with only a little technological advance.[25] In 1919,

---

[21] Wiener, 1948, p. 57.

[22] Dodson A. I. The value of blood transfusion in surgery of the prostate. Annals of surgery. 1925; 82(6), p. 974–977. https://www.ncbi.nlm.nih.gov/pmc/articles/PMC1400355/.

[23] DeGowin E. L. Transfusion Equipment, Chapter 26. In: DeGowin E. L., Hardin R. C., Alsever B. J. Blood transfusion. W.B. Saunders Company Philadelphia & London, 1949, p. 518.

[24] Keynes, 1949, p. 34.

[25] DeGowin, 1949, p. 518.

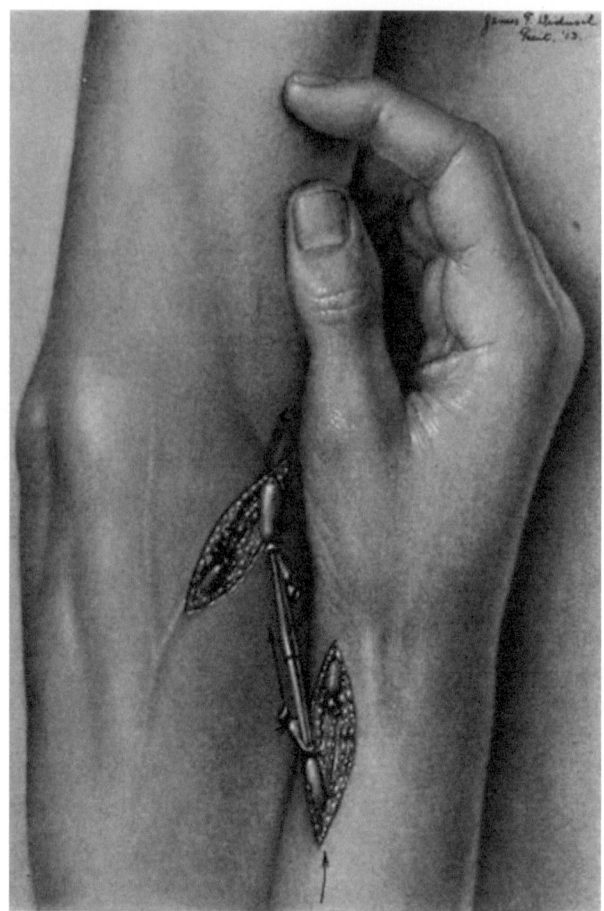

Image 8.4 Arteriovenous blood transfusion by Bernheim. (Source: Arteriovenous blood transfusion by Bernheim. Bernheim B.M. Surgery of the vascular system. Philadelphia, J.B. Lippincott, p. 23; 1913, public domain. The current publisher is Wolters Kluwer. https://archive.org/details/surgeryofvascula00bernuoft/surgeryofvascula00bernuoft/page/18/mode/2up?q=blood transfusion. Accessed 17 Jan 2024)

J. M. Graham experimented with direct blood transfusion using the anastomosis method (Images 8.5 and 8.6), but he concluded that indirect blood transfusion was more useful than direct blood transfusion because this method was difficult to perform.[26]

Anastomosis methods did show that vast amounts of blood could be administered without always having clotting issues. This discovery led to the development of numerous modified pieces of equipment, which helped direct blood transfusions

---

[26] Keynes, 1949, p. 34.

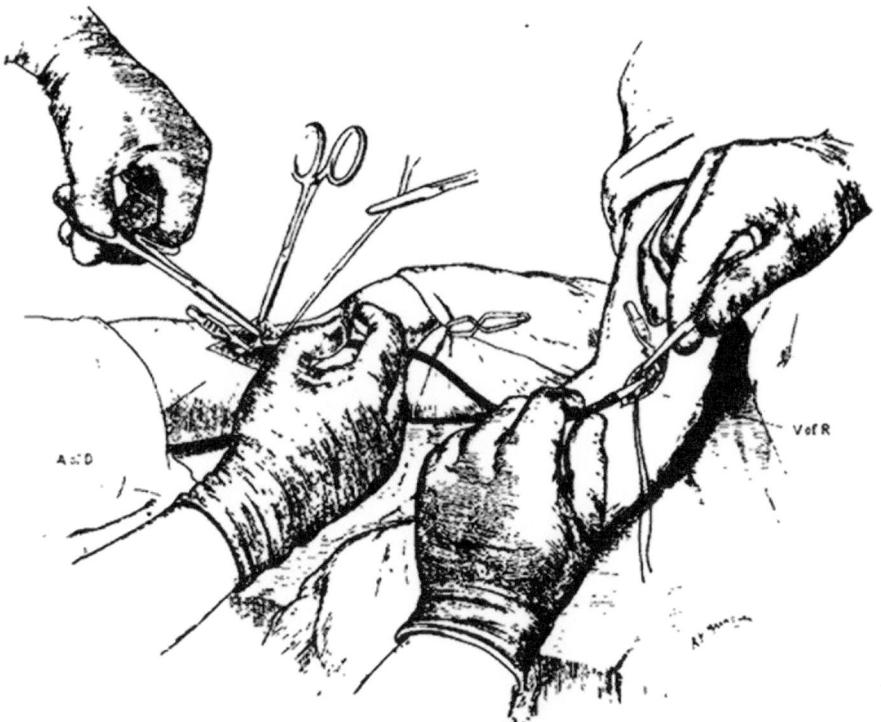

Illustrating the introduction of the cannulæ. A of D, Artery of donor. V of R, Vein of receiver.

Image 8.5 Arteriovenous-anastomosis for the direct blood transfusion. (Source: Arteriovenous-anastomosis for the direct blood transfusion. Fullerton, A., Dreyer, G., & Bazett, H. C. Observations on direct blood transfusion of blood, with a description of a simple method. The Lancet, 1917, 189 (4889), p. 715–719. Permission for usage of this image was granted by the copyright holder, Elsevier, on January 9, 2024. https://www.sciencedirect.com/science/article/abs/pii/S014067360079917X. Accessed 10 Jan 2024)

gain popularity.[27] The direct method of arteriovenous anastomosis was performed in operating rooms in hospitals. They required a trained medical team, and this delicate surgical procedure was often performed in critical emergency conditions, which was time-consuming and presented many challenges, especially taking care of numerous injured patients while also having to find a suitable blood donor who was not dying and could lie close to the patient.[28] Besides problems with blood clotting, there were also other problems. It was impossible to measure the amount of blood that had passed from the blood donor to the patient.[29] Instead, the surgeon had

---

[27] Inwood, 1966, p. 5.
[28] Ibid., p. 212.
[29] Keynes G. Blood transfusion. London, Frowde; 1922, p. 110–111. https://archive.org/details/bloodtransfusion00keynuoft/page/110/mode/2up. Accessed 2 Jan 2024.

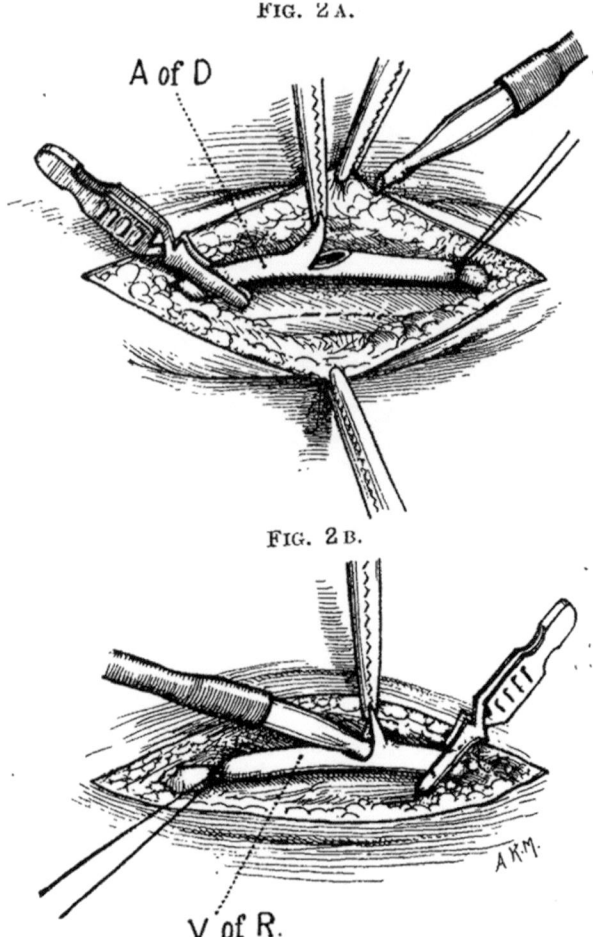

Illustrating on a large scale the introduction of the cannulæ.

Image 8.6 Introduction of the cannula for the direct arteriovenous–anastomosis blood transfusion. (Source: Introduction of the cannula for the direct arteriovenous-anastomosis blood transfusion. Fullerton, A., Dreyer, G., & Bazett, H. C. Observations on direct blood transfusion of blood, with a description of a simple method. The Lancet, 1917, 189 (4889), p. 715–719. Permission for usage of this image was given by the copyright holder, Elsevier, on January 9, 2024. https://www.sciencedirect.com/science/article/abs/pii/S014067360079917X. Accessed 10 Jan 2024)

to guess how much blood was introduced by the blood donor fainting, the patient getting better, or the increase in the patient's weight.[30] Also, the radial artery was exposed through an incision of considerable length and was ligatured at the conclusion of the process. The blood donor was permanently scarred and could not under

---

[30] Horsley Riddell V., 1939, p. 192. https://www.woodlibrarymuseum.org/rare-book/riddell-vh-blood-transfusion-1939/. Accessed 12 Nov 2021.

any circumstances be used for blood transfusion more than twice. It was required that the blood donor and the patient lay side by side, their hands pressed closely. It was nearly essential that both be on appropriately sized operating tables. The bleeding patient, who could not be moved from the bed, presented another issue, though, which made the direct blood transfusion process much more challenging. Additionally, some individuals had radial arteries of very small caliber, making it nearly impossible to proceed when the artery was exposed.[31]

8.3 Syringe Methods During the War

To solve the problems that anastomosis had, Lindemann used the multiple syringe method (Images 8.7 and 8.8) in 1913. His method called for the employment of a unique set of invaginated cylindrical cannulas, twelve 20-cc syringes, and a skilled team. Lindemann, as an example, had a trained team consisting of himself, an assistant (a doctor), and three nurses.[32, 33] In the multiple-syringe method, needles were

---

[31] Keynes G. Blood transfusion, 1922, p. 110–111. https://archive.org/details/bloodtransfusion00keynuoft/page/110/mode/2up. Accessed 2 Jan 2024.
[32] Inwood, 1966, p. 5.
[33] Unger L. J. Blood transfusion—1914 model. Haematologia (Budap). 1972;6(1):47–57.

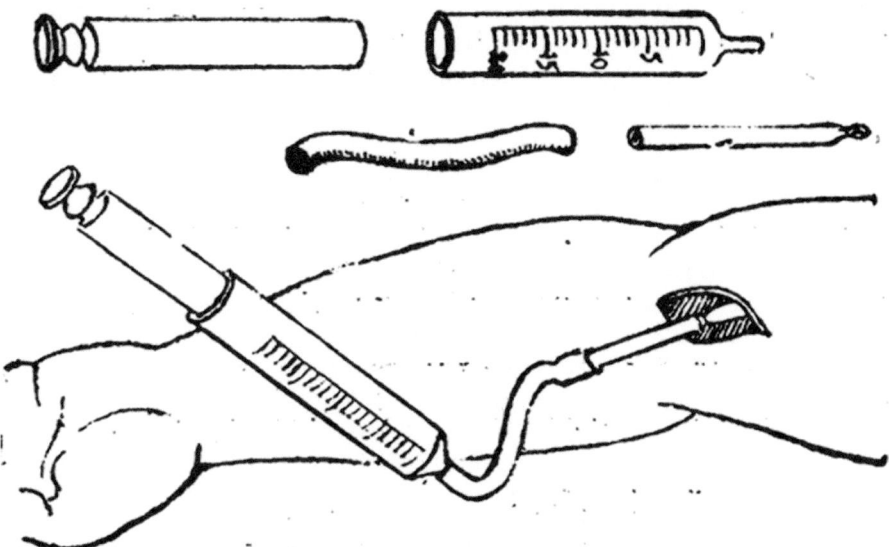

Image 8.7 The syringe method. (Source: The syringe method. Primrose A., Ryerson E. S., The direct blood transfusion of blood: its value in hemorrhage and shock in the treatment of the wounded in war, Br Med J. 1916; 2: p. 384. Permission for usage of this image was granted by the copyright holder BMJ on January 10, 2024. https://www.bmj.com/content/2/2907/384. Accessed 11 Jan 2024)

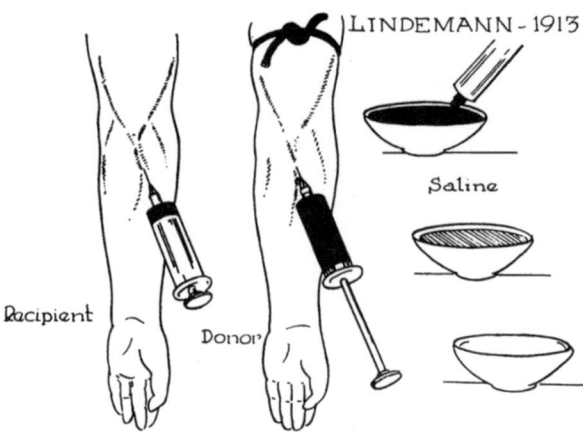

Image 8.8 Lindemann method of blood transfusion (1913). (Source: Lindemann method of blood transfusion (1913). Chapter XV methods and technique of blood transfusion. In: Kilduffe, R. A., DeBakey, M. E. The blood bank and the technique and therapeutics of blood transfusions. Mosby, St. Louis, 1942, p. 402. Permission for usage of the image was granted by the copyright holder, Elsevier, on January 23, 2024. https://babel.hathitrust.org/cgi/pt?id=uc1.$b595310&seq=1. Accessed 28 Jan 2024)

inserted in both the blood donor and the patient. The blood donor needle was connected to a glass syringe that could also have been 50 mL, which was then filled with blood. After this was done, the syringe with blood was separated from the blood donor needle, and then it was connected to the needle inserted in the patient. The blood from the syringe was forced into the patient's vein. At the same time, an assistant prepared another syringe that was immediately ready for use. This method was useful when small quantities of fresh blood were needed, for example, in infants. The blood was transfused rapidly to prevent clotting. To prevent coagulation, sodium citrate could be injected into the syringe before the procedure started, washed, and used with a sterile saline solution.[34, 35] The multiple-syringe method had its disadvantages. It was an open method, and there was an existing danger of bacterial contamination. At times, blood is clotted in the cannulas or in the syringe. When the blood was forced in from the syringe, it would loosen from the cannula, and blood squirted all over the entire room and everyone in it. An orderly was prepared with pails of water, sponges, and a tall ladder to clean up this unwanted mess. It was also time-consuming since it required several syringes and more than one assistant, and because the syringes had to be washed with saline in order to prevent blood from clotting.[36, 37]

---

[34] DeGowin, 1949, p. 519.
[35] Keynes, 1949, p. 36.
[36] Unger, 1972, p. 49–50.
[37] Keynes, 1949, p. 36.

After Lindemann, more blood transfusion apparatuses were invented (1913–1918) that advanced blood transfusion procedures.

The early blood transfusion apparatuses were invented because of the prejudice against citrated blood (Images 8.9, 8.10, 8.11, 8.12 and 8.13).[38] However, these apparatuses, as well as others that were manufactured later, used sodium citrate for direct vein-to-vein blood transfusion.

One of the earliest apparatuses was from Freund in 1913, with a two-way stopcock connected to a 20-cc syringe (Image 8.9).[39] Unger began his work in 1914 with a new method, and in 1915, he employed a four-way stopcock apparatus. He named his work the *"Unger method of blood transfusion."* In Unger's apparatus (Image 8.9), two rubber tubes were used for connection between the blood donor and a patient. One rubber tube connected a needle to the vein of the blood donor from one outlet. The second rubber tube connected another needle in the vein of the patient from another outlet. During the procedure, part of the instrument that was not used at the moment was rinsed with a saline solution to prevent blood from remaining stagnant, and this way, clotting was avoided for a short time before the outlet was used again. Simultaneously, a nurse sprayed ether onto the blood syringe barrel. By evaporating, the ether reduced the blood's temperature as it came into contact with the blood syringe's glass wall, stopping even the earliest signs of the clotting process.[40, 41] In 1923, it was reported that Unger, for his method with his apparatus, always used sodium citrate, if not even before.[42]

8.4 Introduction of Sodium Citrate as an Anticoagulant

The compounds studied in defibrinated blood to prevent coagulation during blood transfusions were ammonia, sodium phosphate, various oxalates, hirudin, and peptone. Although these substances prevented clotting, they produced such toxic symptoms that each was quickly abandoned. Nonetheless, the discovery of sodium citrate, which proved to be a secure and efficient anticoagulant, was a great development.[43] Sodium citrate was a simple, inexpensive, relatively nontoxic chemical substance that simplified the technique of blood transfusion.[44]

The first to use the new sodium citrate method in clinical practice was Belgian surgeon Albert Hustin (1882–1967) on March 27, 1914. He performed a blood

---

[38] DeGowin 1949, p. 518.

[39] Kilduffe, DeBakey, 1942, p. 371.

[40] Inwood, 1966, p. 5.

[41] Unger, 1972, p. 48–50.

[42] Copher G.H. Blood transfusion: a study of two hundred and forty-five cases. Arch surg. 1923;7(1):125–153. https://jamanetwork.com/journals/jamasurgery/article-abstract/536614.

[43] Bird 1971, p. 42.

[44] DeGowin E.L. Historical perspective, Chapter I. In: DeGowin E. L., Hardin R. C., Alsever B. J. Blood transfusion. W.B. Saunders Company Philadelphia & London, 1949, p. 3.

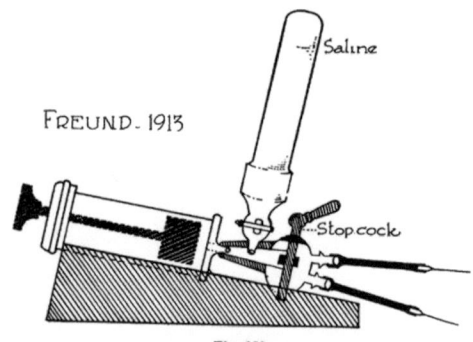

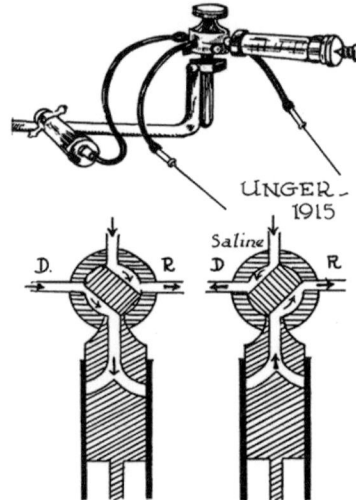

Figs. 152-175.—Syringe valve methods of transfusion in which some type of valve is used for changing direction of flow from donor to recipient. Figs. 152-158 show apparatuses utilizing a valve mechanism which consists of some type of stopcock.

Image 8.9 Freund (1913) and Unger (1915). Blood transfusion apparatus. (Source: Freund (1913) and Unger (1915) blood transfusion apparatus. Chapter XV methods and technique of blood transfusion. In: Kilduffe, R. A., DeBakey, M. E. The blood bank and the technique and therapeutics of blood transfusions. Mosby, St. Louis, 1942, p. 403. Permission for usage of the image was granted by the copyright holder, Elsevier, on January 23, 2024. https://babel.hathitrust.org/cgi/pt?id=uc1.$b595310&seq=1. Accessed 28 Jan 2024)

transfusion from one patient to another with glucose solution and sodium citrate.[45] The method with a small amount of citrated blood was tested by Dr. Luis Agote (September 22, 1868 to November 12, 1954) from Buenos Aires on November 9, 1914, and Dr. Richard Lewisohn (July 12, 1875 to August 11, 1961), a

---

[45] Van Hee R. The Development of Blood Transfusion: The Role of Albert Hustin and the Influence of World War I., Acta Chirurgica Belgica.2015; 115(3), p. 247–255. https://www.researchgate.net/publication/279989937_The_Development_of_Blood_Transfusion_the_Role_of_Albert_Hustin_and_the_Influence_of_World_War_I.

8.4 Introduction of Sodium Citrate as an Anticoagulant

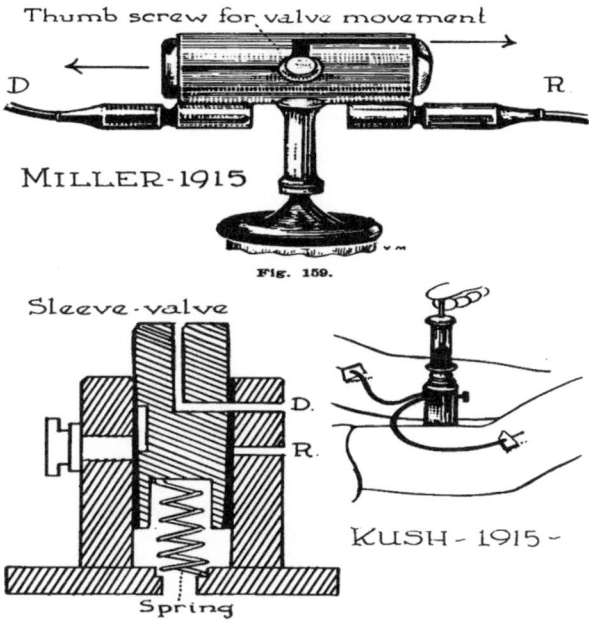

Image 8.10 Miller (1915) and Kush (1915). Blood transfusion apparatuses. (Source: Miller (1915) and Kush (1915) blood transfusion apparatuses. Chapter XV methods and technique of blood transfusion. In: Kilduffe, R. A., DeBakey, M. E. The blood bank and the technique and therapeutics of blood transfusions. Mosby, St. Louis, 1942, p. 408. Permission for usage of the image was granted by the copyright holder, Elsevier, on January 23, 2024. https://babel.hathitrust.org/cgi/pt?id=uc1.$b595310&seq=1. Accessed 28 Jan 2024)

German-American surgeon in New York, on January 23, 1915.[46, 47] They all came to the same conclusion that adding sodium citrate to the blood would effectively hinder its clotting and that a sufficient amount would not harm the patient.[48] In 1915, Richard Weil described that one of the many advantages of sodium citrate was that it was always easily obtainable in comparison to hirudin. He advocated the use of sodium citrate mixed with blood, among others, for different hemorrhagic conditions.[49] In 1915, Dr. Lewisohn demonstrated the viability of storing blood preserved with sodium citrate in the refrigerator (Images 8.14 and 8.15).[50] The new

---

[46] Ibid., p. 251.

[47] Lewisohn R., Blood transfusion by the citrate method. Am J Med. 1952; 13(5), p. 550–555. https://pubmed.ncbi.nlm.nih.gov/12996530/.

[48] Pelis K., Edward Archibald's notes on blood transfusion in war surgery—a commentary. Wilderness Environ Med. Fall. 2002; 13(3), p. 212–213. https://pubmed.ncbi.nlm.nih.gov/12353599/.

[49] Weil R. sodium citrate in the transfusion of blood. *JAMA*. 1915; LXIV (5):425–426. https://jamanetwork.com/journals/jama/article-abstract/439690.

[50] Thompson, P., & Strandenes, G. The history of fluid resuscitation for bleeding. Damage Control Resuscitation,2019, p. 3–29. https://www.ncbi.nlm.nih.gov/pmc/articles/PMC7123228/. Accessed 14 Dec 2021.

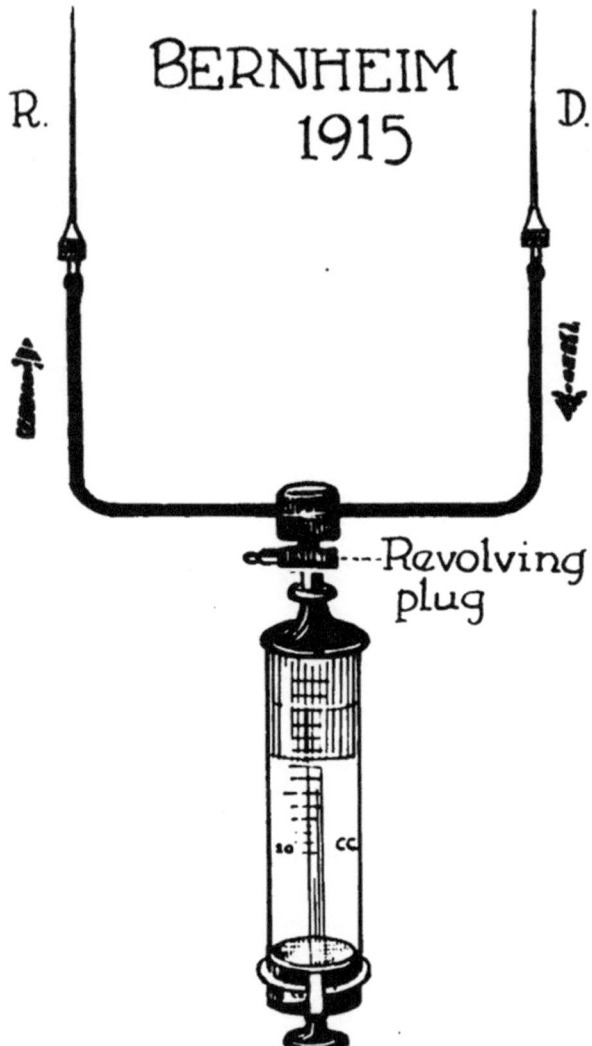

Image 8.11 Bernheim (1915) apparatus for blood transfusion. (Source: Bernheim (1915) apparatus for blood transfusion. Chapter XV methods and technique of blood transfusion. In: Kilduffe, R. A., DeBakey, M. E. The blood bank and the technique and therapeutics of blood transfusions. Mosby, St. Louis, 1942, p. 409. Permission for usage of the image was granted by the copyright holder, Elsevier, on January 23, 2024. https://babel.hathitrust.org/cgi/pt?id=uc1.$b595310&seq=1. Accessed 28 Jan 2024)

8.4 Introduction of Sodium Citrate as an Anticoagulant

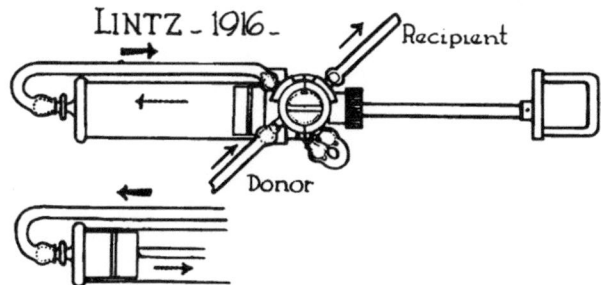

Image 8.12 Lintz (1916) apparatus for blood transfusion. (Source: Lintz (1916) apparatus for blood transfusion. Chapter XV methods and technique of blood transfusion. In: Kilduffe, R. A., DeBakey, M. E. The blood bank and the technique and therapeutics of blood transfusions. Mosby, St. Louis, 1942, p. 404. Permission for usage of the image was granted by the copyright holder, Elsevier, on January 23, 2024. https://babel.hathitrust.org/cgi/pt?id=uc1.$b595310&seq=1. Accessed 28 Jan 2024)

anticoagulant avoided the necessity for the blood donor and patient to be in the same room.[51] Francis Peyton Rous and J. R. Turner (1916) of the Rockefeller Institute had their solution (the Rous-Turner solution) of sodium citrate and glucose that could keep the red cell intact for up to 4 weeks.[52] Their solution served as both an anticoagulant and a preservative for the red cells during refrigeration. The Rous-Turner solution's and its variations' drawback was the need for a high solution-to-blood volume ratio, which diluted the collected blood.[53, 54] Although this solution was used in 1917–1918, in the Second World War, it was replaced by citrate-glucose solutions of much smaller volume, only after the efficacy of glucose as a red cell preservative had been confirmed by red cell survival measurements.[55]

Sodium citrate was an effective method of preventing blood coagulation, but clinicians were at first reluctant to use this method in everyday practice. This was due to the belief that sodium citrate caused post-transfusion chills.

The method of using sodium citrate gained popularity in 1922.[56] In 1923, Florence Seibert discovered the pyrogens. He discovered heat-stable products from bacteria growing in distilled water. Following this discovery, certain precautions

---

[51] Pierce S. R. Blood transfusion in the First World War. KU Medical Center. https://www.kumc.edu/school-of-medicine/academics/departments/history-and-philosophy-of-medicine/archives/wwi/essays/medicine/blood-transfusion.html. Accessed 7 Jan 2024.

[52] Mollison PL. The introduction of citrate as an anticoagulant for transfusion and of glucose as a red cell preservative, Br J Haematol. 2000; 108(1), p. 13–18. https://pubmed.ncbi.nlm.nih.gov/10651719/.

[53] Curling, Goss, Bertolini, 2012, p. 4.

[54] Rous, P., & Turner, J. R. (1916). The preservation of living RBC in vitro: ii. the transfusion of kept cells. The Journal of experimental medicine. 1916; 23(2), 239–248. https://www.ncbi.nlm.nih.gov/pmc/articles/PMC2125395/.

[55] Mollison, 13–18.

[56] Horsley J. S, Vaughan W. T., Dodson A. I. direct transfusion of blood: report of cases. Archives of surgery, 1922, 5.2: 301–313. https://ia800708.us.archive.org/view_archive.php?archive=/28/

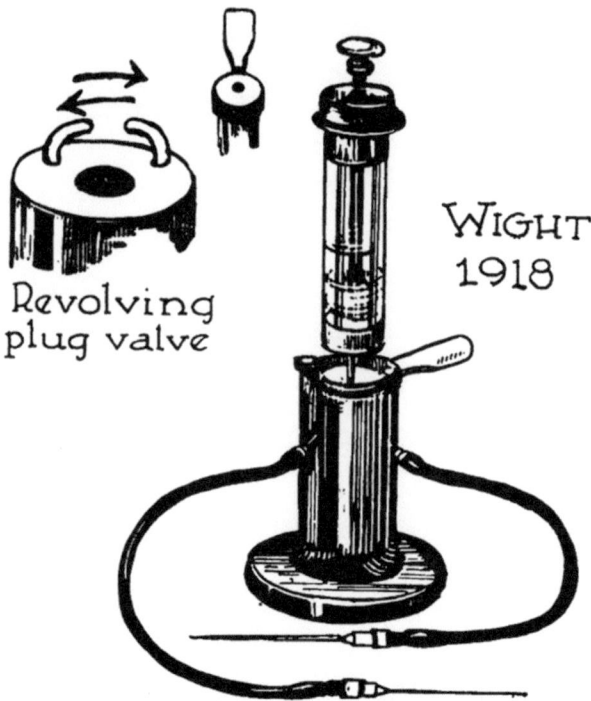

Image 8.13 Wight (1918) apparatus for blood transfusion (1918). (Source: Wight (1918) apparatus for blood transfusion. Chapter XV methods and technique of blood transfusion. In: Kilduffe, R. A., DeBakey, M. E. The blood bank and the technique and therapeutics of blood transfusions. Mosby, St. Louis, 1942, p. 410. Permission for usage of the image was granted by the copyright holder, Elsevier, on January 23, 2024. https://babel.hathitrust.org/cgi/pt?id=uc1.$b595310&seq=1. Accessed 28 Jan 2024)

were introduced to protect against the contamination of fluids with pyrogens. Because of this injection, solutions or blood were given with minimal risk of occurrence of chills and fever. This further proved that sodium citrate was a safe method to use.[57] Eventually conducted studies by 1933 confirmed that sodium citrate was not the reason for post-blood transfusion chills and that there was no obstacle to using solutions[58] in clinical practice. The problems with chills were actually caused by the increased usage of intravenous medication in the form of dextrose infusions or blood transfusions as a preoperative and postoperative procedure. Chills and reactions following intravenous therapy were due to the presence of foreign proteins, which were either extraneous matter present in the distilled water or the

---

items/crossref-pre-1923-scholarly-works/10.1001%252Farchpedi.1921.01910340093008.zip&file=10.1001%252Farchsurg.1922.01110140087003.pdf

[57] DeGowin, 1949, p.3.

[58] Solutions (sodium citrate and a physiologic solution of sodium chloride prepared with triple distilled water).

Image 8.14 Instruments for Lewisohn's citrate method of blood transfusion. (Source: Instruments for Lewisohn's citrate method of blood transfusion. Wiener, A. S. Blood groups and blood transfusion. Charles C. Thomas publisher, 1948, p. 96, public domain)

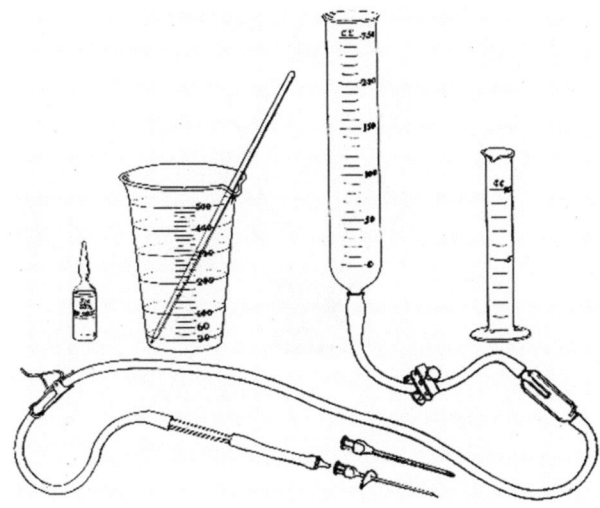

remains of changed blood proteins from a previous intravenous injection. To avoid these problems, special care was advised when cleaning the instruments immediately after a blood transfusion because blood clots and other foreign matter remained in the apparatus. It was also important that the solutions were prepared without the presence of a foreign protein that would cause later problems.[59] In 1935, Marriot and Kekwick additionally confirmed that a large amount of sodium citrate applied to patients did not harm the patient. Studies conducted in 1941 concluded that the incidence of chills and fever with blood transfusions of fresh citrated blood was not higher than compared with cases of blood transfusion of unmodified blood.[60]

Indirect methods using different syringes, tubes, and cannulas were not always present in adequate supply, and the problem of blood contamination still remained. Testing of blood compatibility between the blood donor and patient was mostly considered unnecessary, mainly because of the critical circumstances under which the blood transfusion was performed.[61] Instead, they would rather risk the occurrence of blood transfusion reactions.[62, 63]

Geoffrey Keynes (1887–1982) from Britain; Oswald Hope Robertson (1886–1966), a medical scientist from America; and Lawrence Bruce Robertson

---

[59] Lewisohn R, Rosenthal N. Prevention of chills following transfusion of citrated blood. Jama. 1933;100(7):466–469. https://jamanetwork.com/journals/jama/article-abstract/241639.

[60] Wiener, 1948, p. 59.

[61] Aymard JP, Renaudier P. Blood transfusion during World War I (1914–1918), Hist Sci Med. Jul. 2006; 50(3), p. 353–366. https://pubmed.ncbi.nlm.nih.gov/30005457/.

[62] Stansbury L.G., Hess J.R. Blood transfusion in World War I: the roles of Lawrence Bruce Robertson and Oswald Hope Robertson in the "most important medical advance of the war." Transfus Med Rev. 2009; 23(3), p. 232–236. https://pubmed.ncbi.nlm.nih.gov/19539877/.

[63] Aymard, Renaudier, 2016, p. 353–366.

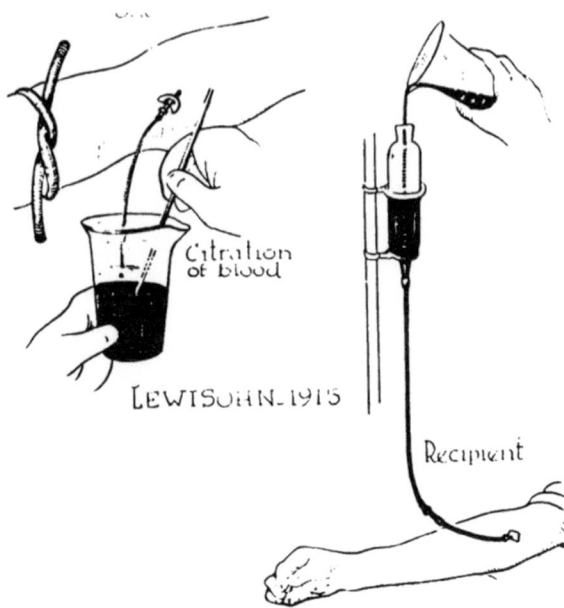

Image 8.15 Lewisohn's method of blood transfusion with citrated blood (1915). (Source: Lewisohn's method of blood transfusion with citrated blood. Chapter 15 methods and technique of blood transfusion. In: Kilduffe, R. A., DeBakey, M. E. The blood bank and the technique and therapeutics of blood transfusions. Mosby, St. Louis, 1942, p. 378. Permission for usage of the image was granted by the copyright holder, Elsevier, on January 23, 2024. https://babel.hathitrust.org/cgi/pt?id=uc1.$b595310&seq=1. Accessed 28 Jan 2024)

(1885–1923) from Canada developed different methods for indirect blood transfusion. The two Robertson's were not related.

Surgeon Geoffrey Keynes developed blood transfusion equipment that enabled blood transfusion to be carried out on the battlefield instead of just at medical bases. On the battlefield, his equipment made it possible to control the blood flow between the blood donor, who was a soldier, and the patient.[64] Major Lawrence Bruce Robertson, of the Canadian Army Medical Corps and a surgeon, learned from Lindemann the multiple syringe method for blood transfusion of uncrossed whole blood. He advocated blood transfusion instead of the use of saline for badly injured soldiers.[65, 66] Captain Oswald Hope Robertson and the physician of the US Army fifth Base Station Hospital had advanced methods of collecting and storing blood. Instead of relying on anastomosis as a method of performing direct artery-to-vein blood transfusions, Robertson organized drawing blood by venipuncture and storing

---

[64] Thompson, Strandenes, 2020, p. 10.
[65] Stansbury, Hess, 2009, p. 232.
[66] Hess, J.R. and Schmidt, P.J. The first blood banker: Oswald Hope Robertson. Transfusion. 2000; 40(1): 112. https://onlinelibrary.wiley.com/doi/abs/10.1046/j.1537-2995.2000.40010110.x.

8.4 Introduction of Sodium Citrate as an Anticoagulant

it for blood transfusion for up to 26 days.[67, 68] Most blood transfusions were, however, given within 10–14 days. The collected blood from blood donors of blood group O was mixed with solutions of sodium citrate with added glucose (1.2 L to 500 mL of blood).[69] Robertson was the first to use citrated blood in glass bottles known as Robertson's bottles,[70, 71, 72] which had three tubes. Blood flowed into the bottle and was mixed with the citrate sodium by rotating the bottle. Through the second tube, blood passed into the patient, and the third tube was attached to a syringe to produce negative or positive pressure inside the bottle.[73] The Robertson bottle was, in fact, a Boston round bottle (or Winchester bottle), a strong, heavy glass bottle that is commonly used in the pharmaceutical industry. It is cylindrical in shape with a short, curved shoulder and a narrow neck, which is usually threaded for a screw cap.[74] Robertson used it for storing blood and ice. The box was made of wood, double-walled with an air space between. Two packing cases, one fitting inside the other, served the purpose well. The space between the two boxes was filled with sawdust or some such "non-conducting material." A tight fitting door or lid was necessary. It was good to line the inside of the box with tin, and one end of this space was fenced off to contain the ice.[75] Robertson was influenced by Rous and Turner and used their solution for blood transfusions in the British Army.[76] Robertson also demonstrated the use and safety of stored universal blood donors or "cross-matched" blood.[77] By the end of 1918, willing blood donors were easily found, often from lightly wounded men, and 700–1000 mL of blood was sometimes taken (Images 8.16 and 8.17).[78]

The American influence was also in the blood grouping.[79] In November 1917, Major Roger Irving Lee defined a simple and rapid method for the selection of suitable blood donors for blood transfusion by the determination of blood groups. Lee essentially used a minimal procedure for testing agglutination between the blood donor's cells and the patient's serum. A small amount of blood was collected from a patient (1 cc) from the ear or the finger, which was then allowed to clot. After this, the serum was obtained. One drop of this serum was placed on a slide. It was mixed

---

[67] Hess, Schmidt, 2000, p. 110–111.

[68] Robertson O.H. Transfusion with preserved RBC. british medical journal.1918; 1(2999): 691. https://www.ncbi.nlm.nih.gov/pmc/articles/PMC2340627/.

[69] Boulton, Roberts, 2014, p. 329–333.

[70] Lbid.

[71] Keynes, 1949, p. 37–38.

[72] Hess, Schmidt, 2000, p. 110–111.

[73] Ibid.

[74] Plascene. What Is a Boston Round Bottle? https://www.plascene.com/what-the-heck-is-a-boston-round-bottle. Accessed 24 March 2024.

[75] Robertson, 1918, p. 692.

[76] DeGowin, 1949, p.3.

[77] Stansbury 2009, p. 232.

[78] Boulton, Roberts, 2014, p. 329–333.

[79] Boulton, Roberts, 2014, p. 329–333.

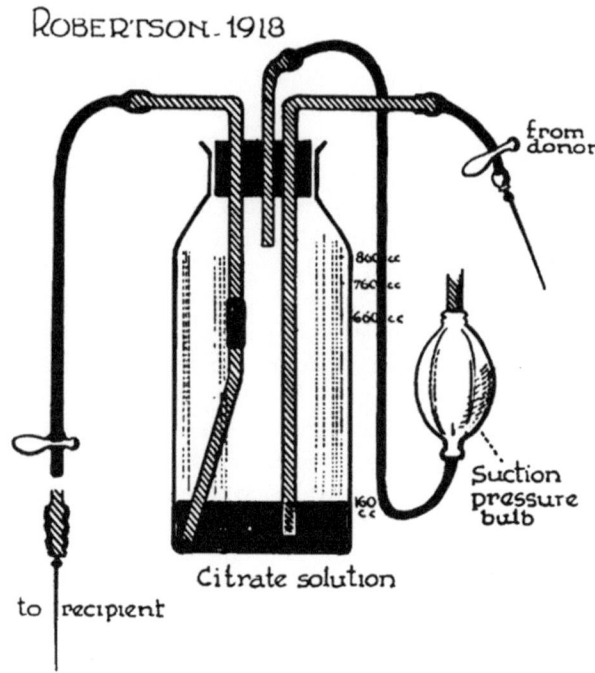

Image 8.16 Robertson bottle (1918). (Source: Robertson bottle (1918). Chapter 15 methods and technique of blood transfusion. In: Kilduffe, R. A., DeBakey, M. E. The blood bank and the technique and therapeutics of blood transfusions. Mosby, St. Louis, 1942, p. 380. Permission for usage of the image was granted by the copyright holder, Elsevier, on January 23, 2024. https://babel.hathitrust.org/cgi/pt?id=uc1.$b595310&seq=1. Accessed 28 Jan 2024)

with a drop of a suspension of blood from the blood donor, taken directly into a 1.5% citrate solution, and shaken. It was important that this mixture was not partially coagulated. The results of the procedure appeared in just a few moments. They were also best examined under a microscope. A positive test resulted in agglutination. They also constantly had a supply of serums known to be Group II, Group III, and Group IV.[80] These techniques allowed preliminary blood grouping in the later stages of the war. However, in emergencies where neither the facilities nor the time for laboratory work were available, a test injection of 15–20 mL of blood donor blood was used to rule out at least partially hemolytic blood transfusion reactions. Blood donors were from pre-selected group O. The British Army rewarded such blood donors with extra leave, much to the envy of their non-group O colleagues who never had a chance to earn such rewards.[81] The blood donors during the war were mostly soldiers. In the later stages of the war, from 1917 to 1918, blood

---

[80] Lee R. I. A simple and rapid method for the selection of suitable blood donors for transfusion by the determination of blood groups. Br Med J. 1917; 24;2(2969):684–685. https://pubmed.ncbi.nlm.nih.gov/20768818/.

[81] Boulton, Roberts, 2014, p. 329–333.

8.4 Introduction of Sodium Citrate as an Anticoagulant

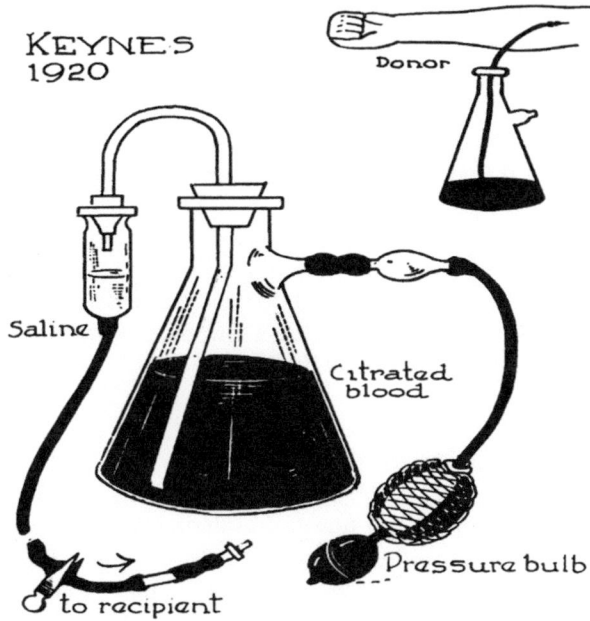

Image 8.17 Keynes flask (1920). (Source: Keynes flask (1920). Chapter XV methods and technique of blood transfusion. In: Kilduffe, R. A., DeBakey, M. E. The blood bank and the technique and therapeutics of blood transfusions. Mosby, St. Louis, 1942, p. 382. Permission for usage of the image was granted by the copyright holder, Elsevier, on January 23, 2024. https://babel.hathitrust.org/cgi/pt?id=uc1.$b595310&seq=1. Accessed 28 Jan 2024)

transfusion was more frequent, with better outcomes and much safer methods and improvements for the safety of a patient.

Blood could be transported in an ambulance over rough terrain. Resuscitation teams, or nursing sisters and orderlies, were established to find blood donors and carry out blood transfusions before and after operations to allow surgeons to operate without the distraction of organizing and executing resuscitation.[82] Specially trained shock teams administered morphine, blankets, and hot tea in so-called resuscitation wards. They also administered and performed blood transfusions because sodium citrate simplified the procedure. Canadian surgeon Edward Archibald also used citrated blood because of the simplified method. The blood donor could be bled by a junior medical officer with the instruments in a separate room. The surgeon could then perform the blood transfusion by himself, with blood at hand when he needed it. Furthermore, he could use that blood without fear that clots would clog syringes or ruin whole paraffin-coated tubes full of blood. The Germans also performed blood transfusions. In 1916, the German surgeon Leo Eloesser (1881–1976) performed direct blood transfusions with tubes irrigated with citrate. When the war ended, blood transfusion with citrate was not only an integral part of the

---

[82] Lbid.

resuscitation of patients in shock but was also an important component in the extension of blood transfusion itself.[83] Also worthy of mentioning is that Rous and Wilson proposed the use of plasma as a replacement for whole blood in 1918.[84]

8.5   Interesting Cases of Blood Donation during World War I

During this difficult period, there were many people who realized the importance of donating blood to others. It was not uncommon for their stories to be published in local newspapers as motivation to help others. Besides the soldiers and other staff, civilians also donated blood. Here are a few, but nevertheless important, stories of humane solidarity from 1914 to 1917.

8.5.1   Blood Transfusion on the Battlefield

One of the earliest cases of blood transfusion during the war was in the French Army on October 16, 1914. A doctor named Emile Jeanbrau performed the blood transfusion on a 25-year-old soldier who had been injured by heavy bombardment and had previously required a right above-the-knee amputation. The blood donor was also a soldier who had been wounded in the leg by shrapnel. An unknown direct blood transfusion method was conducted, notably without compatibility testing. By the end of 1914, the French Army had seen 44 blood transfusions.[85]

8.5.2   Remarkable Operation

Professor Carroll of the Rockefeller Institute in New York performed a blood transfusion operation at the Hotel Dieu military hospital in Lyon, France, in 1914. His patient was a French soldier named Raviot of the 256th Infantry Regiment who had been wounded in Alsace, France. After removing the bullet and a piece of bone, the French soldier's life was in danger due to bleeding until the French doctor Gélibert offered to donate the required amount of blood for his comrade. The operation was successfully performed.[86]

---

[83] Pelis, 2002, p. 213.

[84] Alberton E.C. Fatality due to transfusion of unpooled plasma. American Journal of Clinical Pathology. 1945; 15 (4), p 128–134. https://academic.oup.com/ajcp/article-abstract/15/4/128/1766102?redirectedFrom=PDF.

[85] Boulton, F., & Roberts, D. J., Blood transfusion at the time of the First World War - practice and promise at the birth of transfusion medicine, Transfusion Medicine. 2014; 24(6), p. 325–334. https://pubmed.ncbi.nlm.nih.gov/25586955/.

[86] Anon. A remarkable operation, Sheffield daily telegraph. 1914; October 24, p. 6. https://www.britishnewspaperarchive.co.uk. Accessed 10 Jan 2022.

8.5.3 A Courageous Wife

In 1915, a French officer, Adjutant Aubert, was seriously wounded at Mametz, France. After a successful operation, five bullets were removed from his body. However, a few days later, he started bleeding, with little chance of recovery. Only a blood transfusion could save him. His wife donated her blood to him. The blood transfusion was successful, and the officer Aubert received a medal for his bravery. However, he was even more proud of his wife, who saved him from death. Mrs. Aubert became the heroine of the Red Cross Hospital in the Boulevard de Châteaudun at Amiens.[87]

8.5.4 Heroic Soldier

A British soldier, Drummer Wharton, bravely rescued a wounded soldier from no man's land at the front. He was also injured during the rescue. When he was hospitalized, doctors looked for a volunteer for a blood transfusion among able-bodied patients. Private Wharton came forward and selflessly donated almost four ounces (about 118 mL) of blood to a patient who had been wounded in the chest. Wharton was decorated for his bravery at the front and in the hospital.[88]

8.5.5 Blood Transfusion for a Wounded Captain

Private Sapper James Dodds was hospitalized when a doctor woke him up in the middle of the night and asked if he would donate blood for the wounded captain, whose left leg had been torn off in the bombing. Surprised at first, Private Dodds immediately consented to the blood transfusion, and the critically endangered captain's life was saved.[89]

Experiences in World War I were crucial for the development of blood transfusion medicine in later years. During the war itself, many important discoveries were made that were beneficial to surgery, blood transfusion medicine, and both blood donors and patients. In this period, solidarity between voluntary blood donors was unquestionable.

---

[87] Anon. Brave wife's sacrifice, Loughborough Echo. 1915; 22 January, p.6. https://www.britishnewspaperarchive.co.uk/. Accessed 10 Jan 2022.

[88] Anon. Drummer Wharton, The Observer. 1916; September 29, 1916, p. 5. https://www.britishnewspaperarchive.co.uk/. Accessed 10 Jan 2022.

[89] Anon. Helensburgh soldier's heroic sacrifice, The post Sunday special. 1917; November 11, 1917, p. 5.
 https://www.britishnewspaperarchive.co.uk/, Accessed 10 Jan 2022.

References

1. Anon. A remarkable operation, Sheffield daily telegraph. 1914; October 24, p. 6. https://www.britishnewspaperarchive.co.uk. Accessed 10 Jan 2022.
2. Anon. Brave wife's sacrifice, Loughborough Echo. 1915; 22 January, p.6. https://www.britishnewspaperarchive.co.uk/. Accessed 10 Jan 2022.
3. Anon. Drummer Wharton, The Observer. 1916; September 29, 1916, p. 5. https://www.britishnewspaperarchive.co.uk/. Accessed 10 Jan 2022.
4. Anon. Helensburgh soldier's heroic sacrifice, The post Sunday special. 1917; November 11, 1917, p. 5. https://www.britishnewspaperarchive.co.uk/. Accessed 10 Jan 2022.
5. Alberton EC. Fatality due to blood transfusion of unpooled plasma. Am J Clin Pathol. 1945;15(4):128–34. https://academic.oup.com/ajcp/article-abstract/15/4/128/1766102?redirectedFrom=PDF
6. Aymard JP, Renaudier P. Blood transfusion during world war I (1914–1918). Hist Sci Med. 2006;50(3):353–66. https://pubmed.ncbi.nlm.nih.gov/30005457/
7. Boulton F, Roberts DJ. Blood transfusion at the time of the first world war—practice and promise at the birth of blood transfusion medicine. Blood Transfus Med. 2014;24(6):325–34. https://pubmed.ncbi.nlm.nih.gov/25586955/
8. Carrel A. Results of the transplantation of blood vessels, organs and limbs. JAMA J Am Med Assoc. 1908;51(20):1662–7. https://jamanetwork.com/journals/jama/article-abstract/428456
9. Chandler JG, Chin TL, Wohlauer MV. Direct blood transfusions. J Vasc Surg. 2012;56(4):1173–7. https://www.ncbi.nlm.nih.gov/pmc/articles/PMC4065715/
10. Cramer W, Pringle H. On the coagulation of blood. Exp Physiol. 1913;6:8. https://physoc.onlinelibrary.wiley.com/action/showCitFormats?doi=10.1113%2Fexpphysiol.1913.sp000127
11. Copher GH. Blood transfusion: a study of two hundred and forty-five cases. Arch Surg. 1923;7(1):125–53. https://jamanetwork.com/journals/jamasurgery/article-abstract/536614
12. Dodson AI. The value of blood transfusion in surgery of the prostate. Ann Surg. 1925;82(6):974–7. https://www.ncbi.nlm.nih.gov/pmc/articles/PMC1400355/
13. DeGowin EL. Historical perspective, chapter I. In: DeGowin EL, Hardin RC, Alsever BJ, editors. Blood transfusion. Philadelphia & London: W.B. Saunders Company; 1949. p. 3.
14. DeGowin EL. Transfusion Equipment, chapter 26. In: DeGowin EL, Hardin RC, Alsever BJ, editors. Blood transfusion. Philadelphia & London: W.B. Saunders Company; 1949. p. 518.
15. Horsley Riddell V. Blood transfusion. London: Oxford University Press; 1939. p. 192–7, London: Humphrey Milford. https://www.woodlibrarymuseum.org/rare-book/riddell-vh-blood-blood transfusion-1939/. Accessed 12 Nov 2021
16. Horsley JS, Vaughan WT, Dodson AI. Direct blood transfusion of blood: report of cases. Arch Surg. 1922;5.2:301–13. https://ia800708.us.archive.org/view_archive.php?archive=/28/items/crossref-pre-1923-scholarly-works/10.1001%252Farchpedi.1921.01910340093008.zip&file=10.1001%252Farchsurg.1922.01110140087003.pdf
17. Hess JR, Schmidt PJ. The first blood banker: Oswald Hope Robertson. Blood Transfus. 2000;40(1):112. https://doi.org/10.1046/j.1537-2995.2000.40010110.x.
18. Hakkarainen S. A life-saving soda bottle, Helsinki University Museum. https://blogs.helsinki.fi/hum-object-of-the-month/2023/01/25/a-life-saving-soda-bottle/. Accessed 4 March 2024.
19. Keynes G. Blood transfusion. London, Frowde; 1922, p.110–111. https://archive.org/details/bloodblood transfusion00keynuoft/page/110/mode/2up. Accessed 2 Jan 2024.
20. Kilduffe RA, DeBakey ME. Chapter I, history. In: The blood bank and the technique and therapeutics of blood transfusions. St. Louis: Mosby; 1942. p. 28. https://babel.hathitrust.org/cgi/pt?id=uc1.$b595310&seq=7. Accessed 28 Jan 2024.
21. Kilduffe RA, DeBakey ME. Chapter XV, methods and technique of blood transfusion. In: The blood bank and the technique and therapeutics of blood transfusions. St. Louis: Mosby; 1942. p. 371–99. https://babel.hathitrust.org/cgi/pt?id=uc1.$b595310&seq=1. Accessed 27 Jan 2024.

22. LeBlanc HJ. To what extent did blood transfusion systems and technologies modernize during world war II? Young Historians Conference. 2016;10:1–6. https://pdxscholar.library.pdx.edu/younghistorians/2016/oralpres/10/. Accessed 11 Dec 2021
23. Lewisohn R. Twenty years' experience with the citrate method of blood transfusion. Ann Surg. 1937;105(4):602–9. https://www.ncbi.nlm.nih.gov/pmc/articles/PMC1390374/
24. Lewisohn R, Rosenthal N. Prevention of chills following blood transfusion of citrated blood. JAMA. 1933;100(7):466–9. https://jamanetwork.com/journals/jama/article-abstract/241639
25. Lewisohn R. Blood transfusion by the citrate method. Am J Med. 1952;13(5):550–5. https://pubmed.ncbi.nlm.nih.gov/12996530/
26. Lee RI. A simple and rapid method for the selection of suitable blood donors for blood transfusion by the determination of blood groups. Br Med J. 1917;2(2969):684–5. https://pubmed.ncbi.nlm.nih.gov/20768818/
27. Mollison PL. The introduction of citrate as an anticoagulant for blood transfusion and of glucose as a red cell preservative. Br J Haematol. 2000;108(1):13–8. https://pubmed.ncbi.nlm.nih.gov/10651719/
28. Nathoo N, Lautzenheiser FK, Barnett GH. The first direct human blood transfusion. Oper Neurosurg. 2009;64(3):20–7. https://pubmed.ncbi.nlm.nih.gov/19240569/
29. Pelis K. Edward Archibald's notes on blood transfusionin war surgery—a commentary. Wilderness Environ Med Fall. 2002;13(3):212–3. https://pubmed.ncbi.nlm.nih.gov/12353599/
30. Pierce SR. Blood transfusion in the First World War. KU Medical Center. https://www.kumc.edu/school-of-medicine/academics/departments/history-and-philosophy-of-medicine/archives/wwi/essays/medicine/blood-blood transfusion.html. Accessed 7 Jan 2024.
31. Plascene. What is a Boston round bottle? https://www.plascene.com/what-the-heck-is-a--boston-round-bottle. Accessed 24 March 2024.
32. Rous P, Turner JR. The preservation of living RBC in vitro: ii. The blood transfusion of kept cells. J Exp Med. 1916;23(2):239–48. https://www.ncbi.nlm.nih.gov/pmc/articles/PMC2125395/
33. Robertson OH. Blood transfusion with preserved RBC. Br Med J. 1918;1(2999):691. https://www.ncbi.nlm.nih.gov/pmc/articles/PMC2340627/
34. Stansbury LG, Hess JR. Blood transfusion in World War I: the roles of Lawrence Bruce Robertson and Oswald Hope Robertson in the "most important medical advance of the war,". Transfus Med Rev. 2009;23(3):232–6. https://pubmed.ncbi.nlm.nih.gov/19539877/
35. Till A. The technique of blood transfusion, section VI. In: Brewer HF, Ellis R, Greaves RIN, Keynes G, Mills FW, Bodley Scott R, Till A, Whitby L, editors. Blood transfusion. Bristol: John Wright & sons LTD. London: Simpkin Marshall (1941). LTD.; 1949. p. 420.
36. Thompson P, Strandenes G. The history of fluid resuscitation for bleeding. Damage control. Resuscitation. 2019:3–29. https://www.ncbi.nlm.nih.gov/pmc/articles/PMC7123228/. Accessed 14 Dec 2021
37. Unger LJ. Blood transfusion—1914 model. Haematologia (Budap). 1972;6(1):47–57.
38. Van Hee R. The development of blood transfusion: the role of Albert Hustin and the influence of World War I. Acta Chir Belg. 2015;115(3):247–55. https://www.researchgate.net/publication/279989937_The_Development_of_Blood_Bloodtransfusion_the_Role_of_Albert_Hustin_and_the_Influence_of_World_War_I
39. Weil R. Sodium citrate in the blood transfusion of blood. JAMA. 1915;LXIV(5):425–6. https://jamanetwork.com/journals/jama/article-abstract/439690

Image Sources

Chapter. 15 methods and technique of blood transfusion. In: Kilduffe RA, DeBakey ME. The blood bank and the technique and therapeutics of blood transfusions. St. Louis: Mosby; 1942. p. 400. Permission for usage of the image was granted by the copyright holder, Elsevier, on January 23, 2024. https://babel.hathitrust.org/cgi/pt?id=uc1.$b595310&seq=1. Accessed 28 Jan 2024.

Chapter 15 methods and technique of blood transfusion. In: Kilduffe RA, DeBakey ME. The blood bank and the technique and therapeutics of blood transfusions. St. Louis: Mosby; 1942. p. 400. Permission for usage of the image was granted by the copyright holder, Elsevier, on January 23, 2024. https://babel.hathitrust.org/cgi/pt?id=uc1.$b595310&seq=1. Accessed 28 Jan 2024.

Chapter 15 methods and technique of blood transfusion. In: Kilduffe RA, DeBakey ME. The blood bank and the technique and therapeutics of blood transfusions. St. Louis: Mosby; 1942. p. 401. Permission for usage of the image was granted by the copyright holder, Elsevier, on January 23, 2024. https://babel.hathitrust.org/cgi/pt?id=uc1.$b595310&seq=1. Accessed 28 Jan 2024.

Bernheim BM. Surgery of the vascular system. Philadelphia: J.B. Lippincott; 1913. p. 23. public domain. The current copyright holder is Wolters Kluwer. https://archive.org/details/surgeryofvascula00bernuoft/surgeryofvascula00bernuoft/page/18/mode/2up?q=blood transfusion. Accessed 17 Jan 2024

Fullerton A, Dreyer G, Bazett HC. Observations on direct blood transfusion of blood, with a description of a simple method. The Lancet. 1917;189(4889):715–9. Permission for usage of this image was granted by the copyright holder, Elsevier on January 9, 2024. https://www.sciencedirect.com/science/article/abs/pii/S014067360079917X. Accessed 10 Jan 2024

Fullerton A, Dreyer G, Bazett HC. Observations on direct blood transfusion of blood, with a description of a simple method. The Lancet. 1917;189(4889):715–9. Permission for usage of this image was given by the copyright holder, Elsevier on January 9, 2024. https://www.sciencedirect.com/science/article/abs/pii/S014067360079917X. Accessed 10 Jan 2024

Primrose A, Ryerson ES. The direct blood transfusion of blood: its value in hemorrhage and shock in the treatment of the wounded in war. Br Med J. 1916;2:384. Permission for usage of this image was granted by the copyright holder, BMJ on January 10, 2024. https://www.bmj.com/content/2/2907/384. Accessed 11 Jan 2024

Chapter 15 methods and technique of blood transfusion. In: Kilduffe RA, DeBakey ME. The blood bank and the technique and therapeutics of blood transfusions. Mosby, St. Louis, 1942, p. 402. Permission for usage of the image was granted by the copyright holder, Elsevier, on January 23, 2024. https://babel.hathitrust.org/cgi/pt?id=uc1.$b595310&seq=1. Accessed 28 Jan 2024.

Chapter XV methods and technique of blood transfusion. In: Kilduffe RA, DeBakey ME. The blood bank and the technique and therapeutics of blood transfusions. St. Louis: Mosby, 1942, p. 403. Permission for usage of the image was granted by the copyright holder, Elsevier, on January 23, 2024. https://babel.hathitrust.org/cgi/pt?id=uc1.$b595310&seq=1. Accessed 28 Jan 2024.

Chapter XV methods and technique of blood transfusion. In: Kilduffe RA, DeBakey ME. The blood bank and the technique and therapeutics of blood transfusions. St. Louis: Mosby, 1942, p. 408. Permission for usage of the image was granted by the copyright holder, Elsevier, on January 23, 2024. https://babel.hathitrust.org/cgi/pt?id=uc1.$b595310&seq=1. Accessed 28 Jan 2024.

Chapter XV methods and technique of blood transfusion. In: Kilduffe RA, DeBakey ME. The blood bank and the technique and therapeutics of blood transfusions. St. Louis: Mosby, 1942, p. 409. Permission for usage of the image was granted by the copyright holder, Elsevier, on January 23, 2024. https://babel.hathitrust.org/cgi/pt?id=uc1.$b595310&seq=1. Accessed 28 Jan 2024.

Chapter XV methods and technique of blood transfusion. In: Kilduffe RA, DeBakey ME. The blood bank and the technique and therapeutics of blood transfusions. St. Louis: Mosby, 1942, p. 404. Permission for usage of the image was granted by the copyright holder, Elsevier, on January 23, 2024. https://babel.hathitrust.org/cgi/pt?id=uc1.$b595310&seq=1. Accessed 28 Jan 2024.

Chapter XV methods and technique of blood transfusion. In: Kilduffe RA, DeBakey ME. The blood bank and the technique and therapeutics of blood transfusions. St. Louis: Mosby, 1942, p. 410. Permission for usage of the image was granted by the copyright holder, Elsevier, on January 23, 2024. https://babel.hathitrust.org/cgi/pt?id=uc1.$b595310&seq=1. Accessed 28 Jan 2024.

Image Sources

Apparatus for Lewisohn's citrate method of blood transfusion. Wiener, A. S. Blood groups and blood transfusion. Charles C. Thomas publisher, 1948, p. 96, public domain.

Chapter 15 methods and technique of blood transfusion. In: Kilduffe RA, DeBakey ME. The blood bank and the technique and therapeutics of blood transfusions. St. Louis: Mosby, 1942, p. 378. Permission for usage of the image was granted by the copyright holder, Elsevier, on January 23, 2024. https://babel.hathitrust.org/cgi/pt?id=uc1.$b595310&seq=1. Accessed 28 Jan 2024.

Chapter XV methods and technique of blood transfusion. In: Kilduffe RA, DeBakey ME. The blood bank and the technique and therapeutics of blood transfusions. St. Louis: Mosby, 1942, p. 382. Permission for usage of the image was granted by the copyright holder, Elsevier, on January 23, 2024. https://babel.hathitrust.org/cgi/pt?id=uc1.$b595310&seq=1. Accessed 28 Jan 2024.

Different Methods of Blood Transfusion by the Twentieth Century

Contents

9.1 Difference Between Direct and Indirect Blood Transfusion..... 107
    9.1.1 Classification of Blood Transfusion Methods (1929–1949)..... 108
9.2 Blood Transfusion Apparatuses for Direct Blood Transfusion in the Twentieth Century..... 110
    9.2.1 The Images of Different Apparatuses for Direct Blood Transfusion (1920–1941)..... 114
9.3 Indirect Methods of Blood Transfusion..... 117
    9.3.1 Defibrinated Blood for Blood Transfusion..... 117
    9.3.2 Sodium Citrate for Blood Transfusion..... 118
9.4 Venesection and Venipuncture Technique..... 120
    9.4.1 Venesection Procedure..... 122
9.5 Dosage and Rate of Blood Transfusion..... 125
References..... 139

9.1 Difference Between Direct and Indirect Blood Transfusion

There were a few fundamental differences between the direct and indirect methods of blood transfusion, which in the literature had different definitions until the indirect method of blood transfusion completely replaced the direct method. Sometimes the indirect method is referred to as direct or otherwise. For comparison, the classifications of blood transfusion methods are shown with similarities from the years 1929 and 1949. This classification demonstrates that new methods and instruments were constantly invented and applied in clinical practice, as it is today. Different authors also had different opinions on the definition of the methods that were used.

© The Author(s), under exclusive license to Springer Nature Switzerland AG 2024
Z. Kvržić, *History of Blood Donation and Transfusion Medicine*, https://doi.org/10.1007/978-3-031-68715-0_9

Direct blood transfusion required blood donor–patient proximity and relied on quick transference to mitigate clotting. Blood transfusion from a blood donor artery to a patient's vein occurred spontaneously upon connection, whereas vein-to-vein direct blood transfusion required energizing, which was accomplished by gravity, pumping, or withdrawal into a delivery device for prompt infusion. Authors have sometimes referred the last as indirect transfusing, but the term indirect should be reserved for procedures that do not require immediate blood donor presence and include physical (defibrination) or chemical coagulation control for storage, no matter how brief.[1] In today's modern world, we use indirect blood transfusions. This means that the donated blood is processed into blood components, tested, stored, delivered to hospitals, and transfused to a patient. In some cases, whole blood at the battlefront is still used to prevent shock in emergency cases or in autotransfusion. Because of a shortage of blood components, whole blood is still used in poor countries, such as in Sub-Saharan African countries. Whole blood is also used in neonatal exchange blood transfusion, and for this procedure syringes are used.

There were several methods that were used for blood transfusion (Image 9.1). As a comparison between the differences in the definition of indirect and direct blood transfusion, Gjukić (1929) states a reflecting definition from today's point of view, as provided by Chandler, Chin, and Wohlauer (2012). Gjukić divided blood transfusion methods simply into direct (with apparatuses) and indirect (defibrinated blood and sodium citrate). While DeBakey and Kilduffe (1942) refer to direct blood transfusion as the surgical anastomosis (artery to vein) and the usage of cannulas, in their definition of indirect blood transfusion, opposite of Gjukić, they include in it the usage of different apparatuses as unmodified blood methods. DeGowin (1949), as Gjukić, includes vein-to-vein blood transfusion methods as direct or immediate, as he stated. These confusing differences can also be found in different articles and books by different authors.

9.1.1 Classification of Blood Transfusion Methods (1929–1949)

Classification of Blood Transfusion Methods in 1929

1. **Indirect Blood Transfusion:**
   (a) Defibrinated blood.
   (b) Blood transfusion with sodium citrate.
2. **Direct Blood Transfusion:**
   (a) Vein to vein with different blood transfusion apparatuses with attached glass syringes and methods.[2]
   Classification of Blood Transfusion Methods in 1942

---

[1] Chandler, Chin, Wohlauer, 2012.
[2] Gjukić, 1929, p. 269.

9.1 Difference Between Direct and Indirect Blood Transfusion

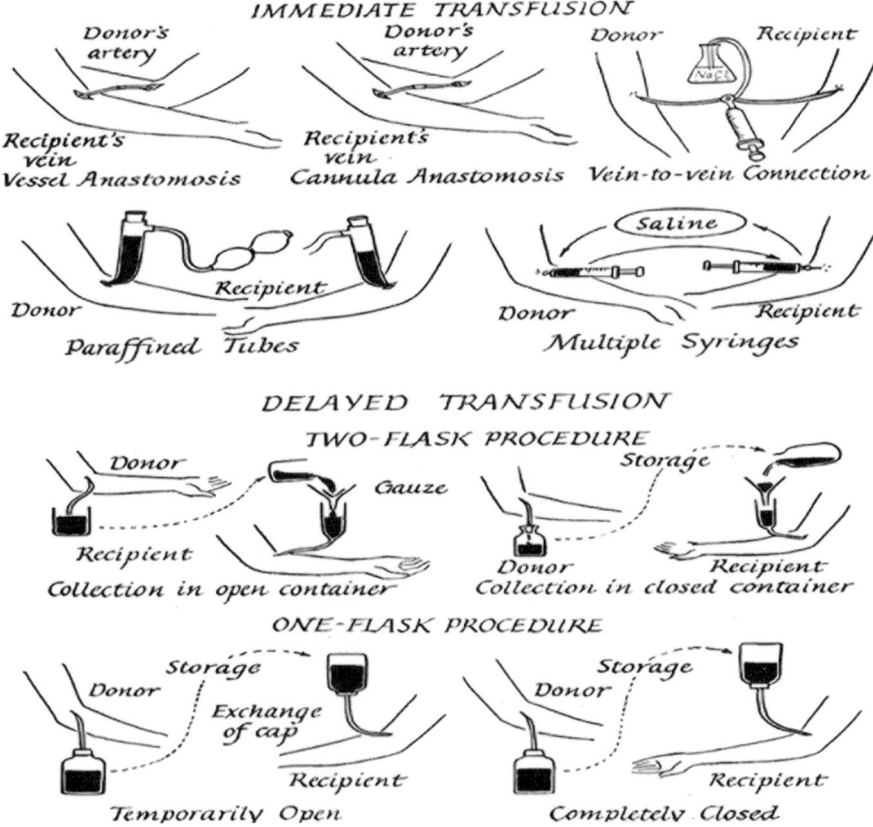

Image 9.1 Blood Transfusion Methods in 1949. (Source: Blood transfusion methods in 1949. DeGowin E. L. Blood transfusion Equipment, part IX. In: DeGowin E. L., Hardin R. C., Alsever B. J. Blood transfusion. W.B. Saunders Company Philadelphia & London, 1949, p. 517. Permission for the use of the image was granted by the copyright holder Elsevier on 6 Dec 2023)

1. **Direct Blood Transfusion:**
   (a) Vessel anastomosis.
   (b) Cannula anastomosis.
2. **Indirect Blood Transfusion:**
   (a) Modified blood (defibrinated, anticoagulants, stored plasma, or serum).
   (b) Unmodified blood (paraffinized containers, athrombit, multiple syringes, syringe-valve, continuous flow).[3]

Classification of Blood Transfusion Methods in 1949.
Direct (Immediate) Blood Transfusion:

- Vessel anastomosis.

---

[3] Kilduffe, DeBakey, 1942, p. 371.

- Cannula anastomosis.
- Vein-to-vein connection by tubing and valve or pump.
- Paraffined tube method.
- Multiple syringe method.

Indirect (Delayed) Blood Transfusion:

- Two flask procedure.
- Collection of blood in open container.
- Collection of blood in closed container.
- One flask procedure.
- Temporarily open systems.
- Completely closed systems.[4]

9.2 Blood Transfusion Apparatuses for Direct Blood Transfusion in the Twentieth Century

After World War I, many apparatuses for blood transfusion and other instruments were developed for vein-to-vein connection by tubing, valves, or pumps for direct blood transfusion. They were similar in their function and, a lot of times, in their design.

With these apparatuses, the veins of both the blood donor and the patient were connected by tubing. Blood flow was directed into the tubing using a valve in the tubing, which alternately directed the flow of blood from the blood donor to the device and from the device to the patient, or by a pump or compressor in the tubing, which forced the blood toward the patient's vein.[5] There were basic differences between them regarding which type of valve was used for managing the direction of flow. In some cases, the direction of flow from the blood donor to the patient was changed with the valve mechanism. In others, this occurred automatically by means of a ball valve.[6]

As an example, in 1929 there were different variations of different methods with different apparatuses, but the basic methods for clinical practice were as follows: *The Oehlecker method*, *the Percy method*, *the Unger method*, *the Jüngling method*, *the Schiller method*, *the Beck method*, and *the Bécart method*. Blood transfusions in 1929 were used in surgery, gynecology and obstetrics, internal medicine, pediatrics, etc. The ideal blood donors in 1929 were thought to be healthy individuals between the ages of 20 and 40.[7] For comparison by the 1948 blood transfusion was used more widely and more frequently already in emergency cases: hemorrhage (traumatic, secondary to local disease, secondary to surgical operations), traumatic

---

[4] DeGowin, 1949, p. 516.
[5] DeGowin 1949, p. 518.
[6] Kilduffe, DeBakey, 1942, p. 405.
[7] Gjukić, 1929, p. 276–286.

shock, preparatory to operation, hemorrhagic diseases, various blood diseases, certain poisonings, infectious diseases, and miscellaneous conditions.[8] By 1949, the recommended age for blood donors was 18–65.[9] The same age is still applicable today. Also, healthy individuals of both sexes can donate blood and blood components within a certain time interval.

The first two methods of direct blood transfusion, from Franz Oehlecker and Nelson Mortimer Percy, were the most commonly used by 1929, with over 30 variations of the two methods. The Oehlecker method was more commonly utilized in Europe than the Percy method was in the USA.[10] The Percy method known also as Brown-Percy because of its adaptation of the Robertson-Brown flask was still widely used in Europe by 1939, but it was no longer the most widely used blood transfusion technique in the USA, where it was developed.[11] Both methods were widely used because of their great results. There were several differences between the two apparatuses, and the main principles are explained as follows: The principle of the Oehlecker method (1916) consisted of the simple transfer of blood from vein to vein using one pump (a syringe) and one faucet with two openings. After the tap was turned, the suctioned blood of the blood donor was injected into the patient, and for such a short time, coagulation was excluded. The faucet was then turned off, and with the help of another syringe, both sides of the apparatus were cleaned so that the glass cannulas were again filled with the table saline and were completely transparent. A saline (sodium chloride solution) without any additives was sufficient for rinsing. After rinsing the device with saline, the blood was again transfused into the other person's bloodstream. The principle of the Percy method was that the entire amount of blood was taken from the blood donor at once using one glass cylinder, and the blood taken using the same cylinder was given to the patient, who did not have to be with the blood donor at the same time.[12] There were also other apparatuses used such as Soresi's apparatus, the Baker transfuser, Pennel blood transfusion apparatus, Jubé's syringe, Rotanda, and others (Images 9.2, 9.3, 9.4, 9.5, 9.6, 9.7, 9.8, 9.9, 9.10, 9.11, 9.12, 9.13, 9.14, 9.15, 9.16, 9.17, 9.18, 9.19, 9.20, 9.21, 9.22, 9.23, 9.24, 9.25, 9.26, 9.27 and 9.28).[13, 14, 15, 16]

---

[8] Wiener A. S. Chap. VI: Indications for and results of transfusion. In: Blood groups and transfusion. Charles C. Thomas publisher; 1948, p. 77.

[9] Brewer H. F. The blood donor, section V-A. In: Brewer H.F., Ellis R., Greaves R. I. N., Keynes G., Mills F. W., Bodley Scott R., Till A., Whitby L. Blood transfusion. Bristol: John Wright & sons LTD. London: Simpkin Marshall (1941). LTD.;1949, p. 335.

[10] Gjukić, 1929, p. 270–280.

[11] Horsley Riddell, 1939, p. 196.

[12] Ibid.

[13] Grífols, J.R. The contribution of Dr. Duran-Jorda to the advancement and development of European blood transfusion. ISBT Science Series2. 2007; 2, p. 134.

[14] Wiener A. S. 1948, p. 102–107.

[15] Grífols, J.R. The contribution of Dr. Duran-Jorda to the advancement and development of European blood transfusion. ISBT Science Series2. 2007; 2, p. 134.

[16] Kvržić Z. Odvzem polne krvi pri krvodajalcu skozi različna zgodovinska obdobja (1875–2023). Utrip: informativni bilten Zbornice zdravstvene nege Slovenije.—ISSN 1318-5470. 2023; 31 (4),

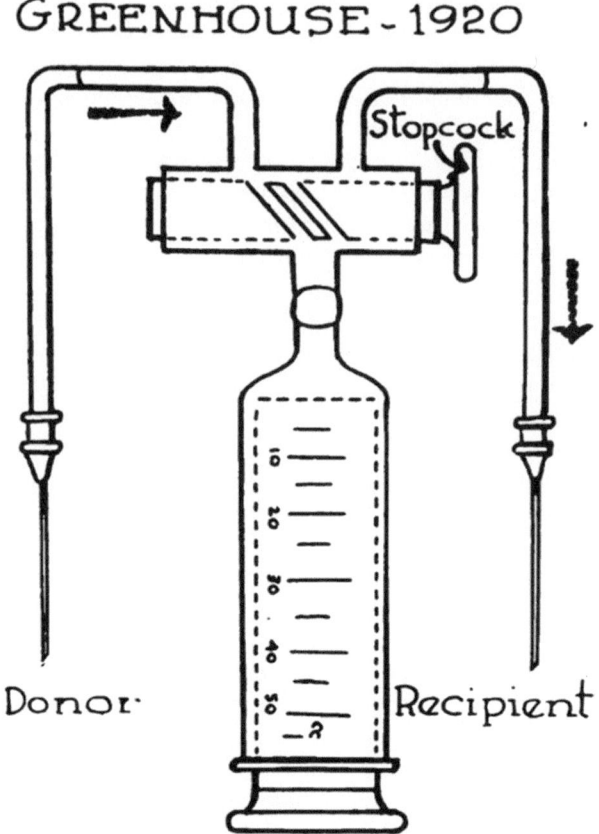

Image 9.2 Greenhouse Apparatus (1920). (Source: Greenhouse apparatus 1920. Chap. XV methods and technique of blood transfusion. In: Kilduffe, R. A., DeBakey, M. E. The blood bank and the technique and therapeutics of blood transfusions. Mosby, St. Louis, 1942, p. 404. Permission for usage of the image was granted by the copyright holder, Elsevier, on January 23, 2024. https://babel.hathitrust.org/cgi/pt?id=uc1.$b595310&seq=1 Accessed 1 Feb 2024)

The syringe valve method for direct blood transfusion of unmodified blood could have been done without assistance, and with some apparatuses, it was simple to operate.[17] However, the use of blood transfusion apparatuses posed both technical and medical challenges. The apparatuses were generally expensive and difficult to maintain. These included the possibility of malfunctions because valves often became stuck, dose restrictions, the potential for overdosing the patient, delayed blood transfusions, and the impossibility of small or large-volume drip blood

---

2023, p. 17–21. https://www.zbornica-zveza.si/wp-content/uploads/2023/08/UTRIP_Avgust-September_2023_SPLET-1.pdf. Accessed 3 Jan 2024.

[17] Wiener A. S. Chap. VII: Technic of transfusion of fresh blood. In: Blood groups and transfusion. Charles C. Thomas publisher; 1948, p. 108–111.

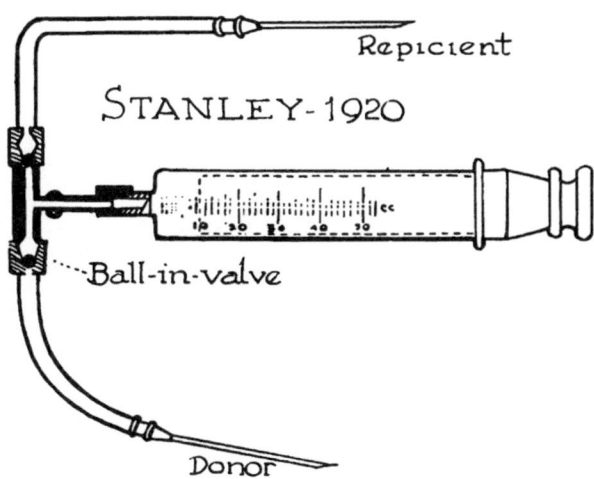

Image 9.3 Stanley Apparatus (1920). (Source: Stanley apparatus (1920). Chap. XV methods and technique of blood transfusion. In: Kilduffe, R. A., DeBakey, M. E. The blood bank and the technique and therapeutics of blood transfusions. Mosby, St. Louis, 1942, p. 413. Permission for usage of the image was granted by the copyright holder, Elsevier, on January 23, 2024. https://babel.hathitrust.org/cgi/pt?id=uc1.$b595310&seq=1 Accessed 1 Feb 2024)

transfusions.[18] Another problem occurred if the operator was inexperienced or lacked familiarity with the instrument.[19] Some valves have transmitted infections[20] if the blood donor was infectious from syphilis, malaria, or tuberculosis.[21] If, in a septicemic situation, patient blood accidentally ran back into the syringe and was subsequently injected into the blood donor, there was a danger that the blood donor might get infected. If the patient had become extremely ill and required multiple blood transfusions, etc., there were no more accessible superficial veins.[22] DeBakey and Kilduffe (1942) state that in this period, the different apparatuses were more or less obsolete.[23] Wiener stated that by 1948, the safety of stored citrated blood and plasma for blood transfusion had been established and that the blood transfusion of unmodified blood was used in minor cases.[24] Because of this, experts have rather used indirect methods of blood transfusion. Interesting facts are that evidence for the usage of these apparatuses was found to have been used in the late 1950s. The rotary pumps for direct exchange of blood were used in Australia in the late 1960s.

---

[18] Horsley Riddell, 1939, p. 193–194.
[19] Kilduffe, DeBakey, 1942, p. 399.
[20] DeGowin 1949, p. 518.
[21] Gjukić, 1929, p. 267.
[22] Horsley Riddell, 1939, p. 193–194.
[23] Kilduffe, DeBakey, 1942, p. 399.
[24] Wiener, 1948, p. 59.

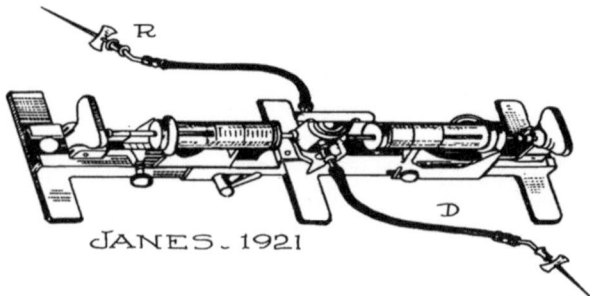

Image 9.4 Janes Apparatus (1921). (Source: Janes apparatus (1921). Chap. XV methods and technique of blood transfusion. In: Kilduffe, R. A., DeBakey, M. E. The blood bank and the technique and therapeutics of blood transfusions. Mosby, St. Louis, 1942, p. 405. Permission for usage of the image was granted by the copyright holder, Elsevier, on January 23, 2024. https://babel.hathitrust.org/cgi/pt?id=uc1.$b595310&seq=1 Accessed 1 Feb 2024)

9.2.1 The Images of Different Apparatuses for Direct Blood Transfusion (1920–1941)

The introduction of the syringe-valve methods marked another advance in the simplification of the technical difficulties of blood transfusion. The essential features of this method consisted of the utilization of a syringe and some type of valve for the change in the direction of flow from the donor to the recipient. Among the earliest of these syringe valve apparatuses were those of Freund, Unger, Bernheim, Kush, and Miller. Subsequently, a multitudinous variety of modifications were devised and advocated, but the majority are basically the same. The method in principle has continued to enjoy a wide popularity because of its obvious advantage in transfusing unmodified blood.

Among the earliest syringe valve apparatuses from 1913 to 1918 were those of Freund, Unger, Bernheim, Kush, Miller, and Wight. Later, from 1920 to 1940, came the development of a multitudinous variety of other valves and modifications (Rotanda, Feinblatt, Bergenstein, Rudder, Stanley, Moore, Koster, Soresi, Hirsch, Jube, Head, Bécart, and Touvet). From these apparatuses utilizing a valve mechanism that consisted of some type of stopcock were Lintz, Greenhouse, Janes, Scannell, and Tzanck. Apparatus utilizing valve mechanisms based on a rotating disk or revolving plug principle were Bernheim, Rotanda, Feinblatt, Bergenstein, and Rudder. Apparatuses utilizing grooved pistons for changing the direction of the flow were Head and Jubé. Bécart apparatus utilized a rotary valve based on the piston-cylinder principle. Touvet apparatus used pincer clamps that compressed rubber tubes and which could be opened and closed by turning the crank. Apparatuses utilizing ball-valve principle were Stanley, Moore, Koster, Soresi, and Hirsch.[25] The Scannel apparatus set was developed by John Matthew Scannell, Jr. The wooden case contains the various syringes, cannulas, etc. for Scannell's blood transfusion procedure.

The Rotanda was constructed by Otto Adolf Jüngling (1884–1944). Wilhelm Haselmeier from Stuttgart manufactured it.[26] This was a modification of the Oehlecker

---

[25] Kilduffe, DeBakey, 1942, p. 405–418.
[26] Kvržić, 2023. p. 17–21.

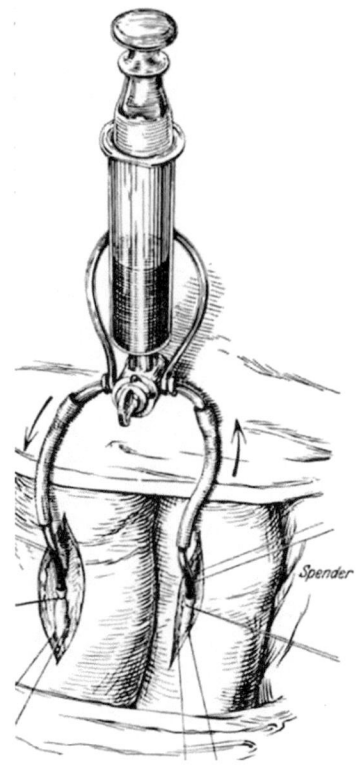

Image 9.5 Oehlecker Apparatus and Direct Blood Transfusion from a Blood Donor to a Patient. With permission from: Oehlecker apparatus and direct blood transfusion from a blood donor to a patient. Schiff F. Die Blutgruppen und ihre Anwendungsgebiete. Berlin, Verlag von Julius, Springer; 1933, p. 133

method. Jüngling constructed this apparatus in order to avoid the regular replacement of syringes. This was a three-way syringe.[27] One of the ways Rotanda was operated was to fill the entire syringe with sodium citrate. Then they inserted one needle into the blood donor's vein and one into the patient's vein. This was followed by the injection of 5 mL of sodium citrate into the blood donor vein, then the same amount into the patient's vein. Then 10 mL of the blood donor's blood was injected into the patient's vein, and the syringe was washed twice in a row with sodium citrate. Then 5 mL of sodium citrate was injected into the blood donor's vein again, and the same amount was also injected into the patient's vein. This was followed by a second blood transfusion. After transfusing a sufficient volume of blood, the syringe was washed again with sodium citrate. Then 5 mL of sodium citrate was re-injected into both the blood donor and the patient. The blood was transfused again, and the procedure continued in the same order until the direct blood transfusion was completed. At the end of the procedure, saline was injected into the blood donor's vein. Up to 800 mL of blood could be transfused in this way. The syringe was sterilized after use. Switching between the three different directions (pumping, returning, and rinsing) of the chambers was made possible by a rotating glass cylinder in the Rotanda.[28] The development of dependable technology, sterilization, and the discovery of blood groups in the early twentieth century made whole blood transfusions safe and therapeutic. Infectious

---

[27] Gjukić, 1929, p. 277.
[28] Kvržić Z., 2023, p. 18.

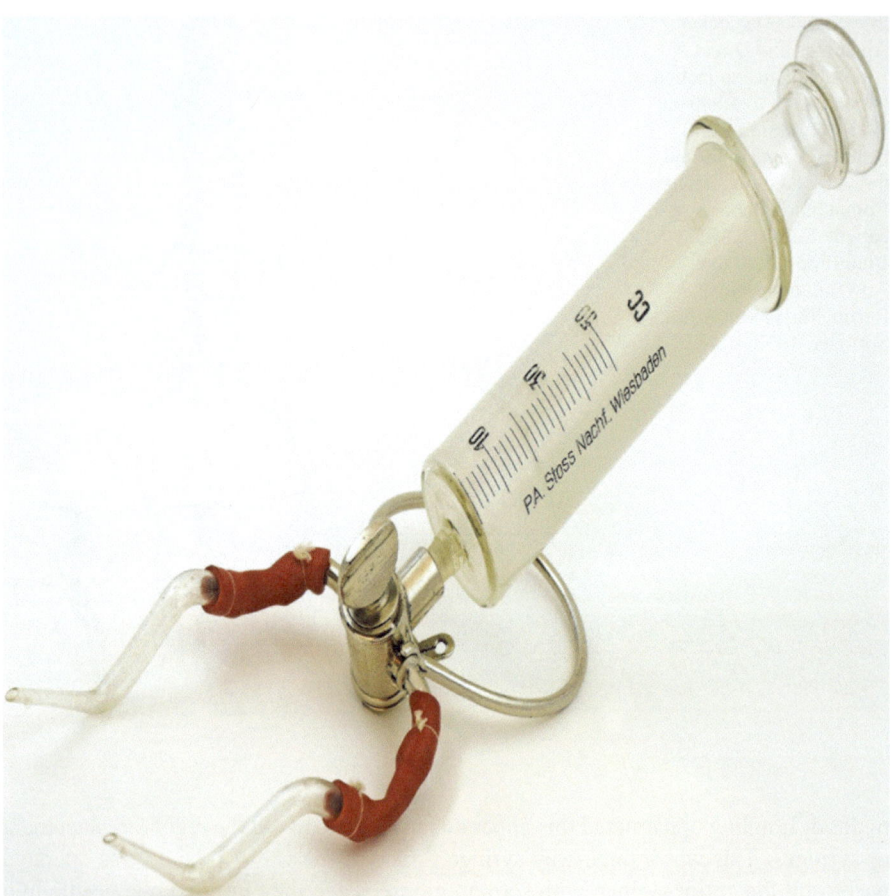

Image 9.6 Oehlecker Apparatus (1922). (Source: Gütebier T. Oehlecker apparatus (1922). Medicinhistoriska museet, VGR (CC BY). Permission for usage of the image was granted by the item holder on January 26, 2024. https://medicinhistoriska.sahlgrenska.se/utstallningar/manadens-foremal/2018/ Accessed 25 Jan 2024)

diseases, blood fractionation, and economic opportunities all contributed to the shift from whole blood transfusion to blood component therapy throughout the 1970s.[29]

The inventors of Beck apparatus were Alfred Beck and Ernst Pohl. This apparatus was known as Beck apparatus, Satrans blood transfusion apparatus, and blood mill.[30,31]

Rotary pumps were designed by Julian Smith (1941). For better blood flow, the rubber tubing was replaced by polyvinyl tubing, which was translucent. The rotary

---

[29] Carmichael S.P. second, Lin N, Evangelista M.E., Holcomb J.B. The Story of Blood for Shock Resuscitation: How the Pendulum Swings. J. Am. Coll. Surg. 2021; 233(5), p. 644–653. https://pubmed.ncbi.nlm.nih.gov/34390843/.

[30] Medicinhistoriska museet. Juni 2019: Blodkvarn. https://medicinhistoriska.sahlgrenska.se/utstallningar/manadens-foremal/2019/. Accessed 3 Feb 2024.

[31] Kilduffe, DeBakey, 1942, p. 422.

9.3 Indirect Methods of Blood Transfusion

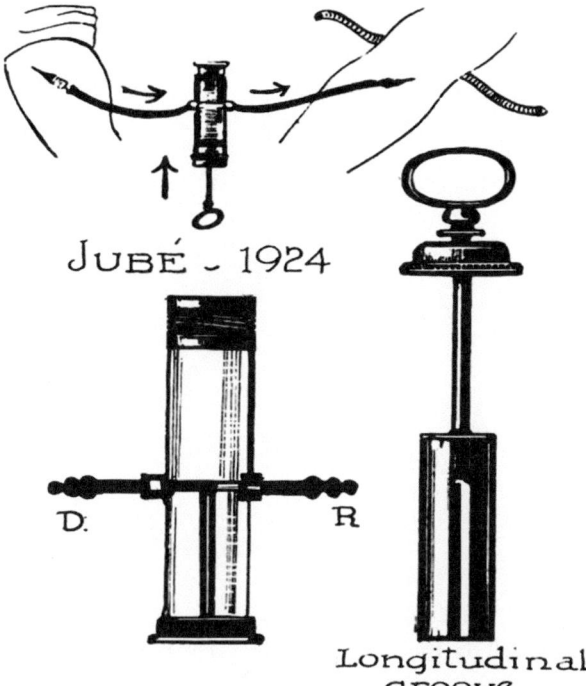

Image 9.7 Jubé Apparatus (1924). (Source: Jubé apparatus (1924). Chap. XV methods and technique of blood transfusion. In: Kilduffe, R. A., DeBakey, M. E. The blood bank and the technique and therapeutics of blood transfusions. Mosby, St. Louis, 1942, p. 416. Permission for usage of the image was granted by the copyright holder, Elsevier, on January 23, 2024. https://babel.hathitrust.org/cgi/pt?id=uc1.$b595310&seq=1 Accessed 1 Feb 2024)

pumps for direct exchange of blood in the treatment of hepatic coma were used in Australia in the late 1960s.[32] In this country, it is reported that in at least one case of acute leukemia, they used both indirect and direct blood transfusions. After the direct blood transfusions, the value of hemoglobin increased, and the patient was in remission, which lasted for nine years.[33]

9.3 Indirect Methods of Blood Transfusion

9.3.1 Defibrinated Blood for Blood Transfusion

In 1929, for a successful indirect method for using defibrinated blood for blood transfusion, blood was released from the blood donor's vein using a paraffin-coated cannula into a sterile vessel, placed in a water bath of 39–40°, in the amount that was to

---

[32] McLean JA, Luke HA. Direct exchange blood transfusion in treatment of hepatic coma. Brit Med J 1967;4: 78–80.

[33] McLean JA. Direct blood transfusion. Its history, with special reference to the Alfred Hospital, Melbourne. Med J Aust 1979;2: 625–628.

Image 9.8 Jubé Apparatus (cc. 1935). (Source: Jubé apparatus (1935). Syringe for direct blood transfusion according to Dr. Louis Jubé, cc 1935 (Museum of Science and Technology—Belgrade, Collection of the Museum of the Serbian Medical Society, Inv. No. MST: T:11.7.900). Permission for usage of the image was granted by the item holder on January 12, 2024)

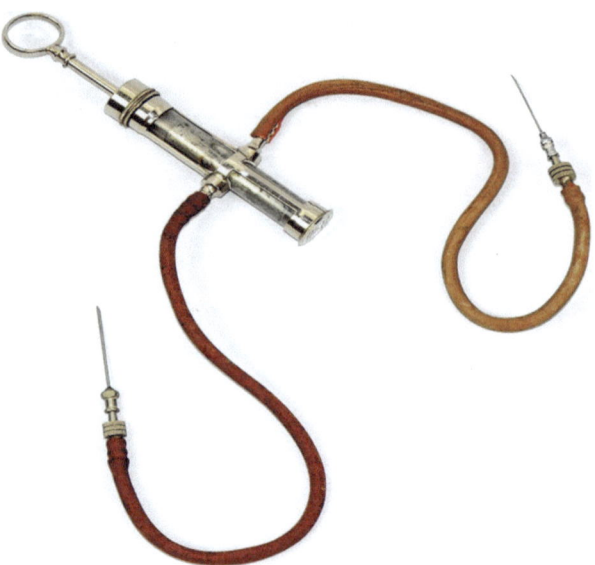

be given to the patient. Then the blood was shaken using a sterile glass rod, tweezers, glass beads, etc. until all the fibrin was separated. The blood was then filtered through multiple layers of sterile gauze, and it could no longer coagulate. It was slowly infused into the patient's vein using a syringe or an irrigator. At the same time, some physiological salt solutions could be added. In order to avoid ferment intoxication and the unpleasant phenomena related to it, it was necessary to leave the blood after defibration at room temperature for half an hour in order to lose the toxic effects of enzymes. After that time, such blood could be introduced into the patient's bloodstream without fear. By 1929, the blood transfusion of defibrinated blood was almost completely abandoned. This method had numerous flaws. Mechanical treatment of blood during the defibrination process not only reduced the number of blood elements but also damaged the majority of the remaining ones, so that they were not capable of a longer life in the patient's body. Elements damaged in this way quickly decayed in the patient's bloodstream, and if a large number of them were to decay at once, unwanted consequences could occur for the patient. Not only do the solid elements of the blood suffer during defibrination, but also, due to mixing, contact of the blood with air, and cooling of the blood, the structure of the serum also suffers. The big disadvantage of this method lies in the fact that the taken blood was not transfused immediately but had to wait for some time in order to avoid "ferment-intoxication."[34]

9.3.2 Sodium Citrate for Blood Transfusion

The method of indirect blood transfusion with sodium citrate as an example in 1929 was as follows: The blood was drawn from the blood donor's vein into a sterile and

---

[34] Gjukić, 1929, p. 269–278.

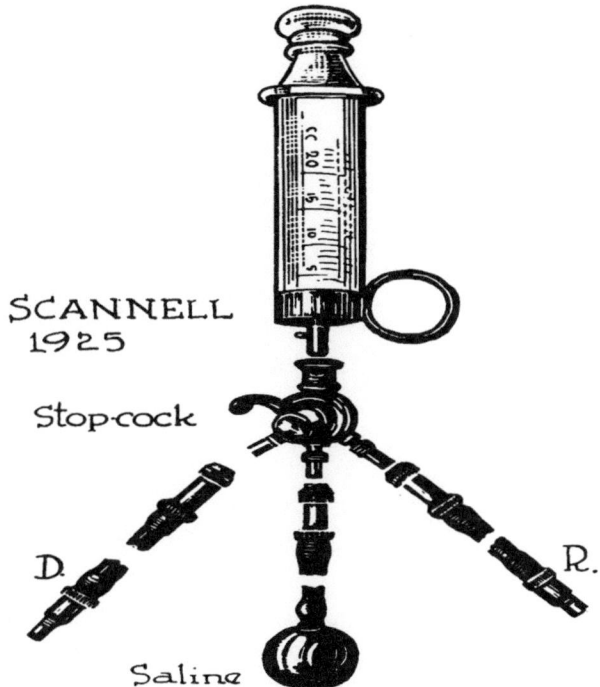

Image 9.9 Scannell Apparatus (1925). (Source: Scannell apparatus (1925). Chap. XV methods and technique of blood transfusion. In: Kilduffe, R. A., DeBakey, M. E. The blood bank and the technique and therapeutics of blood transfusions. Mosby, St. Louis, 1942, p. 406. Permission for usage of the image was granted by the copyright holder, Elsevier, on January 23, 2024. https://babel.hathitrust.org/cgi/pt?id=uc1.$b595310&seq=1 Accessed 1 Feb 2024)

graduated cylinder, which was placed in a 40–41° water bath and mixed with a sodium citrate solution. The percentage of sodium citrate in the blood was reported to be 0.4–0.5% and, according to some authors, even higher. The citrate solution was prepared either in distilled water or in saline. In either case, the solution was freshly prepared, neutral, and sterile. The concentration may have been arbitrary, but it was preferable to have it so that it was convenient to calculate how much solution should be added to the blood, e.g., a 2.5% solution was added to 20 cc at 100 cc of blood and a 10% solution to 10 cc at 2.5 cc of blood. The mixing of the blood with the citrate solution was not done with a stick or anything else but by moving the cylinder itself. After the desired amount of blood has been drawn and the required percentage of citrate has been added, the mixture was mixed and strained through a sterile, reusable gauze, as some coagulum may still remain. The filtrate was then infused intravenously using a funnel or irrigator, which was also pre-washed with citrate solution.[35] The techniques for blood transfusion of citrated blood that were established by 1939 included the gravity method using a tube and funnel, the air-pressure method of injecting blood, the syringe method using a flask and bellows, blood transfusion using a rotary pump, which combined gravity and

---

[35] Ibid., p. 269.

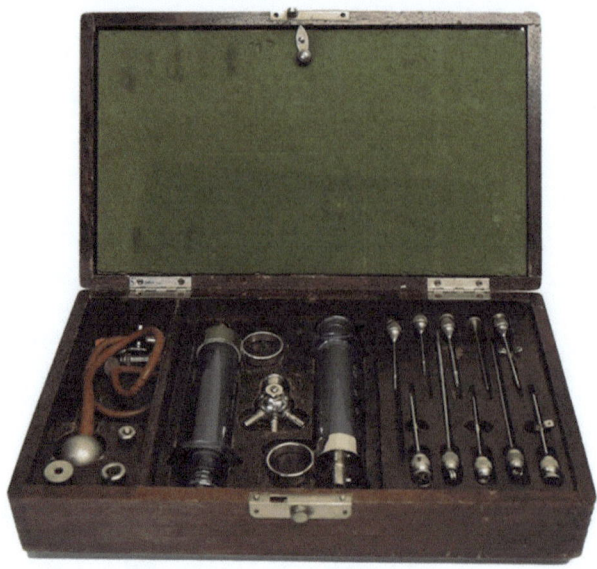

Image 9.10 Scannell Blood Transfusion Apparatus Set. (Source: Scannell blood transfusion apparatus set. Permission for usage of the image was granted by the item holder from his personal archive, Mr. Steven Pierce, on January 10, 2024)

pressure, the athrombit apparatus, the paraffin wax methods, and the multiple syringe method by Lindeman (Images 9.29, 9.30 and 9.31). The multiple syringe method included an operator and two assistants who, in real time, had to transfuse a certain amount of blood and wash the syringe with saline. For this, they had to be skilled. Using the mechanical principles of the Kimpton-Brown tube, the athrombit apparatus consisted of a synthetic amber cylinder. Known as athrombit, the artificial material was transparent, amber in color, boilable, and only broke under extreme pressure. Blood in contact with synthetic amber did not clot for a short time.[36] The glass bottle could also contain sodium citrate, through which the blood flowed, and the blood transfusion after this could have been performed almost immediately, or the bottle could have been stored and later used for blood transfusion. From 1943 onward, new anticoagulants for direct blood transfusions were gradually developed with blood bags that contained additives.

Over time, different equipment from different manufacturers for indirect blood transfusions were invented and applied to provide safe practice in the everyday healthcare environment.

9.4 Venesection and Venipuncture Technique

In blood transfusion medicine, for drawing blood from the blood donor, there were two techniques (venipuncture and venesection) with the use of a sharp needle. Venesection, or cutting the vein, as it was also known, was an unpleasant feeling for the blood donor. In comparison with the venipuncture, blood donors could not donate blood with venesection as much as they could with the venipuncture. The London Blood Transfusion Service even succeeded in prohibiting venesection. Other

---

[36] Horsley Riddell, 1939, p. 195–196.

9.4 Venesection and Venipuncture Technique

Image 9.11 The Rotanda (1925). (Source: Lara Miholič Ilc. The Rotanda (1925). The illustrator Lara Miholič Ilc gave her permission to Zdravko Kvržić for the usage of her illustration of Rotanda for this work on November 28, 2023. Permission to reuse the image from the article Zdravko Kvržić, Odvzem polne krvi pri krvodajalcu skozi različna zgodovinska obdobja (1875–2023). Utrip 31 (4), August–September, p. 17–21, was also given by the Nurses and Midwives Association of Slovenia on November 29, 2023)

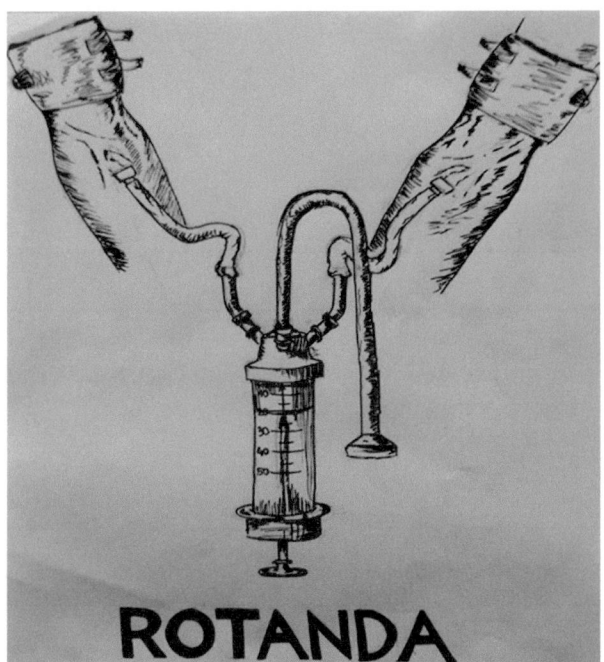

countries gradually shifted from venesection to venipuncture. Today, for drawing blood from the blood donor, we only use venipuncture. The venipuncture itself must be careful and accurate in order to avoid damaging the vein and an unpleasant feeling for the blood donor. Also, the area of the venipuncture must be cleaned with an approved antiseptic solution. Before performing the venipuncture, the area must be dry. The area of venipuncture should not have any scars, injuries, or skin disorders, which could make the venipuncture difficult and could transfer different impurities into the collection container. The prepared area for venipuncture should not be touched directly with fingers before needle insertion. It is also important to calm the blood donor and make him comfortable before inserting the needle.

Indications for venesection using cannulas instead of needles were in cases where veins were so small or collapsed, as in cases of severe burns where inserting a needle was virtually impossible. Then, for major operations where there was sudden and severe bleeding and there was no difficulty in immediately correcting the lost blood volume (operations on blood vessels), for blood transfusions where it was anticipated that prolonged intravenous infusions or further blood transfusions would be necessary for several days in hematemesis,[37] in cerebral and thoracic operations where the position, movement, or draping of the patient made it difficult to replace a needle if it was replaced during the operation. Also, the technique was applied in small nursing homes and private houses where skilled medical assistance was not readily available.[38]

---

[37] Hematemesis means vomiting of blood.
[38] Till, 1949, p. 403.

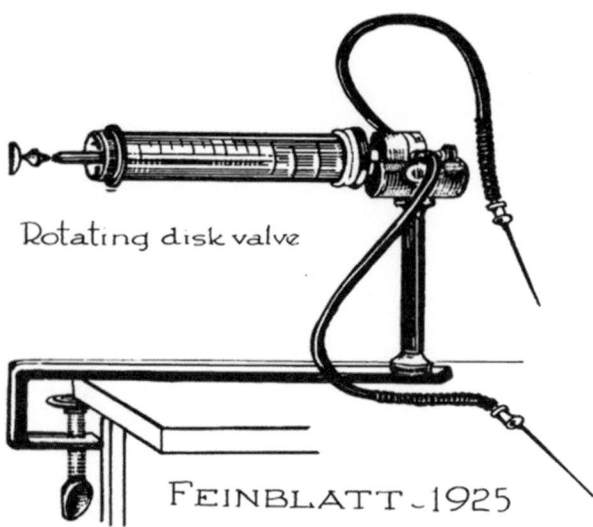

Image 9.12 Feinblatt Apparatus (1925). (Source: Feinblatt apparatus (1925). Chap. XV methods and technique of blood transfusion. In: Kilduffe, R. A., DeBakey, M. E. The blood bank and the technique and therapeutics of blood transfusions. Mosby, St. Louis, 1942, p. 411. Permission for usage of the image was granted by the copyright holder, Elsevier, on January 23, 2024. https://babel.hathitrust.org/cgi/pt?id=uc1.$b595310&seq=1 Accessed 1 Feb 2024)

9.4.1 Venesection Procedure

Venesection itself was a complicated procedure, and it required certain instruments, as follows: Scalpel, stitch scissors, toothed and plain 5-in. dissecting forceps, two mosquito forceps, two plain 5-in. artery forceps, a small aneurysm needle, a 2-cubic centimeter syringe and needle, a piece of narrow rubber tubing, and a roll of fine thread or silk ligature (Image 9.32). This set of instruments, which always had to be sharp and finely pointed, was packed in a folded towel or cellophane wrapping and sterilized by autoclaving. If re-sterilizing was needed in a hurry after use, they could be boiled in the usual manner.[39] With venesection, it was necessary to cut open the veins in both the blood donor and the patient, requiring two procedures. The operator in charge of the procedure had to be very skilled. He had to be focused on both the blood donor and the patient. The operator needed up to two assistants. During the procedure, a certain amount of blood was spilled, which made the procedure look unpleasant.[40] For venipuncture, one drop of 1% procaine on the skin was recommended before the insertion of the needle. For venesection, 0.5% procaine hydrochloride solution to 1–2 c.c. of 2% procaine solution was injected subcutaneously, and a sharp scalpel was used for the skin incision of 1–1.5 cm in length. A skin incision was made at a right angle to the vein and was freed from surrounding

---

[39] Ibid., p. 396.
[40] Horsley Riddell, 1939, p. 193–194.

9.4 Venesection and Venipuncture Technique

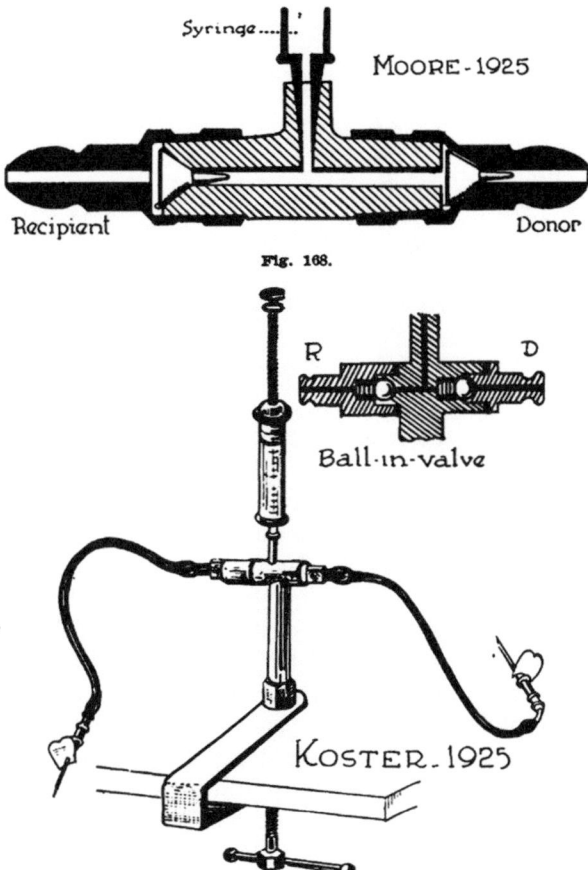

Image 9.13 Moore and Koster Apparatus (1925). (Source: Moore and Koster apparatus (1925). Chap. XV methods and technique of blood transfusion. In: Kilduffe, R. A., DeBakey, M. E. The blood bank and the technique and therapeutics of blood transfusions. Mosby, St. Louis, 1942, p. 414. Permission for usage of the image was granted by the copyright holder, Elsevier, on January 23, 2024. https://babel.hathitrust.org/cgi/pt?id=uc1.$b595310&seq=1 Accessed 1 Feb 2024)

fat and subcutaneous tissue with small, curved hemostats. The vein was delivered into the wound by placing a fine aneurysm needle around it. This greatly facilitated freeing the vein above and below for the desired distance. Two ligatures were placed around the vein, proximally and distally, about 1 cm apart. The distal ligature was tied and used for traction, and one untightened knot was placed in the proximal ligature, also to be used for traction. The vein was nicked between these two ligatures with scissors or bistoury at an oblique angle. Small hemostats with fine tips were then used to grasp the cut wall on either side and, if necessary, also the apex of the cut flap of the vein wall, thus separating the collapsed wall and enlarging the

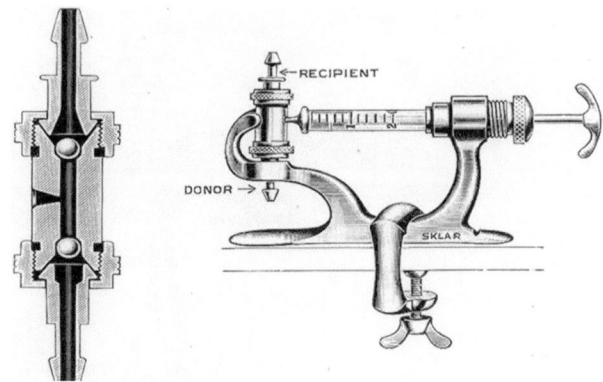

Image 9.14 Soresi's Apparatus (1925). (Source: Soresi's apparatus (1925). Wiener A. S. Blood groups and blood transfusion. Charles C. Thomas publisher; 1948, p. 109, public domain. Accessed 8 Jan 2024)

opening into the lumen of the vein. The cannula was then easily inserted between the forceps (Image 9.33).[41,42]

Compared to venesection, venipuncture offered two significant advantages (Image 9.36). The vein was relatively unharmed, which was a crucial aspect if more than one blood transfusion was planned. The technical process was also much faster. It was suggested as the preferred technique for high-volume blood transfusions—blood transfusions involving 1000 cubic centimeters or less—that were not anticipated to take more than eight hours.[43] For blood transfusion in adults, veins from the neck, arms, and legs were used, but most veins were used from the antecubital fossa. In infants, the veins of the dorsum of the hands were frequently used.[44]

Many techniques and methods were developed that were indeed of the most significance during a certain period, but for practical usage, venipuncture for blood donation and the indirect method of blood transfusion proved to be the best choices for safe blood transfusion medicine.

In cases in which the cannula had to remain for several hours or longer, the proximal ligature was tied with a fine bow knot (Image 9.34).[45]

If the blood donor fainted during the procedure, the circuit was immediately flushed with saline to displace the stagnant blood and prevent clotting until the blood donor recovered. For the same reason, the blood donor was never allowed to assume the sitting position, but he or she always lay down in the dorsal or supine position (Image 9.35).[46]

---

[41] Till, 1949, p. 398.

[42] Kilduffe, DeBakey, 1942, p. 446.

[43] Horsley Riddell, 1939, p. 262.

[44] Hardin R. C. The recipient and the administration of blood, part V. In: DeGowin E. L., Hardin R. C., Alsever B. J. Blood transfusion. W.B. Saunders Company Philadelphia & London, 1949, p. 250–253.

[45] Kilduffe, DeBakey, 1942, p. 447.

[46] Ibid, p. 451.

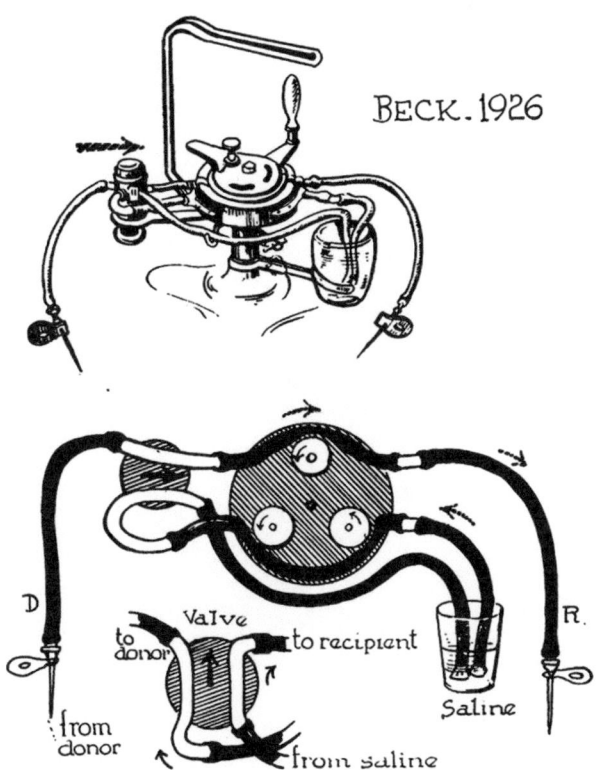

Image 9.15 Beck Apparatus (1926). (Source: Beck apparatus (1926). Chap. XV methods and technique of blood transfusion. In: Kilduffe, R. A., DeBakey, M. E. The blood bank and the technique and therapeutics of blood transfusions. Mosby, St. Louis, 1942, p. 422. Permission for usage of the image was granted by the copyright holder, Elsevier, on January 23, 2024. https://babel.hathitrust.org/cgi/pt?id=uc1.$b595310&seq=1 Accessed 1 Feb 2024)

9.5 Dosage and Rate of Blood Transfusion

In direct blood transfusions of unmodified blood in adults, the blood was injected at a rate of 50–100 c.c. per minute. In severe hemorrhage, it was allowed for blood to be injected at higher rates. In cases where the blood was required to be given slowly (definite myocardial disease or patients with marked secondary anemia), the sodium citrate method was used at a rate of 10 c.c. per minute. In 1942, it was discussed that some investigators believed that the rate of blood transfusion flow would be slow. The investigators stated that because of the temporary increase in circulating blood volume, there was a possibility of overloading the cardiovascular system, especially in patients who were not in a state of fluid depletion. They refer to this situation as "speed shock." But Kilduffe and DeBakey stated that in more than 5000 cases of unmodified blood transfusions, this reaction has never been observed. They also stated that, in the average adult, a transfusion of 500 cc. could be safely transfused

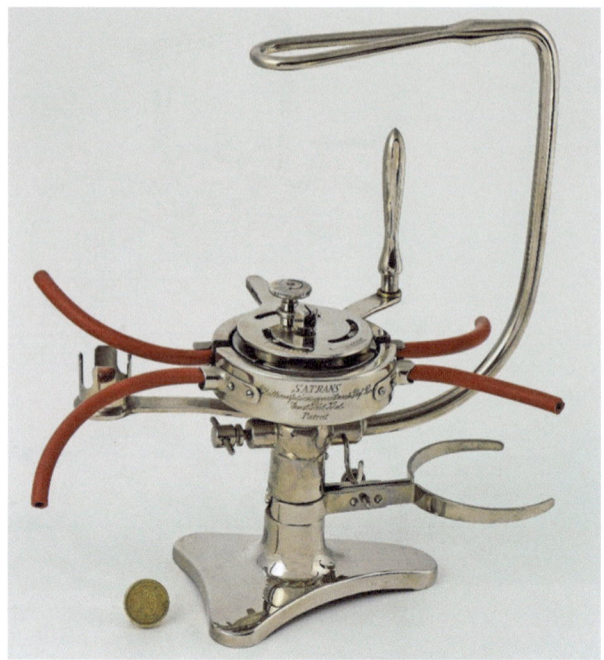

Image 9.16 Beck Apparatus, Also Known as Satrans Blood Transfusion Apparatus. (Source: Gütebier T. Beck apparatus, also known as Satrans blood transfusion apparatus. Permission for usage of the image was granted by the item holder on January 26, 2024. Medicinhistoriska museet, VGR (CC BY). https://medicinhistoriska.sahlgrenska.se/utstallningar/manadens-foremal/2019/ Accessed 25 Jan 2024)

at a rate of 1 cc. per second. In urgent cases, such as peripheral circulatory failure, blood, in their opinion, could be transfused at an even faster rate. In such cases, they stated that they frequently gave as much as 600 cc. of blood in less than 5 min. On the other hand, in patients with definite myocardial disease or patients with marked secondary anemia in whom impairment of the myocardium was probably present because of the chronic anemia, considerable care was exercised in blood transfusion. They considered that the efficiency of the heart musculature in such cases was obviously diminished and that sudden overburdening was entirely feasible. For this reason, they claimed that it was desirable in these cases to administer the blood slowly, preferably by the drip method, during which the patient should be carefully watched for any signs of cardiac embarrassment. A safe rule in these cases was to administer the blood steadily at a rate of about 1 cc. per minute and not more than 75 cc. per hour.[47,48] The standards for blood transfusions eventually changed in order to avoid even the slightest possibility of accidentally overloading the circulatory system. In transfusion medicine, comprehensive protocols have been established to address this issue. It is possible that in more than the 5000 cases mentioned, they simply didn't pay much attention to reactions related to the overload of the circulatory system, and as a result, they were not reported or they didn't connect the reactions as a consequence of overloading the circulatory system and in connection to blood transfusion reactions. Even today, there are cases where rapid transfusions are

---

[47] Wiener, 1948, p. 112.
[48] Kilduffe, DeBakey, 1942, p. 452–458.

9.5 Dosage and Rate of Blood Transfusion

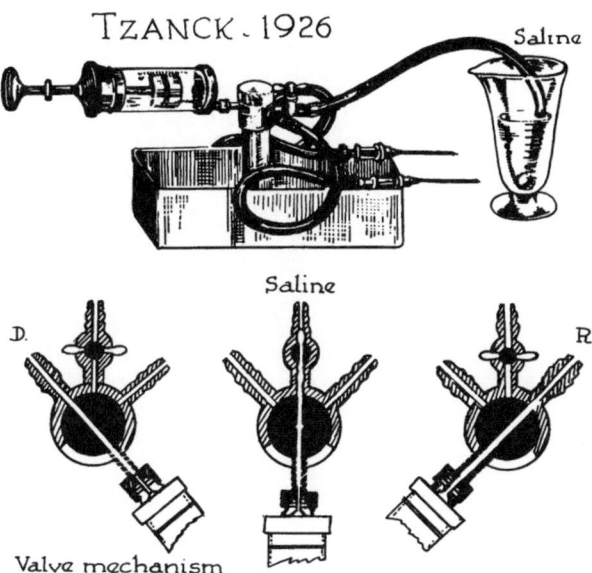

Image 9.17 Tzanck Apparatus (1926). (Source: Tzanck apparatus (1926). Chap. XV methods and technique of blood transfusion. In: Kilduffe, R. A., DeBakey, M. E. The blood bank and the technique and therapeutics of blood transfusions. Mosby, St. Louis, 1942, p. 407. Permission for usage of the image was granted by the copyright holder, Elsevier, on January 23, 2024. https://babel.hathitrust.org/cgi/pt?id=uc1.$b595310&seq=1 Accessed 1 Feb 2024)

required. This is in the case of massive transfusions in cases of trauma-related bleeding, obstetrical hemorrhage, surgery, and gastrointestinal bleeding. Massive transfusions involve administering 10 or more units of whole blood or packed red blood cells (PRBCs) within 24 h. An ultra-massive transfusion is defined as using more than 20 units of PRBCs within a 24-to 48-h period. The primary objective of a massive transfusion is to prevent fatal outcomes resulting from critical hypoperfusion-related complications while striving to attain hemostasis, the mechanism that leads to the cessation of bleeding from a blood vessel.[49, 50] In these cases, special protocols are applied, but these rapid methods are still safer than in the past, when experts transfused blood in only a couple of minutes.

Today, in general, the blood transfusion for the first 15 min starts slowly to be certain that there are no reactions, and then after about 15 min, the rate increases. The RBC transfusion in adults of 350 mL lasts for almost 2 h and up to 4 h, while the plasma transfusion of 200–250 mL can last 30–60 min (maximum 4 h), the

---

[49] Jennings L.K., Watson S. Massive Transfusion. [Updated 2023 Oct 29]. In: StatPearls [Internet]. Treasure Island (FL): StatPearls Publishing; 2024 Jan-. Available from: https://www.ncbi.nlm.nih.gov/books/NBK499929/. Accessed 1 April 2024.

[50] LaPelusa A, Dave HD. Physiology, Hemostasis. [Updated 2023 May 1]. In: StatPearls [Internet]. Treasure Island (FL): StatPearls Publishing; 2024 Jan-. Available from: https://www.ncbi.nlm.nih.gov/books/NBK545263/. Accessed 1 April 2024.

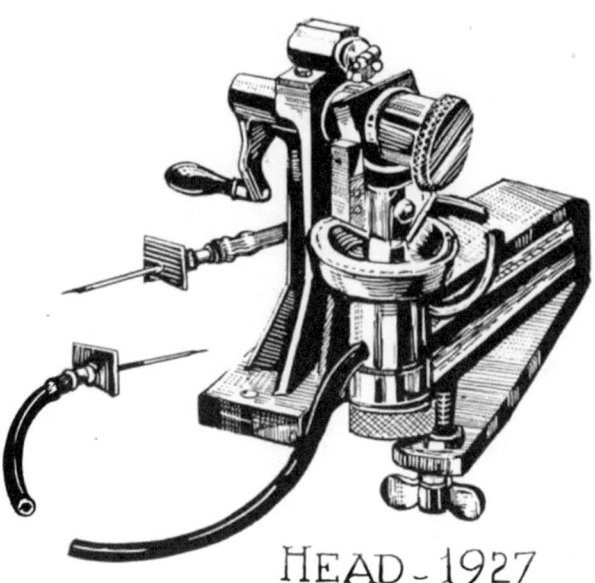

Image 9.18 Head Apparatus (1927). (Source: Head apparatus (1927). Chap. XV methods and technique of blood transfusion. In: Kilduffe, R. A., DeBakey, M. E. The blood bank and the technique and therapeutics of blood transfusions. Mosby, St. Louis, 1942, p. 416. Permission for usage of the image was granted by the copyright holder, Elsevier, on January 23, 2024. https://babel.hathitrust.org/cgi/pt?id=uc1.$b595310&seq=1 Accessed 1 Feb 2024)

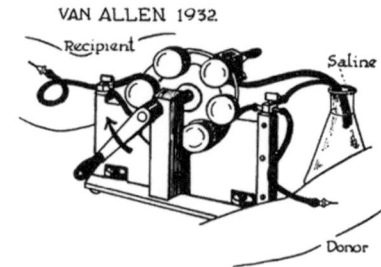

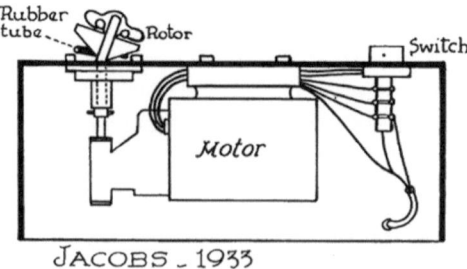

Image 9.19 Van Allen (1932) and Jacobs Apparatus (1933). (Source: Van Allen (1932) and Jacobs apparatus (1933). Chap. XV methods and technique of blood transfusion. In: Kilduffe, R. A., DeBakey, M. E. The blood bank and the technique and therapeutics of blood transfusions. Mosby, St. Louis, 1942, p. 423. Permission for usage of the image was granted by the copyright holder, Elsevier, on January 23, 2024. https://babel.hathitrust.org/cgi/pt?id=uc1.$b595310&seq=1 Accessed 1 Feb 2024)

9.5 Dosage and Rate of Blood Transfusion

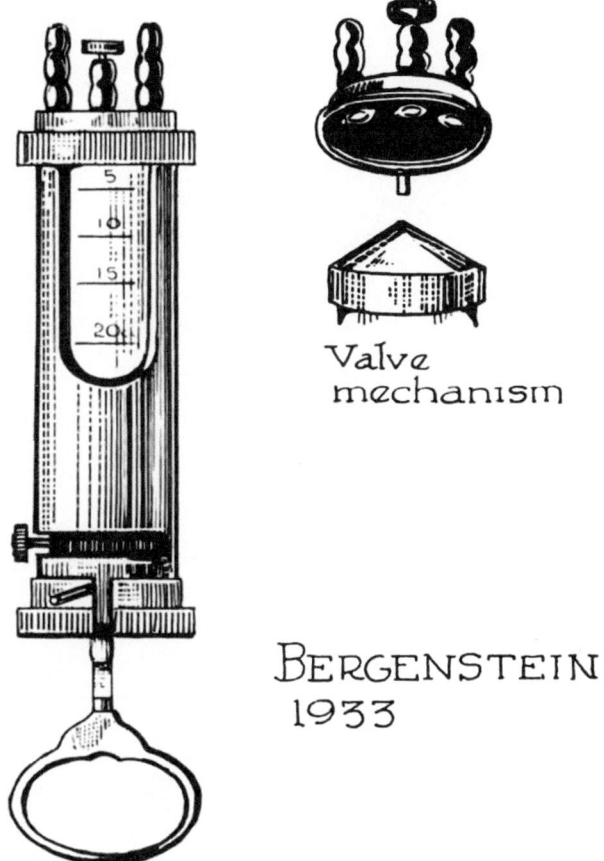

Image 9.20 Bergenstein Apparatus (1933). (Source: Bergenstein apparatus (1933). Chap. XV methods and technique of blood transfusion. In: Kilduffe, R. A., DeBakey, M. E. The blood bank and the technique and therapeutics of blood transfusions. Mosby, St. Louis, 1942, p. 412. Permission for usage of the image was granted by the copyright holder, Elsevier, on January 23, 2024. https://babel.hathitrust.org/cgi/pt?id=uc1.$b595310&seq=1 Accessed 1 Feb 2024)

transfusion of cryoprecipitate of 90–120 mL takes about 15–30 min, and granulocytes of 220–450 mL take up to 1–2 h.[51,52] The rate and the dosages may vary depending on whether the patient is a child or an adult, the amount of blood that must be transfused, etc.

---

[51] BloodWorks Northwest. Typical rates, volumes, and duration. https://www.bloodworksnw.org/medical-services/transfusion-medicine/rates-volumes-duration-transfusions. Accessed 1 April 2024.

[52] American Cancer Society. Transfusion Steps and Possible Side Effects. https://www.cancer.org/cancer/managing-cancer/treatment-types/blood-transfusion-and-donation/how-blood-transfusions-are-done.html#written_by. Accessed 1 April 2024.

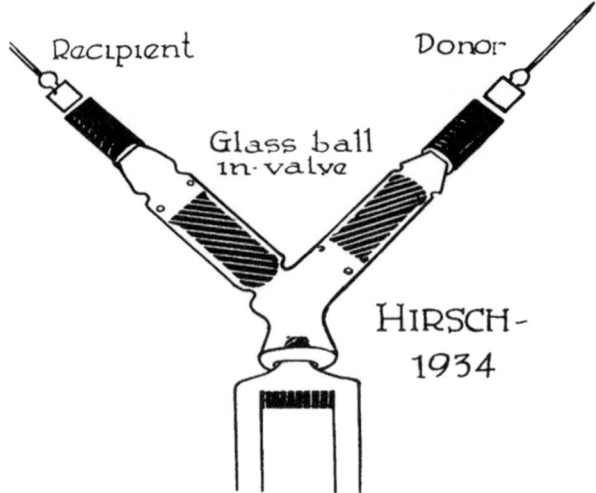

Image 9.21 Hirsch Apparatus (1934). (Source: Hirsch apparatus (1934). Chap. XV methods and technique of blood transfusion. In: Kilduffe, R. A., DeBakey, M. E. The blood bank and the technique and therapeutics of blood transfusions. Mosby, St. Louis, 1942, p. 415. Permission for usage of the image was granted by the copyright holder, Elsevier, on January 23, 2024. https://babel.hathitrust.org/cgi/pt?id=uc1.$b595310&seq=1 Accessed 1 Feb 2024)

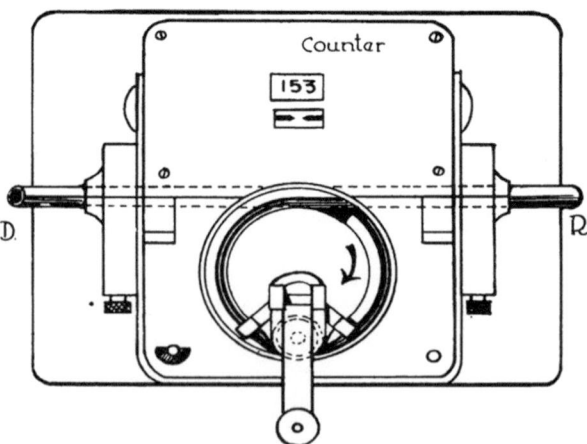

Image 9.22 Henry-Jouvelet Apparatus (1934). (Source: Henry-Jouvelet apparatus (1934). Chap. XV methods and technique of blood transfusion. In: Kilduffe, R. A., DeBakey, M. E. The blood bank and the technique and therapeutics of blood transfusions. Mosby, St. Louis, 1942, p. 424. Permission for usage of the image was granted by the copyright holder, Elsevier, on January 23, 2024. https://babel.hathitrust.org/cgi/pt?id=uc1.$b595310&seq=1 Accessed 1 Feb 2024)

9.5 Dosage and Rate of Blood Transfusion

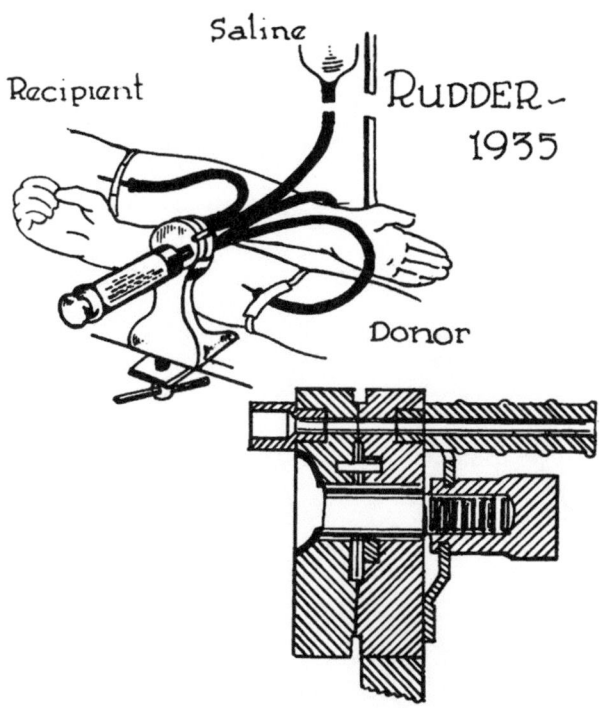

Image 9.23 Rudder Apparatus (1935). (Source: Rudder apparatus (1935). Chap. XV methods and technique of blood transfusion. In: Kilduffe, R. A., DeBakey, M. E. The blood bank and the technique and therapeutics of blood transfusions. Mosby, St. Louis, 1942, p. 413. Permission for usage of the image was granted by the copyright holder, Elsevier, on January 23, 2024. https://babel.hathitrust.org/cgi/pt?id=uc1.$b595310&seq=1 Accessed 1 Feb 2024)

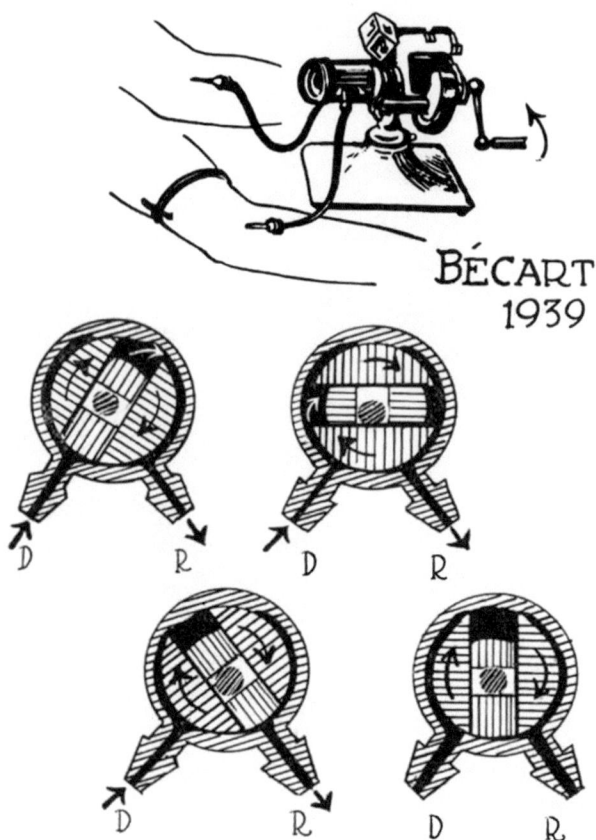

Image 9.24 Bécart Apparatus (1939). (Source: Bécart apparatus (1939). Chap. XV methods and technique of blood transfusion. In: Kilduffe, R. A., DeBakey, M. E. The blood bank and the technique and therapeutics of blood transfusions. Mosby, St. Louis, 1942, p. 417. Permission for usage of the image was granted by the copyright holder, Elsevier, on January 23, 2024. https://babel.hathitrust.org/cgi/pt?id=uc1.$b595310&seq=1 Accessed 1 Feb 2024)

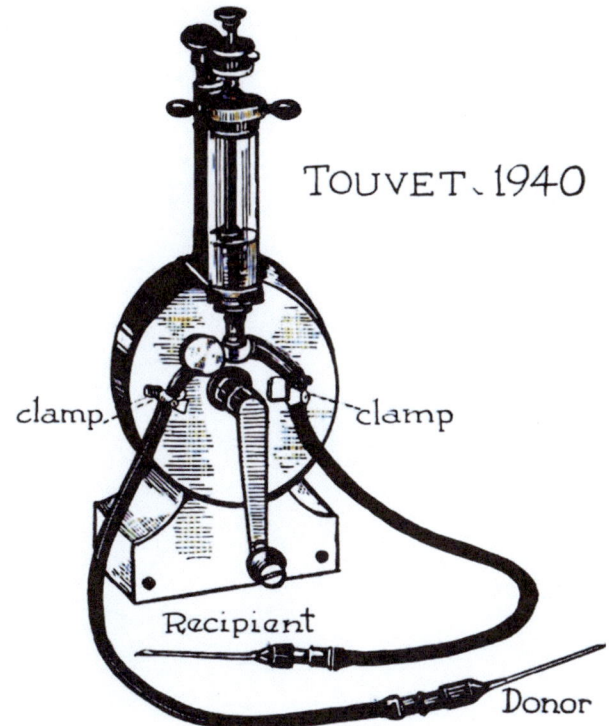

Image 9.25 Touvet Apparatus (1940). (Source: Touvet apparatus (1940). Chap. XV methods and technique of blood transfusion. In: Kilduffe, R. A., DeBakey, M. E. The blood bank and the technique and therapeutics of blood transfusions. Mosby, St. Louis, 1942, p. 418. Permission for usage of the image was granted by the copyright holder, Elsevier, on January 23, 2024. https://babel.hathitrust.org/cgi/pt?id=uc1.$b595310&seq=1 Accessed 1 Feb 2024)

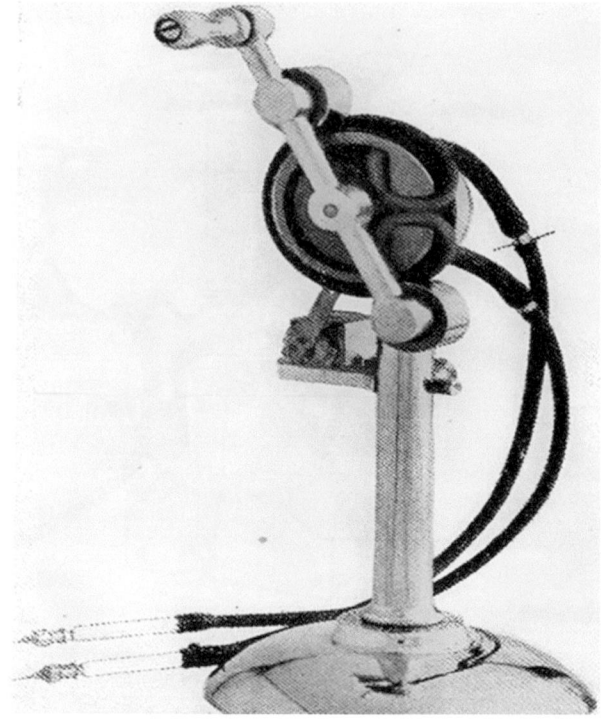

Image 9.26 Cashman Baker Transfuser (1936). (Source: The Cashman Baker Transfuser (1936). Wiener A. S. Blood groups and blood transfusion. Charles C. Thomas publisher; 1948, p. 110, public domain. Accessed 8 Jan 2024)

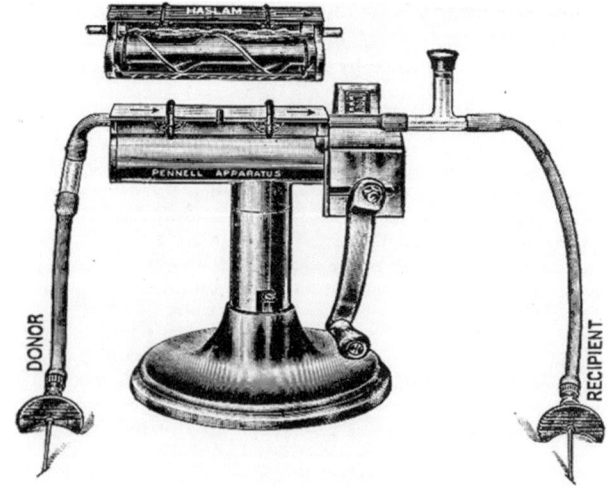

Image 9.27 Pennell Apparatus (1939). (Source: Pennell apparatus (1939). Wiener A. S. Blood groups and blood transfusion. Charles C. Thomas publisher; 1948, p. 111, public domain. Accessed 8 Jan 2024)

9.5 Dosage and Rate of Blood Transfusion

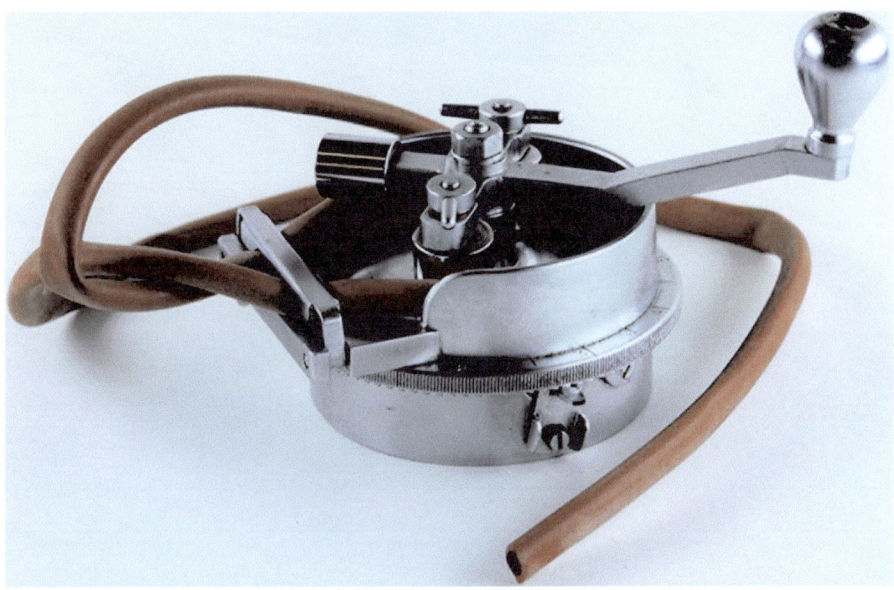

Image 9.28 Rotary Blood Pump (1940s). (Source: Blood pump—Julian Smith Rotary Pump, circa 1940s. Source: Museums Victoria Copyright Museums Victoria/CC BY (licensed as attribution 4.0 international). https://collections.museumsvictoria.com.au/items/2006501)

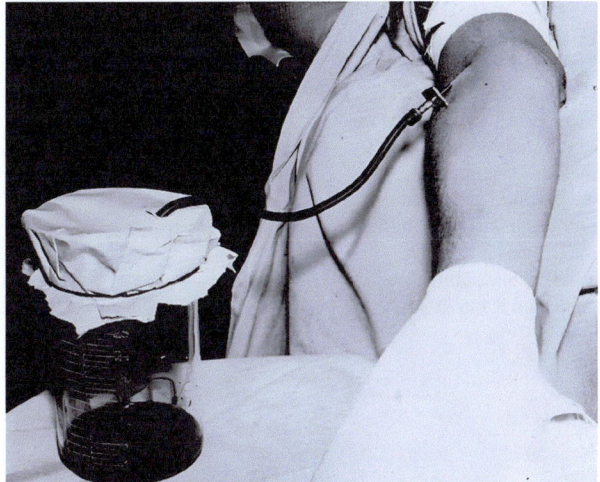

Image 9.29 Drawing Blood from Blood Donor (Citrate Method). (Source: Drawing blood from blood donor (citrate method). Wiener A. S. Blood groups and blood transfusion. Charles C. Thomas publisher; 1948, p. 97, public domain. Accessed 8 Jan 2024)

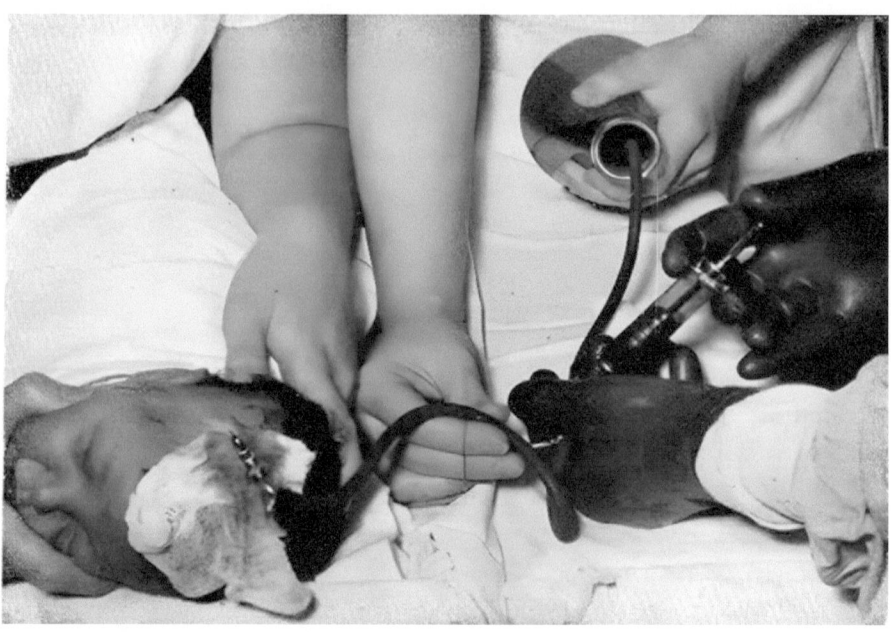

Image 9.30 Blood Transfusion of Citrated Blood by Syringe-Valve Method. (Source: Blood transfusion of citrated blood by syringe-valve method. Wiener A. S. Blood groups and blood transfusion. Charles C. Thomas publisher; 1948, p. 99, public domain. Accessed 8 Jan 2024)

Image 9.31 Blood Transfusion of Citrated Blood by Gravity Method. (Source: Blood transfusion of citrated blood by gravity method. Wiener A. S. Blood groups and blood transfusion. Charles C. Thomas publisher; 1948, p. 98, public domain. Accessed 8 Jan 2024)

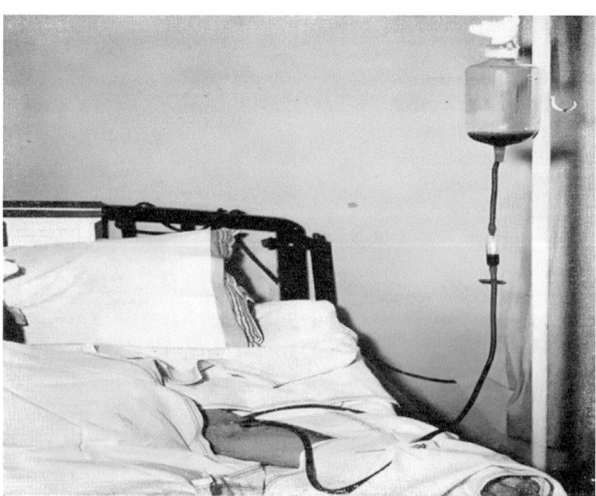

9.5 Dosage and Rate of Blood Transfusion

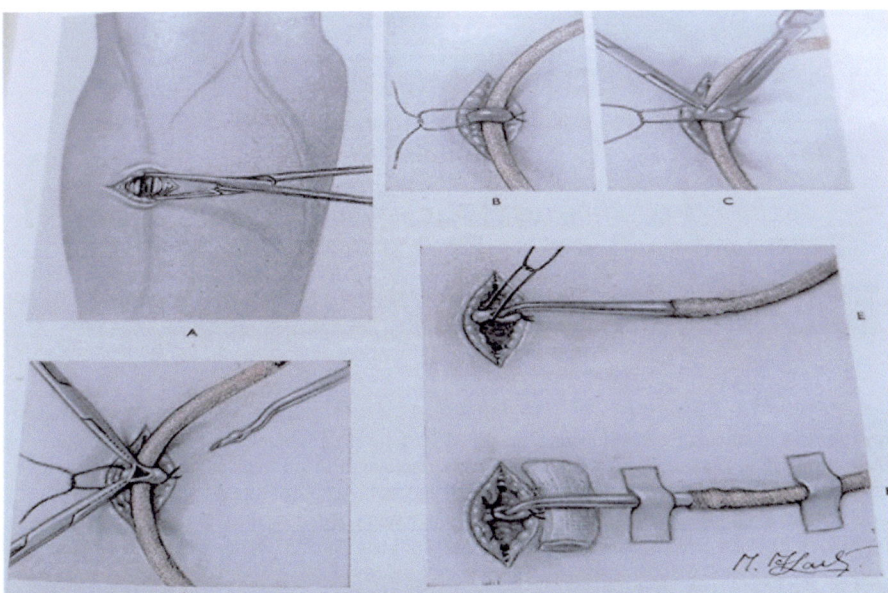

Image 9.32 Venesection Technique. (Source: Venesection technique. Till A. The technique of blood transfusion, section VI. In: Brewer H.F., Ellis R., Greaves R. I. N., Keynes G., Mills F. W., Bodley Scott R., Till A., Whitby L. Blood transfusion. Bristol: John Wright & sons LTD. London: Simpkin Marshall (1941). LTD.;1949, p. 397. Permission for usage of the image was granted by the copyright holder, Elsevier, on February 7, 2024)

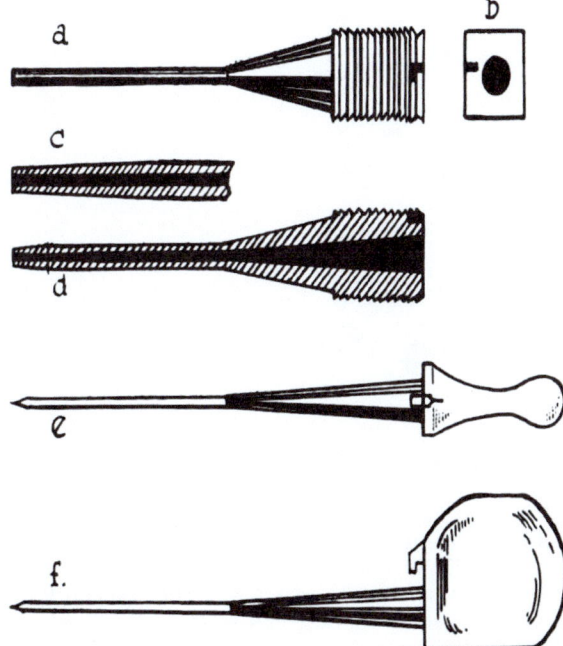

Image 9.33 Needle and Cannula for Blood Transfusion (1942). (Source: Needle and cannula for blood transfusion (1942). Chap. XV methods and technique of blood transfusion. In: Kilduffe, R. A., DeBakey, M. E. The blood bank and the technique and therapeutics of blood transfusions. Mosby, St. Louis, 1942, p. 436. Permission for usage of the image was granted by the copyright holder, Elsevier, on January 23, 2024. https://babel.hathitrust.org/cgi/pt?id=uc1.$b595310&seq=1 Accessed 1 Feb 2024)

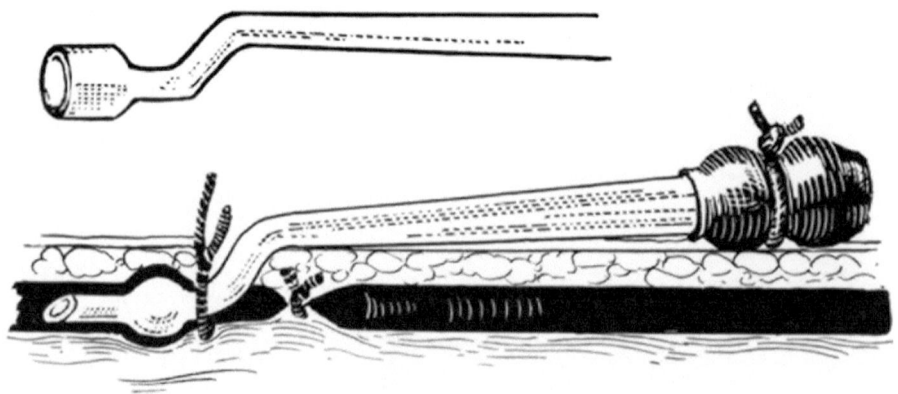

Image 9.34 Cannula for Continuous Drip Blood Transfusion. (Source: Cannula for continuous drip blood transfusion (1942). Chap. XV methods and technique of blood transfusion. In: Kilduffe, R. A., DeBakey, M. E. The blood bank and the technique and therapeutics of blood transfusions. Mosby, St. Louis, 1942, p. 447. Permission for usage of the image was granted by the copyright holder, Elsevier, on January 23, 2024. https://babel.hathitrust.org/cgi/pt?id=uc1.$b595310&seq=1 Accessed 1 Feb 2024)

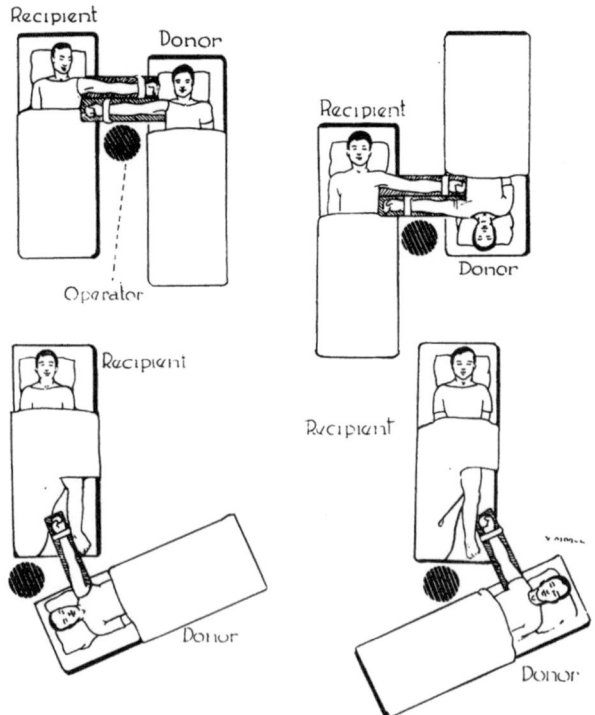

Image 9.35 Position of a Blood Donor and a Patient for Direct Blood Transfusion (1942). (Source: Position of a blood donor and a patient for direct blood transfusion (1942). Chap. XV methods and technique of blood transfusion. In: Kilduffe, R. A., DeBakey, M. E. The blood bank and the technique and therapeutics of blood transfusions. Mosby, St. Louis, 1942, p. 449. Permission for usage of the image was granted by the copyright holder, Elsevier, on January 23, 2024. https://babel.hathitrust.org/cgi/pt?id=uc1.$b595310&seq=1 Accessed 1 Feb 2024)

Image 9.36 Modern Blood donation with Venipuncture Technique. (Source: Modern blood donation with the venipuncture technique. Permission for the use of the photograph in this book was granted by the Center for Public Relations and Marketing and the Center for Transfusion Medicine Maribor on February 28, 2024, both of the University Medical Center Maribor. The owner of the photograph is the University Clinical Center Maribor Archive)

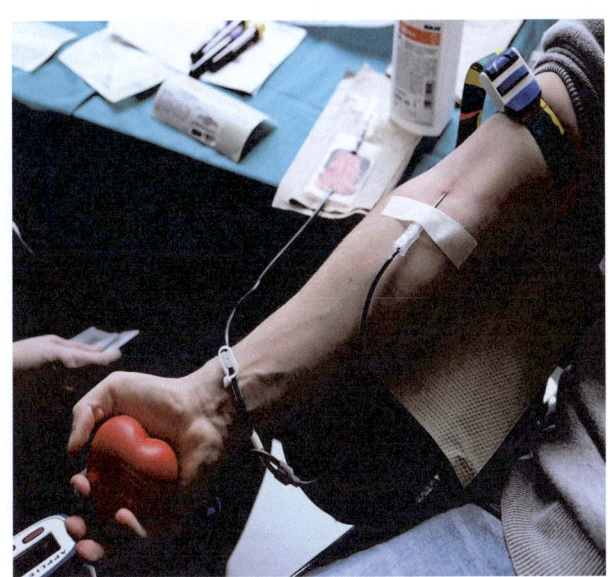

References

1. American Cancer Society. Transfusion Steps and Possible Side Effects. https://www.cancer.org/cancer/managing-cancer/treatment-types/blood-transfusion-and-donation/how-blood-transfusions-are-done.html#written_by. Accessed 1 Apr 2024.
2. BloodWorks Northwest. Typical rates, volumes, and duration. https://www.bloodworksnw.org/medical-services/transfusion-medicine/rates-volumes-duration-transfusions. Accessed 1 Apr 2024.
3. Brewer HF. The blood donor, section V - a. In: Brewer HF, Ellis R, Greaves RIN, Keynes G, Mills FW, Bodley Scott R, Till A, Whitby L, editors. Blood transfusion. Bristol: John Wright & sons LTD. London: Simpkin Marshall (1941). LTD; 1949. p. 335.
4. Carmichael SP 2nd, Lin N, Evangelista ME, Holcomb JB. The story of blood for shock resuscitation: how the pendulum swings. J Am Coll Surg. 2021;233(5):644–53. https://pubmed.ncbi.nlm.nih.gov/34390843/.
5. Jennings LK, Watson S. Massive transfusion. [updated 2023 Oct 29]. In: StatPearls [internet]. Treasure Island (FL): StatPearls Publishing; 2024. https://www.ncbi.nlm.nih.gov/books/NBK499929/. Accessed 1 April 2024.
6. LaPelusa A, Dave HD. Physiology, hemostasis. [updated 2023 may 1]. In: StatPearls [internet]. Treasure Island (FL): StatPearls Publishing; 2024. https://www.ncbi.nlm.nih.gov/books/NBK545263/. Accessed 1 April 2024.
7. Grífols JR. The contribution of Dr. Duran-Jorda to the advancement and development of European blood transfusion. ISBT Sci Ser. 2007;2:134.
8. Hardin RC. The recipient and the administration of blood, part V. In: DeGowin EL, Hardin RC, Alsever BJ, editors. Blood transfusion. Philadelphia & London: W.B. Saunders Company; 1949. p. 250–3.
9. Medicinhistoriska museet: Blodkvarn. 2019. https://medicinhistoriskasahlgrenskase/utstallningar/manadens-foremal/2019/. Accessed 3 Feb 2024.
10. McLean JA, Luke HA. Direct exchange blood transfusion in treatment of hepatic coma. Brit Med J. 1967;4:78–80.
11. McLean JA. Direct blood transfusion. Its history, with special reference to the Alfred Hospital, Melbourne. Med J Aust. 1979;2:625–8.

12. Kvržić Z. Odvzem polne krvi pri krvodajalcu skozi različna zgodovinska obdobja (1875–2023). Utrip: informativni bilten Zbornice zdravstvene in babiške nege Slovenije. 2023;31(4):17–21. https://www.zbornica-zveza.si/wp-content/uploads/2023/08/Odvzem-polne-krvi-pri-krvodajalcu-skozi-razlicna-zgodovinska-obdobja-1875-2023-Kvrzic-Avgust-September-2023.pdf.
13. Wiener AS. Indications for and results of blood transfusion. In: Blood groups and blood transfusion. Springfield: Charles C. Thomas publisher; 1948. p. 77.
14. Wiener AS. Technic of blood transfusion of fresh blood. In: Blood groups and blood transfusion. Springfield: Charles C Thomas publisher; 1948. p. 108–11.

Image Source

Blood transfusion methods in 1949, DeGowin EL. Blood transfusion Equipment, part IX. In: Degowin EL, Hardin RC, Alsever BJ, editors. Blood transfusion. Philadelphia & London: W.B. Saunders Company; 1949. p. 517. Permission for the use of the image was granted by the copyright holder Elsevier on 6 Dec 2023.
Greenhouse apparatus 1920. Chapter XV methods and technique of blood transfusion. In: Kilduffe RA, DeBakey ME, editors. The blood bank and the technique and therapeutics of blood transfusions. St. Louis: Mosby; 1942. p. 404. Permission for usage of the image was granted by the copyright holder, Elsevier, on January 23, 2024. https://babel.hathitrust.org/cgi/pt?id=uc1.$b595310&seq=1 Accessed 1 Feb 2024.
Stanley apparatus (1920). Chapter XV methods and technique of blood transfusion. In: Kilduffe RA, DeBakey ME, editors. The blood bank and the technique and therapeutics of blood transfusions. St. Louis: Mosby; 1942. p. 413. Permission for usage of the image was granted by the copyright holder, Elsevier, on January 23, 2024. https://babel.hathitrust.org/cgi/pt?id=uc1.$b595310&seq=1 Accessed 1 Feb 2024.
Janes apparatus (1921). Chapter XV methods and technique of blood transfusion. In: Kilduffe RA, DeBakey ME, editors. The blood bank and the technique and therapeutics of blood transfusions. St. Louis: Mosby; 1942. p. 405. Permission for usage of the image was granted by the copyright holder, Elsevier, on January 23, 2024. https://babel.hathitrust.org/cgi/pt?id=uc1.$b595310&seq=1. Accessed 1 Feb 2024.
Oehlecker apparatus and direct blood transfusion from a blood donor to a patient, Schiff F. Die Blutgruppen und ihre Anwendungsgebiete. Berlin: Springer; 1933. p. 133. With permission.
Gütebier T. Oehlecker apparatus (1922). Medicinhistoriska museet, VGR (CC BY). Permission for usage of the image was granted by the item holder on January 26, 2024. https://medicinhistoriska.sahlgrenska.se/utstallningar/manadens-foremal/2018/. Accessed 25 Jan 2024.
Jubé apparatus (1924). Chapter XV methods and technique of blood transfusion. In: Kilduffe RA, DeBakey ME, editors. The blood bank and the technique and therapeutics of blood transfusions. St. Louis: Mosby; 1942. p. 416. Permission for usage of the image was granted by the copyright holder, Elsevier, on January 23, 2024. https://babel.hathitrust.org/cgi/pt?id=uc1.$b595310&seq=1 Accessed 1 Feb 2024.
Jubé apparatus (1935). Syringe for direct blood transfusion according to Dr. Louis Jubé, cc 1935 (Museum of Science and Technology—Belgrade, Collection of the Museum of the Serbian Medical Society, Inv. No. MST: T:11.7.900). Permission for usage of the image was granted by the item holder on January 12, 2024.
Scannell apparatus (1925). Chapter XV methods and technique of blood transfusion. In: Kilduffe RA, DeBakey ME, editors. The blood bank and the technique and therapeutics of blood transfusions. St. Louis: Mosby; 1942. p. 406. Permission for usage of the image was granted by the copyright holder, Elsevier, on January 23, 2024. https://babel.hathitrust.org/cgi/pt?id=uc1.$b595310&seq=1. Accessed 1 Feb 2024.
Scannell blood transfusion apparatus set. Permission for usage of the image was granted by the item holder from his personal archive, Mr. Steven Pierce, on January 10, 2024.
Lara Miholič Ilc. The Rotanda (1925). The illustrator Lara Miholič Ilc gave her permission to Zdravko Kvržić for the usage of her illustration of Rotanda for this work on November 28,

2023. Permission to reuse the image from the article Zdravko Kvržić, Odvzem polne krvi pri krvodajalcu skozi različna zgodovinska obdobja (1875–2023). Utrip. 2023;31(4):17–21, was also given by the Nurses and Midwives Association of Slovenia on November 29, 2023

Feinblatt apparatus (1925). Chapter XV methods and technique of blood transfusion. In: Kilduffe RA, DeBakey ME, editors. The blood bank and the technique and therapeutics of blood transfusions. St. Louis: Mosby; 1942. p. 411. Permission for usage of the image was granted by the copyright holder, Elsevier, on January 23, 2024. https://babel.hathitrust.org/cgi/pt?id=uc1.$b595310&seq=1. Accessed 1 Feb 2024.

Moore and Koster apparatus (1925). Chapter XV methods and technique of blood transfusion. In: Kilduffe RA, DeBakey ME, editors. The blood bank and the technique and therapeutics of blood transfusions. St. Louis: Mosby; 1942. p. 414. Permission for usage of the image was granted by the copyright holder, Elsevier, on January 23, 2024. https://babel.hathitrust.org/cgi/pt?id=uc1.$b595310&seq=1. Accessed 1 Feb 2024.

Soresi's apparatus (1925), Wiener AS. Blood groups and blood transfusion. Charles C. Thomas publisher; 1948. p. 109. public domain. Accessed 8 Jan 2024.

Beck apparatus (1926). Chapter XV methods and technique of blood transfusion. In: Kilduffe RA, DeBakey ME, editors. The blood bank and the technique and therapeutics of blood transfusions. St. Louis: Mosby; 1942. p. 422. Permission for usage of the image was granted by the copyright holder, Elsevier, on January 23, 2024. https://babel.hathitrust.org/cgi/pt?id=uc1.$b595310&seq=1. Accessed 1 Feb 2024.

Gütebier T. Beck apparatus, also known as Satrans blood transfusion apparatus. Permission for usage of the image was granted by the item holder on January 26, 2024. Medicinhistoriska museet, VGR (CC BY). https://medicinhistoriska.sahlgrenska.se/utstallningar/manadens-foremal/2019/. Accessed 25 Jan 2024.

Tzanck apparatus (1926). Chapter XV methods and technique of blood transfusion. In: Kilduffe, R. A., DeBakey, M. E. The blood bank and the technique and therapeutics of blood transfusions. Mosby, St. Louis, 1942, p. 407. Permission for usage of the image was granted by the copyright holder, Elsevier, on January 23, 2024. https://babel.hathitrust.org/cgi/pt?id=uc1.$b595310&seq=1 Accessed 1 Feb 2024.

Head apparatus (1927). Chapter XV methods and technique of blood transfusion. In: Kilduffe RA, DeBakey ME, editors. The blood bank and the technique and therapeutics of blood transfusions. St. Louis: Mosby; 1942. p. 416. Permission for usage of the image was granted by the copyright holder, Elsevier, on January 23, 2024. https://babel.hathitrust.org/cgi/pt?id=uc1.$b595310&seq=1. Accessed 1 Feb 2024.

Van Allen (1932) and Jacobs apparatus (1933). Chapter XV methods and technique of blood transfusion. In: Kilduffe RA, DeBakey ME, editors. The blood bank and the technique and therapeutics of blood transfusions. St. Louis: Mosby; 1942. p. 423. Permission for usage of the image was granted by the copyright holder, Elsevier, on January 23, 2024. https://babel.hathitrust.org/cgi/pt?id=uc1.$b595310&seq=1 Accessed 1 Feb 2024.

Bergenstein apparatus (1933). Chapter XV methods and technique of blood transfusion. In: Kilduffe RA, DeBakey ME, editors. The blood bank and the technique and therapeutics of blood transfusions. St. Louis: Mosby; 1942. p. 412. Permission for usage of the image was granted by the copyright holder, Elsevier, on January 23, 2024. https://babel.hathitrust.org/cgi/pt?id=uc1.$b595310&seq=1. Accessed 1 Feb 2024.

Hirsch apparatus (1934). Chapter XV methods and technique of blood transfusion. In: Kilduffe RA, DeBakey ME, editors. The blood bank and the technique and therapeutics of blood transfusions. St. Louis: Mosby; 1942. p. 415. Permission for usage of the image was granted by the copyright holder, Elsevier, on January 23, 2024. https://babel.hathitrust.org/cgi/pt?id=uc1.$b595310&seq=1. Accessed 1 Feb 2024.

Henry-Jouvelet apparatus (1934). Chapter XV methods and technique of blood transfusion. In: Kilduffe RA, DeBakey ME, editors. The blood bank and the technique and therapeutics of blood transfusions. St. Louis: Mosby; 1942. p. 424. Permission for usage of the image was granted by the copyright holder, Elsevier, on January 23, 2024. https://babel.hathitrust.org/cgi/pt?id=uc1.$b595310&seq=1. Accessed 1 Feb 2024.

Rudder apparatus (1935). Chapter XV methods and technique of blood transfusion. In: Kilduffe RA, DeBakey ME, editors. The blood bank and the technique and therapeutics of blood transfusions. St. Louis: Mosby; 1942. p. 413. Permission for usage of the image was granted by the copyright holder, Elsevier, on January 23, 2024. https://babel.hathitrust.org/cgi/pt?id=uc1.$b595310&seq=1. Accessed 1 Feb 2024.

Bécart apparatus (1939). Chapter XV methods and technique of blood transfusion. In: Kilduffe RA, DeBakey ME, editors. The blood bank and the technique and therapeutics of blood transfusions. St. Louis: Mosby; 1942. p. 417. Permission for usage of the image was granted by the copyright holder, Elsevier, on January 23, 2024. https://babel.hathitrust.org/cgi/pt?id=uc1.$b595310&seq=1. Accessed 1 Feb 2024.

Touvet apparatus (1940). Chapter XV methods and technique of blood transfusion. In: Kilduffe RA, DeBakey ME, editors. The blood bank and the technique and therapeutics of blood transfusions. St. Louis: Mosby; 1942. p. 418. Permission for usage of the image was granted by the copyright holder, Elsevier, on January 23, 2024. https://babel.hathitrust.org/cgi/pt?id=uc1.$b595310&seq=1. Accessed 1 Feb 2024.

The Cashman Baker Transfuser (1936), Wiener AS. Blood groups and blood transfusion. Charles C. Thomas publisher; 1948. p. 110. public domain. Accessed 8 Jan 2024.

Pennell apparatus (1939), Wiener AS. Blood groups and blood transfusion. Charles C. Thomas publisher; 1948. p. 111. public domain. Accessed 8 Jan 2024.

Blood pump—Julian Smith Rotary Pump, circa 1940s. Source: Museums Victoria Copyright Museums Victoria/CC BY (licensed as attribution 4.0 international). https://collections.museumsvictoria.com.au/items/2006501.

Drawing blood from blood donor (citrate method), Wiener AS. Blood groups and blood transfusion. Charles C. Thomas publisher; 1948. p. 97. public domain. Accessed 8 Jan 2024.

Blood transfusion of citrated blood by syringe-valve method, Wiener AS. Blood groups and blood transfusion. Charles C. Thomas publisher; 1948. p. 99. public domain. Accessed 8 Jan 2024.

Blood transfusion of citrated blood by gravity method, Wiener AS. Blood groups and blood transfusion. Charles C. Thomas publisher; 1948. p. 98. public domain. Accessed 8 Jan 2024.

Venesection technique, Till A. The technique of blood transfusion, section VI. In: Brewer HF, Ellis R, Greaves RIN, Keynes G, Mills FW, Bodley Scott R, Till A, editors. Whitby L. blood transfusion. Bristol, John Wright & sons LTD. London: Simpkin Marshall (1941). LTD; 1949. p. 397. Permission for usage of the image was granted by the copyright holder, Elsevier, on February 7, 2024.

Needle and cannula for blood transfusion (1942). Chapter XV methods and technique of blood transfusion. In: Kilduffe RA, DeBakey ME, editors. The blood bank and the technique and therapeutics of blood transfusions. St. Louis: Mosby; 1942. p. 436. Permission for usage of the image was granted by the copyright holder, Elsevier, on January 23, 2024. https://babel.hathitrust.org/cgi/pt?id=uc1.$b595310&seq=1 Accessed 1 Feb 2024.

Cannula for continuous drip blood transfusion (1942). Chapter XV methods and technique of blood transfusion. In: Kilduffe RA, Debakey ME, editors. The blood bank and the technique and therapeutics of blood transfusions. Mosby, St. Louis; 1942. p. 447. Permission for usage of the image was granted by the copyright holder, Elsevier, on January 23, 2024. https://babel.hathitrust.org/cgi/pt?id=uc1.$b595310&seq=1. Accessed 1 Feb 2024.

Position of a blood donor and a patient for direct blood transfusion (1942). Chapter XV methods and technique of blood transfusion. In: Kilduffe RA, DeBakey ME, editors. The blood bank and the technique and therapeutics of blood transfusions. St. Louis: Mosby; 1942. p. 449. Permission for usage of the image was granted by the copyright holder, Elsevier, on January 23, 2024. https://babel.hathitrust.org/cgi/pt?id=uc1.$b595310&seq=1. Accessed 1 Feb 2024.

Modern blood donation with the venipuncture technique. Permission for the use of the photograph in this book was granted by the Center for Public Relations and Marketing and the Center for Transfusion Medicine Maribor on February 28, 2024, both of the University Medical Center Maribor. The owner of the photograph is the University Clinical Center Maribor Archive.

The First Voluntary Blood Transfusion Service in the World

Contents

10.1 Percy Lane Oliver.. 143
10.2 Organization of the First Voluntary Blood Transfusion Service......................... 144
References... 147

10.1 Percy Lane Oliver

Percy Lane Oliver was born in 1878. He was an assistant librarian with Camberwell Borough Council in 1893, and in 1901, he was transferred to the Town Hall staff, where he remained until his retirement (Image 10.1). He was a founding member of the Camberwell Division of the Red Cross and was appointed honorary secretary in 1910. During World War I, he served in the Royal Naval Air Service. During his off-duty and leave periods, he and his wife organized and managed four refugee hostels in Camberwell. For this large humanitarian work, he was awarded the Order of the British Empire in 1918. He died in 1944.[1] He was an advocate of voluntary and non-remunerated blood donation, and with his supporters in 1921, he established an honorable altruistic organization that benefited patients.

---

[1] Richards T. Percy Lane Oliver, blood donor extraordinary. The St Ives Times & Echo newspaper in December sixth 1991, p. 6.

© The Author(s), under exclusive license to Springer Nature Switzerland AG 2024
Z. Kvržić, *History of Blood Donation and Transfusion Medicine*,
https://doi.org/10.1007/978-3-031-68715-0_10

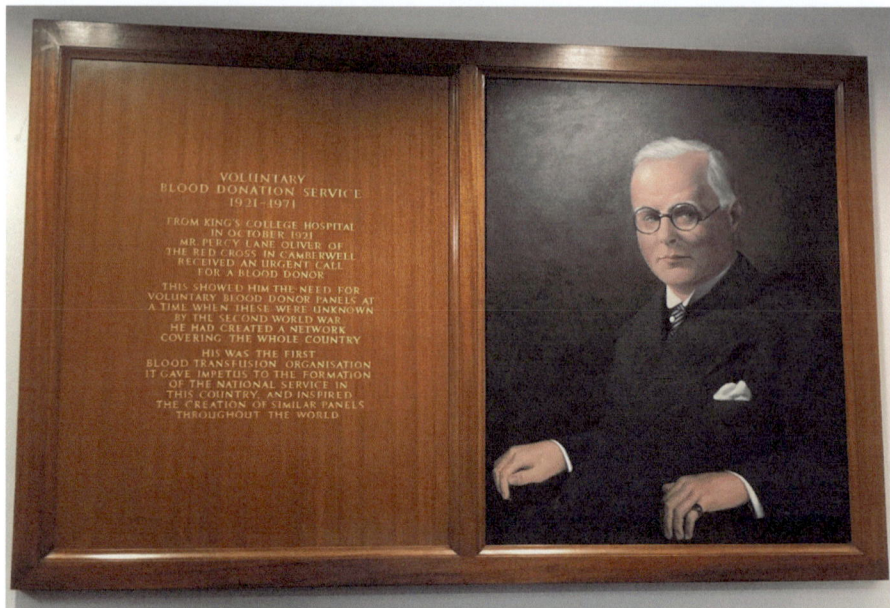

Image 10.1 Percy lane Oliver. (Source: Permission for the use of the image of Percy Lane Oliver for this book was obtained from the Dulwich Society on January 9, 2024, and by the King's College Hospital NHS Foundation Trust on January 10, 2024)

10.2 Organization of the First Voluntary Blood Transfusion Service

For the first time, blood transfusion was widely used during World War I. They were useful in critical cases to save the lives of dying soldiers. Therefore, after the end of the war, hospitals everywhere wanted to have enough blood donors who could respond to their calls in emergency situations.[2] The Camberwell branch of the Red Cross in London received the first call for blood donors from King's College Hospital in December 1920. Although they had available voluntary blood donors, the issue was payment. Mr. Percy Lane Oliver, the Red Cross Branch Manager, stated that if any payment was made, the money should not go to the blood donors but should be retained by the Red Cross Branch to continue funding their work. It is not mentioned if blood donors donated blood at that time. The second appeal came to the Camberwell branch of the Red Cross on an October evening in 1921. They

---

[2] Blood transfusion service. [video], A Ministry of Information film. Made for the Ministry of Health with the cooperation of the Medical Research Council and the Blood Transfusion Units of the Fighting Services. Directed and edited by H.M. Nieter. A Paul Rotha production. 1941. Attribution-NonCommercial 4.0 International (CC BY-NC 4.0). Source: Wellcome Collection. https://wellcomecollection.org/works/hb7wfbuz. [Accessed 10 January 2022].

were called by the secretary of King's College Hospital.[3] At the time of the telephone call, several members of the Red Cross, under the direction of Mr. Percy Lane Oliver, were carrying out their routine work. A telephone call from the secretary of King's College Hospital was answered by Mr. Oliver, who was asked by the secretary if he had a blood donor available that he could refer to the hospital. Mr. Oliver replied that his request was impossible, as everyone was busy with work and no one could afford to miss work. The secretary replied that the blood donor would only be needed for a few minutes. After a quick reflection, Mr. Oliver personally responded to the call, and he was immediately joined by staff who worked with him.[4] After arriving at the hospital, the blood was donated by a nurse with the surname Linstead, whose blood was compatible with the patients'. She reported that she was impressed by the blood donation itself because it was a painless and professional experience and that her blood helped the patient.[5]

Oliver's organization was called the London Blood Transfusion Service. It was, however, a blood donor service, not a blood transfusion service in the modern sense.[6] It was officially recognized for its outstanding work by the British Red Cross in 1925/1926. In this period, they also took over this organization. Mr. Oliver was elected honorary secretary and secretary of the British Red Cross. A committee was established, consisting of doctors, hospital representatives, and blood donors.[7, 8] Each blood donor had his own card, on which was written the blood donor's name, home address, and blood group, along with the dates and places where the blood donor donated blood. Blood donors were not allowed to accept money for their service. This was a strict rule, and upon any suspicion that someone had done that, they were immediately crossed off the blood donor panel.[9] The London blood transfusion service was conducted from the private house of Mr. Oliver.[10] Charitable

---

[3] Pelis, K. (2007). 'A Band of Lunatics down Camberwell Way': Percy Lane Oliver and Voluntary Blood Donation in Interwar Britain. In: Bivins, R., Pickstone, J.V., editors. Medicine, Madness and Social History. Palgrave Macmillan, London. London 2016, p. 148–158.

[4] Blood transfusion service [video], 1941.

[5] Gunson H. H, Dodsworth H. Towards a national blood transfusion service in England and Wales 1940–1946- chapter 2, In: Anstee D.J., Barbara J. A. J., Lincoln P. J., McClelland D. B. L., Voak D., editors. Fifty Years of Blood transfusion. Oxford: Blackwell Science. Blood transfusion Medicine. 1996, 6 (1), p. 4–16. https://www.infectedbloodinquiry.org.uk/sites/default/files/2023-06-09%20Oral%20Evidence%20Docs%20-%20Row%202701-2900%20%20copy/2023-06-09%20Oral%20Evidence%20Docs%20-%20Row%202701-2900%20%20copy/NHBT0000028%20-%20Fifty%20Years%20of%20Blood%20Transfusion%20-%2001%20Jan%201996.pdf Accessed 3 March 2024.

[6] Bird G.W. Percy Lane Oliver, OBE (1878–1944): founder of the first voluntary blood donor panel. Transfus Med. 1992; 2 (2), p. 159–60. Available at: https://pubmed.ncbi.nlm.nih.gov/1308211/ [Accessed 15 January 2022].

[7] Gunson, Dodsworth, 1996, p. 7.

[8] Blood transfusion service [video], 1941.

[9] Gunson, Dodsworth, 1996, p. 6.

[10] Mills F. W. The London blood transfusion service and the psychology of blood donors, section V-B. In: Brewer H.F., Ellis R., Greaves R. I. N., Keynes G., Mills F. W., Bodley Scott R., Till A.,

donations were collected to cover administrative costs. Mr. Oliver actively searched for new blood donors. He was assisted by a surgeon, Geoffrey Keynes.[11]

Besides Dr. Keynes, there were also other experts who helped Oliver's organization. In different sources, there are various numbers of calls that are presented about the work of Oliver's blood donor service. Nonetheless, it can be summarized that from one call received by the organization in 1921, this number by 1938 increased by a couple of thousand phone calls per year.

Similar blood services emerged in the following years, and some even paid the blood donors for their donations.[12] Even around the world, several countries later in the 1930s set up blood donor services, but only Denmark and Nederland were the ones that followed the example of Mr. Oliver's organization with voluntary and non-remunerated blood donation.[13]

The service prepared the lists of blood donors, maintained day and night telephone service, and immediately notified the blood donor when he was requested. If it was necessary, a taxi was ordered for the blood donor to take him to the hospital at the hospital's expense.[14] However, not all blood donors had access to a phone, so frequently the police had to let the donor know that he was needed. Women represented almost 20% of the population of the London blood donor service. Blood donors were also recruited through films and lectures.[15] A physical examination was always performed to ensure that the blood donor was healthy. Charitable donations were collected to cover administrative costs. Different regulations were established to ensure that the hospital staff treated blood donors politely and professionally. Hospitals at large had problems accurately determining blood groups. This resulted in several deaths from ABO incompatibility. Some hospitals found solutions by demanding blood donors with blood group O rather than buying reagents for blood group testing.[16] Improvements in drawing blood were also made. Instead of cutting the vein with venesection, the blood was taken by venipuncture in a glass bottle with sodium citrate. This was stirred with a glass rod to ensure adequate anticoagulation. Cutting blood donors' veins was forbidden in 1929.[17] But there is clear evidence that this technique was still practiced later, in 1952, at least in one case. Ward reported that at the Royal Victoria Infirmary in Newcastle, UK, they used a vein-cutting method for exchange transfusion in anemia. He even gives a clear description: "*A vein in the antecubital fossa is incised immediately distal to a venous valve. A transverse skin incision is*

Whitby L. Blood transfusion. Bristol: John Wright & sons LTD. London: Simpkin Marshall (1941). LTD.;1949, p. 346–368.

[11] Giangrande PL. The history of blood transfusion. Br J Haematol. 2000;110 (4), p. 762. https://pubmed.ncbi.nlm.nih.gov/11054057/ Accessed 15 Jan 2022.

[12] Gunson, Dodsworth, 1996, p. 9.

[13] Blood transfusion service [video] 1941.

[14] Lbid, p. 346–368.

[15] Gunson, Dodsworth, 1996, p. 6.

[16] Giangrande, 762.

[17] Gunson, Dodsworth, 1996, p. 8.

made across the vein, the vein is mobilized, ligatures are passed beneath the vein, and the ends are brought out through the skin. A longitudinal incision is made into the vein. When the lumen is opened, the hemorrhage is stopped by passing a hemostasis beneath the vein. (The tension in the vein causes the walls to come together."[18] Besides cutting the veins, there were also painful burns due to the plentiful usage of iodine, especially where iodine swabs were used and bandaged on right after the procedure.[19] Blood donors also received different awards, such as an official Red Cross medal or badge for ten blood transfusions, with bars for each succeeding ten. Blood donors also received certificates as a respectful gesture when they gave blood.[20]

In 1936, Oliver addressed his opinion regarding direct and indirect blood transfusions. He stated that in London, direct transfusion was almost obsolete, but some of its users were emphatic in their praise. Oliver personally saw direct blood transfusions with many drawbacks to their use, and He wanted this practice to be entirely abolished. Oliver stated that there was a certain complication of apparatus; one or both needles were needed to be withdrawn by an involuntary or delirious movement; more staff were required in the limited space available; the attention of the surgeon was divided; the donor had to be kept in an uncomfortable position for too long or the patient received the blood too fast; and important in the case of a voluntary and often hypersensitive donor, the latter may have his feelings unpleasantly exacerbated, possibly leading to fainting, by long proximity to a delirious, moaning, or moribund patient. Should the patient collapse or die during the transfusion, a not-unknown occurrence, the donor would still be further affected by the attempts at resuscitation.[21]

Percy Lane Oliver established a humane, voluntary, and non-remunerated blood donor service that remained loyal to its honorable cause. The blood donors who served under this organization were highly motivated and altruistic. This organization proved that in order to have a substantial number of blood donors, it had to promote the importance of this humanitarian deed with healthy blood donors of all blood groups who were, by demand, willing to selflessly donate their precious blood. Mr. Oliver was a wise, ethical, and moral visionary and expert.

References

1. Blood transfusion service. [video], A Ministry of Information film. Made for the Ministry of Health with the cooperation of the Medical Research Council and the Blood Transfusion Units of the Fighting Services. Directed and edited by H.M. Nieter. A Paul Rotha production. 1941.

---

[18] Ward T. Exchange transfusion in severe anaemia. British Medical Journal. 1952; 1(4759), p. 631. https://www.ncbi.nlm.nih.gov/pmc/articles/PMC2023185/pdf/brmedj03486-0027.pdf.

[19] Mills, 1949, p. 348–349.

[20] Lbid., p. 350.

[21] Oliver P. L. (1936). A plea for a national blood transfusion conference. British medical journal. 1936; 2(3959), p.1032–1033. https://www.ncbi.nlm.nih.gov/pmc/articles/PMC2457902/.

Attribution-NonCommercial 4.0 International (CC BY-NC 4.0). Source: Wellcome Collection. https://wellcomecollection.org/works/hb7wfbuz. Accessed 10 Jan 2022.
2. Bird GW. Percy lane Oliver, OBE (1878-1944): founder of the first voluntary blood donor panel. Transfus Med. 1992;2(2):159–60. https://pubmed.ncbi.nlm.nih.gov/1308211/.
3. Gunson HH, Dodsworth H. Towards a national blood transfusion service in England and Wales 1940–1946. In: Anstee DJ, Barbara JAJ, Lincoln PJ, McClelland DBL, Voak D, editors. Fifty years of blood transfusion. Blood transfusion medicine, vol. 6. Oxford: Blackwell Science; 1996. p. 4–16. https://www.infectedbloodinquiry.org.uk/sites/default/files/2023-06-09%20Oral%20Evidence%20Docs%20-%20Row%20 2701-2900%20%20copy/2023-06-09%20Oral%20Evidence%20Docs%20-%20Row%20 2701-2900%20%20copy/NHBT0000028%20-%20Fifty%20Years%20of%20Blood%20 Transfusion%20-%2001%20Jan%201996.pdf Accessed 3 March 2024.
4. Giangrande PL. The history of blood transfusion. Br J Haematol. 2000;110(4):762. https://pubmed.ncbi.nlm.nih.gov/11054057/. Accessed 15 Jan 2022.
5. Mills FW. The London blood transfusion service and the psychology of blood donors, section V - B. In: Brewer HF, Ellis R, Greaves RIN, Keynes G, Mills FW, Bodley Scott R, Till A, Whitby L, editors. Blood transfusion. Bristol: John Wright & sons LTD. London: Simpkin Marshall (1941). LTD.; 1949. p. 346–68.
6. Oliver PL. A plea for a national blood transfusion conference. Br Med J. 1936;2(3959):1032–3. https://www.ncbi.nlm.nih.gov/pmc/articles/PMC2457902/.
7. Pelis K. 'A band of lunatics down Camberwell way': Percy lane Oliver and Voluntary blood donation in interwar Britain. In: Bivins R, Pickstone JV, editors. Medicine, madness and social history, vol. 2016. London: Palgrave Macmillan; 2007. p. 148–58.
8. Richards T. Percy lane Oliver, blood donor extraordinary. The St Ives Times & Echo Newspaper; 1991. p. 6.
9. Ward T. Exchange transfusion in severe anaemia. Br Med J. 1952;1(4759):631. https://www.ncbi.nlm.nih.gov/pmc/articles/PMC2023185/pdf/brmedj03486-0027.pdf.

Image Source

Permission for the use of the image of Percy Lane Oliver for this book was obtained from the Dulwich Society on January 9, 2024, and by the King's College Hospital NHS Foundation Trust on January 10, 2024.

The First Blood Banks   11

Contents

11.1 Blood Bank.. 149
11.2 Early Blood Banks... 150
    11.2.1 The First Blood Bank in the Soviet Union..................................... 150
    11.2.2 The First Blood Bank in Spain.. 151
    11.2.3 The First Blood Bank in the USA.. 152
References.. 153

11.1 Blood Bank

There are different definitions of blood bank with similarities in terminology, but it is common that the blood bank is usually a department within a hospital that is responsible for storing and distributing blood components. The term blood banking commonly refers to the process of collecting, separating, and storing blood. Other definitions expand its activity to include testing and distributing.

There are different types of blood banks. Community blood banks (blood centers and hospitals) collect blood in a reasonably contiguous area and supply the hospitals within the blood collection area. The blood center may or may not supply the total needs of the hospitals in its area or may supply hospitals in other areas as well. Hospital blood banks usually collect blood only for use in that hospital and do not supply other hospitals.[1]

---

[1] Institute of Medicine (US) Committee to Study HIV Transmission Through Blood and Blood Products; Leveton LB, Sox HC Jr., Stoto MA, editors, HIV and the blood supply: An Analysis of Crisis Decision making. Washington (DC): National Academies Press (US), 1995, p. 2, The

© The Author(s), under exclusive license to Springer Nature
Switzerland AG 2024
Z. Kvržić, *History of Blood Donation and Transfusion Medicine*,
https://doi.org/10.1007/978-3-031-68715-0_11

11.2 Early Blood Banks

The early period of blood storage started in World War I and later in the 1930s, but at first, it was only in a few countries (Soviet Union, USA, and Spain) up to 1936. From 1937 onward, blood banks in other countries started slowly to emerge.

During the period of WW1, stored citrated blood was somewhat used in 1916 in the USA by Rous and Turner[2] and by Captain Oswald Hope Robertson in 1917, who is known as the first blood banker.[3] Robertson was the first who, on the battlefront of World War I, used blood transfusions to preserve blood. From 1917 to 1918, he gave 22 blood transfusions.[4] Experts knew that the storage of blood was important in vast countries such as the Soviet Union and the USA because the blood had to be sent long distances.[5] The demand for stored blood also proved to be of important value during the horrific Spanish Civil War.

11.2.1 The First Blood Bank in the Soviet Union

In 1926, Dr. Alexander Bogdanov in Moscow established the Institute of Blood Transfusion.[6] In 1930, the Central Institute for Blood Transfusion in Moscow started to develop the technique of storing blood. In 10 years, they successfully succeeded in developing the technique for storing it.[7] Sergei Yudin (1891–1954), a surgeon, founded the first blood bank in Leningrad (today's Saint Petersburg) in 1932.[8] The Soviets even used cadaveric blood. The idea derived from a surgeon Vladimir Nikolayevich Shamov (1882–1962) in 1928, who experimented on dogs.[9] Shamov reported that cadaveric blood was not toxic and could be transfused from a dead animal to a live one. He also noted and advocated that the blood was sterile for

---

U.S. Blood supply system. https://www.ncbi.nlm.nih.gov/books/NBK232409/ Accessed 9 Feb 2022.

[2] Bird 1971, p. 43.

[3] Hess, Schmidt, 2000, p. 110.

[4] DeGowin, E. L., Harris, J. E., & Plass, E. D. Studies on preserved human blood: I. Various factors influencing hemolysis. Journal of the American Medical Association. 1940; 115 (13), 895. https://jamanetwork.com/journals/jama/article-abstract/307719.

[5] Blood transfusion service [video] 1941.

[6] Huestis D.W. Russia's National Research Center for Hematology: its role in the development of blood banking. Transfusion. 2002; 42, p. 490–494. https://doi.org/10.1046/j.1525-1438.2002.00065.x.

[7] Lbid.

[8] Yudin, S. S. Transfusion of Stored Cadaver Blood: Practical Considerations: The First Thousand Cases. The Lancet. 1937; 230(5946): 362–366. Accessed 11 Feb 2024. https://www.sciencedirect.com/science/article/abs/pii/S0140673600917847.

[9] Kilduffe R.A., DeBakey M. The blood bank, chap. VIII. In: The Blood Bank and the technique and therapeutics of transfusion, St. Louis, USA: C.V. Mosby company, 1942, p. 196–207. Available at: https://babel.hathitrust.org/cgi/pt?id=uc1.$b595310&seq=1 [Accessed 9 February 2022].

several hours and that the toxicity developed later.[10] The first person to employ this method was Yurin in 1930. His patient was a man who had sliced the veins in his wrist in an attempt to commit suicide. At the Sklifosovsky Center, an infusion of corpse blood kept him alive.[11] In 1971, there was additional information about these Soviet experiments. Six hours after a person's death, the Sklifosovsky Institute used their blood. Three liters of blood were drawn from patients with myocardial infarction, hypertension, alcoholism, electric shock, and severe (non-penetrating) head or brain injuries. The blood was then mixed with a glucose-phosphate stabilizer and antibiotics and stored in the refrigerator until necropsy and all necessary laboratory tests were completed.[12] During the Spanish Civil War, Republican government doctor Frederic Durán-Jordà quickly dismissed the use of cadaveric blood because it had been demonstrated that the blood of those who died violently did not coagulate properly and that the problem of cadaveric blood transfusion should be abandoned as unsolvable.[13] In Spain in 1989, experts in their transplant program reported that they used blood not from dead bodies as it was used in the Soviet Union but from patients who were brain and biologically dead. From them, they obtained whole blood from the femoral artery and peripheral arm vein.[14] There were also experiments with placental blood by Howkins and Brewer (1937) and Halbrecht (1939).[15]

11.2.2 The First Blood Bank in Spain

Spanish doctor Frederic Durán-Jordà established the world's first transfusion service, also referred to as the first blood bank in Barcelona, in August 1936 during the early stages of the Spanish Civil War (July 17, 1936 to April 1, 1939).

The blood was stored in refrigerators at 2–4 °C. The Barcelona Institute had its own means of transport to enable the blood to be taken to the required place with the greatest safety. There were two lorries and a railway van, each fitted with a refrigerator. Advanced military posts were provided with refrigerators that functioned well either with electricity, gasoline, or paraffin. For transport to places that could

---

[10] Tarasov M. M., Cadaveric blood transfusion, Ann N Y Acad Sci.1960; 87:512–521. https://pubmed.ncbi.nlm.nih.gov/13836924/.

[11] Yudin, S. S. 1937, p. 362–366.

[12] Bird 1971, p. 43.

[13] Lethbridge, D. "The Blood Fights on in Other Veins:" Norman Bethune and the Transfusion of Cadaver Blood in the Spanish Civil War, Canadian Bulletin of Medical History. 2012;29 (1):69–81. https://pubmed.ncbi.nlm.nih.gov/22849251/.

[14] Vázquez-Valdés E., Marín-López A., Velasco C., Herrera-Martínez E., Pérez-Rojas A., Ortega-Rocha R., Aldama-Romano M., Murray J., Barradas-Guevara D. C., Transfusión de sangre de cadáver [Blood transfusion from cadavers], Rev. Invest. Clin.1989; 41 (1): 11–16. https://pubmed.ncbi.nlm.nih.gov/2727428//.

[15] Whitby L. The storage and preservation of blood and blood derivatives, section VIII. In: In: Brewer H.F., Ellis R., Greaves R. I. N., Keynes G., Mills F. W., Bodley Scott R., Till A., Whitby L. Blood transfusion. Bristol: John Wright & sons LTD. London: Simpkin Marshall (1941). LTD.;1949, p. 457.

not be reached by vehicles, the blood was carried in isothermic cases supplied with a refrigerating mixture.[16] It was also important for the quality of storage and preservation of blood that during transportation there must be a minimum shaking of the refrigerators containing blood and a delivery distance should not exceed 200 km. The growth of anaerobes was prevented by using oxygen. This was achieved with the full oxygenation of the blood under the pressure of two atmospheres of oxygen. The methods from Spain for storing blood had some impact on a few countries, mostly the Soviet Union, prior to World War II.[17]

11.2.3 The First Blood Bank in the USA

Prior to the introduction of blood banking systems in the 1930s, all blood was given by "professional blood donors" or by the friends and relatives of hospital patients.[18] The first blood bank in the USA was in 1935, when Dr. John Silas Lundy started a blood bank for transfusions at the Mayo Clinic, and he wrote reports on the activity in that and the following years. Stored citrated blood was kept in ice boxes for 14 days.[19] In many sources, it is stated that the first blood bank in the USA was established in 1937. But clearly, this was 2 years earlier.

The second blood bank in the USA, often referred to as the first, was founded in 1937 at Cook County Hospital in Chicago. It was founded by Dr. Bernard Fantus (1874–1940).[20] Blood in the USA was contributed to the blood bank by every hospital service that required it. After the test and grouping, it was kept in a refrigerator. When blood was needed for blood transfusion, it was given in a bottle of the blood of the required group. It was depicted on the account of that particular hospital and had to be replaced by another bottle of blood, but not necessarily the same group. This method was gradually copied in other parts of the world.[21] By 1942, in the USA, they already had a system for blood banks that had an organized blood donor registry. The source of the blood for storage was voluntary blood donors, phlebotomy[22] for therapeutic purposes, and placental blood. Some experts advocated placental blood, which was, in their opinion, suitable for blood transfusions because it was free of dietary allergens and because of its increased clotting power. For the storage of blood, they used several different anticoagulants and existing solutions.

---

[16] Jorda, F. D. The Barcelona blood-transfusion service. The Lancet. 1939;233(6031):773–775. https://www.sciencedirect.com/science/article/abs/pii/S0140673600603926.

[17] Whitby L. 1949, p. 457.

[18] LeBlanc, 2016, p. 4.

[19] Moore, S. Breanndan. A brief history of the early years of blood transfusion at the Mayo Clinic: The first blood bank in the United States (1935). Transfusion Medicine Reviews. 2005;19 (4): 241–245. https://www.sciencedirect.com/science/article/abs/pii/S0887796305000179.

[20] Fantus B. Landmark article July 10, 1937: The therapy of the Cook County Hospital. By Bernard Fantus. JAMA. 1984;251 (6):647–649. https://pubmed.ncbi.nlm.nih.gov/6361307/.

[21] Blood transfusion service [video] 1941.

[22] Phlebotomy is a process of drawing blood for diagnostic purposes.

The stored blood, regardless of its origin, was recommended to be stored at a required temperature of 4–6 °C and used for blood transfusion within 10 days. Several preserving solutions for storing blood were used, such as M.I.H. preservative from Moscow, sodium citrate solutions, dextrose-sodium citrate solutions, Rous and Turner solutions, and Maizels and Whittaker.[23]

Without different blood banks and different accredited establishments, storing blood components and using them for blood transfusions would be impossible. These establishments around the world evolved gradually with the same mission of preserving and storing blood. Cadaveric blood is no longer used for blood transfusions because the blood of human voluntary blood donors is the only way to ensure safe blood for dying patients. Each country has its own mandatory set of regulations and directions for blood donation and blood transfusion, as well as organized establishments that are responsible for collecting blood and performing other important tasks.

References

1. DeGowin EL, Harris JE, Plass ED. Studies on preserved human blood: I. various factors influencing hemolysis. JAMA J Am Med Assoc. 1940;115(11):895. https://jamanetwork.com/journals/jama/article-abstract/307719.
2. Huestis DW. Russia's National Research Center for hematology: its role in the development of blood banking. Transfusion. 2002;42:490–4. https://doi.org/10.1046/j.1525-1438.2002.00065.x.
3. Institute of Medicine (US) Committee to Study HIV Transmission Through Blood and Blood Products. In: Leveton LB, Sox Jr HC, Stoto MA, editors. HIV and the blood supply: an analysis of crisis decision making. Washington (DC): National Academies Press; 1995. p. 2. The U.S. Blood supply system. https://www.ncbi.nlm.nih.gov/books/NBK232409/ Accessed 9 Feb 2022.
4. Kilduffe RA, DeBakey M. The blood bank, chapter VIII. In: The blood Bank and the technique and therapeutics of transfusion. St. Louis: C.V. Mosby company; 1942. p. 196–207. https://babel.hathitrust.org/cgi/pt?id=uc1.$b595310&seq=1.
5. Fantus B. Landmark article July 10, 1937: the therapy of the Cook County Hospital By Bernard Fantus. JAMA. 1984;251(5):647–9. https://pubmed.ncbi.nlm.nih.gov/6361307/.
6. Jorda FD. The Barcelona blood-transfusion service. Lancet. 1939;233(6031):773–5. https://www.sciencedirect.com/science/article/abs/pii/S0140673600603926.
7. Lethbridge D. "The blood fights on in other veins:" Norman Bethune and the transfusion of cadaver blood in the Spanish civil war. Can Bull Med Hist. 2012;29(1):69–81. https://pubmed.ncbi.nlm.nih.gov/22849251/.
8. Moore SB. A brief history of the early years of blood transfusion at the Mayo Clinic: the first blood bank in the United States (1935). Transfus Med Rev. 2005;19(3):241–5. https://www.sciencedirect.com/science/article/abs/pii/S0887796305000179.
9. Tarasov MM. Cadaveric blood transfusion. Ann N Y Acad Sci. 1960;87:512–21. https://pubmed.ncbi.nlm.nih.gov/13836924/.
10. The European Directorate for the Quality of Medicines & HealthCare (EDQM). Guide to the preparation, use and quality assurance of blood components. 20th ed. Strasbourg: Council of Europe; 2020. p. 184–252.

---

[23] Kilduffe, DeBakey 1942, p. 196–207.

11. Vázquez-Valdés E, Marín-López A, Velasco C, Herrera-Martínez E, Pérez-Rojas A, Ortega-Rocha R, Aldama-Romano M, Murray J, Barradas-Guevara DC. Transfusión de sangre de cadáver [Blood transfusion from cadavers]. Rev Investig Clin. 1989;41(1):11–6. https://pubmed.ncbi.nlm.nih.gov/2727428//.
12. Whitby L. The storage and preservation of blood and blood derivatives, section VIII. In: Brewer HF, Ellis R, Greaves RIN, Keynes G, Mills FW, Bodley Scott R, Till A, editors. Whitby L. Blood transfusion. Bristol: John Wright & sons LTD. London: Simpkin Marshall (1941). LTD.; 1949. p. 457.
13. Yudin SS. Transfusion of stored cadaver blood: practical considerations: the first thousand cases. Lancet. 1937;230(5946):362–6. https://www.sciencedirect.com/science/article/abs/pii/S0140673600917847.

Blood Organization During the Spanish Civil War

12

Contents

References.. 157

With the first significant aerial bombardment of civilian populations, the Spanish Civil War is regarded as the first conflict in which civilian casualties outnumbered those of combatants. More serious injuries were sustained as a result of the heavy artillery and bombing than during the First World War.[1] During the war, several thousand people donated blood at intervals of between 3 weeks and 1 month. Special refrigerated vehicles transported the blood to the front. The vehicles always had enough stored blood from all blood groups stored in the refrigerators. The cooled blood was usable for up to 18 days. In the first year of the war, 1200 L of blood were sent to the front.[2] Blood donors gave between 300 and 400 mL of blood, which was mixed by medical staff in a 500-mL Erlenmeyer flask with a 0.4% sodium citrate solution, and sometimes a 0.1% glucose solution was added. After usage, empty flasks were rinsed with water and sterilized, ready for reuse. Each donated blood in the flask was tested, and its blood group was determined. It was preferable for blood donors to donate blood in the morning when they hadn't eaten anything. Life was difficult in that period, and infections after ingestion were common due to

---

[1] Palfreeman L. The Development of Blood Transfusion in Spain during the Spanish Civil War (1936–1939): The Contribution of British Doctor, Reginald Saxton, Bulletin of Spanish Studies. 2019; 96(8), p. 1251. https://www.tandfonline.com/doi/citedby/10.1080/14753820.2019.1647996?%20scroll=top&%20needAccess=true&role=tab Accessed 22 Feb 2022.

[2] Blood transfusion service [video] 1941.

© The Author(s), under exclusive license to Springer Nature Switzerland AG 2024
Z. Kvržić, *History of Blood Donation and Transfusion Medicine*,
https://doi.org/10.1007/978-3-031-68715-0_12

contaminated food and poor living conditions.[3] Besides, the nationalists occupied the major food-producing regions; therefore, regions under the control of the Republic were more vulnerable to starvation. The donated blood was tested for syphilis and malaria. With an X-ray apparatus, individuals with tuberculosis were prevented from donating blood.[4] Dr. Frederic Durán-Jordà (1905–1957) was the director of the blood transfusion service of the Republican Army[5] and a pioneer in the development of modern blood transfusion services and blood banking.[6] He drew up preliminary plans for a blood transfusion service with his colleagues, Dr. Wenceslau Dutrem and Dr. Serafina Palma. His superior, Joaquím Trías, supported Dr. Duran-Jordà's ideas.[7] The blood transfusion service in Barcelona began to function in August 1936 and worked until January 1939.[8] It served as a model for similar systems in other parts of Spain.[9] Dr. Durán-Jordà organized and promoted blood donations, replaced direct vein-to-vein blood transfusions with citrated and stored blood, designed a standard 300-mL glass blood bottle that could be transfused at any time, and ensured that the blood was distributed throughout Spain, far from where it was donated.[10] Under the control of the Republic, the Canadian Dr. Norman Bethune (1890–1939) founded the Canadian Blood Transfusion Institute in Madrid in 1936.[11] Dr. Bethune traveled to Paris and London to obtain literature on blood transfusion, as he had little experience in the field of transfusion medicine. He also acquired a caravan, a refrigerator, an incubator, a steam sterilizer, and 1375 other pieces of equipment. Dr. Bethune demonstrated excellent organizational skills during the war (recruiting blood donors, collecting, processing, storing, and systematically transporting blood).[12] Bethune was one of four Canadians on the staff, along with one American and six Spaniards, two of whom were physicians. The doctors and medical students who worked with Bethune were promoted to captain, and Bethune was commissioned with the rank of major. By the end of 1936, the Canadian Blood Service had 1000 registered blood donors, who each gave about 500 mL of blood. In 1937, the staff numbered 100 and the blood donors numbered 3875. Five

---

[3] Grífols, J.R., The contribution of Dr. Duran-Jorda to the advancement and development of European blood transfusion. ISBT Science Series. 2007;2 (1);135–138. https://onlinelibrary.wiley.com/doi/abs/10.1111/j.1751-2824.2007.00078.x#.

[4] Coni N. Medicine and the Spanish Civil War. Journal of the Royal Society of Medicine.2002;95 (3);147–150. https://journals.sagepub.com/doi/abs/10.1177/014107680209500314 Accessed 22 Feb 2022.

[5] Palfreeman, 2019, p. 1251.

[6] Grifols, 2007, p. 138.

[7] Palfreeman, 2019, p. 1253.

[8] Jorda, 1939, p. 773–775.

[9] Lozano M, Cid J., Frederic Duran-Jorda: a transfusion medicine pioneer, Transfus. Med. Rev. 2007;21 (1);75–81. https://pubmed.ncbi.nlm.nih.gov/17256247/.

[10] Grifols, 2007, p. 138.

[11] Lozano, Cid, 2007, p. 75–81.

[12] Pinkerton, P.H. Norman Bethune and Transfusion in the Spanish Civil War, Vox sanguinis.2002; 83 (1);117–120. https://onlinelibrary.wiley.com/doi/abs/10.1111/j.1423-0410.2002.tb05282.x. Accessed 26 Feb 2022.

cars transported blood, and a total of 1900 blood transfusions were performed in 1937. His mobile attendance method, which was founded on the idea of bringing the blood to the wounded rather than the wounded to the blood, was particularly noteworthy. Dr. Bethune personally went to the front and gave blood to soldiers who were being fired upon by the enemy. For his efforts, Bethune was recognized by the Spanish government, which gave him one of the highest degrees given to a foreigner during the conflict.[13]

War destruction resulted in organized blood donation, which supplied the endangered population and the army during the most difficult times. The need for blood has led to significant advances in this area. Durán-Jordà and Norman Bethune are just two of many who recognized transfusion medicine as an extremely important branch of medicine. One of the major advancements was the transportation of blood over long distances, where patients could not come to hospitals. Once again, it was demonstrated that prepared and stored blood was a better solution than direct vein-to-vein transfusion because it did not require the blood donor to be in the patient's vicinity or a large group of blood donors to be present, and the blood was tested and labeled with its blood group prior to blood transfusion. It was also shown that to have large quantities of blood from different blood groups, a blood donation is necessary for recruiting new blood donors.

References

1. Coni N. Medicine and the Spanish civil war. J R Soc Med. 2002;95(3):147–50. https://doi.org/10.1177/014107680209500314.
2. Franco A, Cortes J, Alvarez J, Diz JC. The development of blood transfusion: the contributions of Norman Bethune in the Spanish Civil War (1936–1939). Can J Anaesth. 1996;43(10):1076–8. https://pubmed.ncbi.nlm.nih.gov/8896864/.
3. Grífols JR. The contribution of Dr. Duran-Jorda to the advancement and development of European blood transfusion. ISBT Sci Ser. 2007;2(1):135–8. https://doi.org/10.1111/j.1751-2824.2007.00078.x.
4. Lozano M, Cid J. Frederic Duran-Jorda: a transfusion medicine pioneer. Transfus Med Rev. 2007;21(1):75–81. https://pubmed.ncbi.nlm.nih.gov/17256247/.
5. Palfreeman L. The Development of Blood Transfusion in Spain during the Spanish Civil War (1936–1939): The Contribution of British Doctor, Reginald Saxton. Bull Span Stud. 2019;96(8):1251. https://doi.org/10.1080/14753820.2019.1647996. Accessed 22 Feb 2022.
6. Pinkerton PH. Norman Bethune and transfusion in the Spanish civil war. Vox sanguinis. 2002;83(1):117–20. https://doi.org/10.1111/j.1423-0410.2002.tb05282.x. Accessed 26 Feb 2022

---

[13] Franco, A., Cortes, J., Alvarez, J., & Diz, J. C. The development of blood transfusion: the contributions of Norman Bethune in the Spanish Civil War (1936–1939). Canadian Journal of Anaesthesia. 1996; 43(10);1076–1078. https://pubmed.ncbi.nlm.nih.gov/8896864/.

Transfusion Medicines During World War II

Contents

13.1 The United Kingdom... 159
13.2 The United States of America... 160
    13.2.1 Liquid and Dried Plasma and Serum.......................... 163
    13.2.2 Plasma for Britain... 168
    13.2.3 Race Segregation of Blood Products.......................... 169
13.3 The Soviet Union... 170
13.4 The Third Reich.. 170
References... 171

The actual birth of transfusion medicine in the modern sense occurred during WWII, as more people became aware of the critical role that blood transfusions play in treating hemorrhagic shock.[1]

13.1 The United Kingdom

At the outbreak of WWII, the UK organized large-scale blood donations. Both sexes donated their blood on a larger scale. The working class, such as clerks, typists, housewives, factory workers, shop assistants, and various other workers between the ages of 18 and 65, regularly donated blood to blood transfusion services. When they registered for blood donation, they gave the reception staff their personal details, their residential address, and details of their health. From a donated drop of blood from an ear or finger, the blood group was then determined

---

[1] Högman, 1992, p. 139.

© The Author(s), under exclusive license to Springer Nature Switzerland AG 2024
Z. Kvržić, *History of Blood Donation and Transfusion Medicine*,
https://doi.org/10.1007/978-3-031-68715-0_13

in the laboratory. Blood donors also received their blood donor card, which contained information about their blood group, details of their medical condition, an address where they could be contacted in case of an emergency, and how much blood they had donated. The blood donation service went to the workplaces and took drops of blood for blood grouping from workers who could not attend the blood donations. The blood transfusion service was able to call all the employees to the blood donation in case of an emergency because they had their blood groups determined by this method of visit. They donated blood in a large room, lying on a couch, with a curtain between the couches to ensure the blood donor's privacy. There was a nurse with each blood donor, and a doctor walked to each blood donor, prepared and cleaned the venipuncture site, injected a local anesthetic so that they did not feel pain from the needle, and performed the venipuncture. The blood donation took about 5 min, and about 425 mL of blood was donated. The bottle of blood was labeled and put in the refrigerator. After the blood donation, the blood donor rested for 10 min. Blood donors were given sweet tea and biscuits for refreshment. The blood transfusion services visited many towns and villages where blood donors gave blood. Organized blood donations saved many civilian lives during the Third Reich's air raids on the UK. There was also a military blood transfusion service, which supplied blood to soldiers at the front from civilians. Mobile blood donation teams in villages and towns collected up to a ton of blood a day. The blood was sent to the belligerent country by air, from where it was escorted to the front by van. Blood transfusions were carried out in cases of hemorrhages, when the patient had lost whole blood, and for patients in shock.[2] An important part of the daily routine of the military blood transfusion service was the preparation of blood collection and blood transfusion kits. All the kits were cleaned, and the needles were re-sharpened every day. The systems were connected by rubber tubing. When the kits were finished, the contents were checked, wrapped in cellophane, and placed in sterile tin boxes. The kits were ready for the mobile blood donation teams for the next day. The blood transfusion kits were placed side by side on the bottles for blood collection. Stored blood was sent from the depot to the front by special planes. The blood arrived at the overseas depots, and from there, it was sent to the front by vehicles.[3]

13.2 The United States of America

Voluntary and unpaid blood donation was first offered in selected US cities and hospitals in 1920. The US Red Cross launched a sizable civilian blood donation program in 1941 after the US government formally created a national blood

---

[2] Shock is a state of the body where the blood circulation no longer meets the needs for oxygen and other substances.
[3] Blood transfusion service [video] 1941.

donation program in 1940.[4] At the beginning of the war, doctors began to question whether whole blood was necessary for blood transfusions. In a state of shock, the liquid part of the blood plasma leaks out of the bloodstream into the body tissues. As a result, the body needs more fluid in the bloodstream to replenish the blood cells.[5] Plasma transfusions proved to be very successful during the WWII (Image 13.1).[6] Without the need for blood cross-matching, plasma transfusions helped raise blood volume and helped to cure the dramatic drop in blood pressure brought on by shock.[7] Cross-matching with plasma transfusion was not necessary because the RBCs were removed from the plasma.[8] In the USA, plasma collection establishments were established as a result of the use of plasma in shock management. In 1935, two biochemists, Earl William Flosdorf and Stuart Mudd, developed the process of lyophilization, or freeze drying, in which water is removed from a product after it is frozen and placed under a vacuum, allowing the ice to change directly from solid to vapor without passing through a liquid phase. The process consists of three separate, unique, and interdependent processes: freezing, primary drying (sublimation), and secondary drying (desorption). Their research was devoted to the drying and packaging of human blood serum, a medical technique that was later developed and used in WWII.[9, 10] This, along with the introduction of ABO-independent "universal" plasma produced by pooling several thousand units of plasma, facilitated efficient long-term storage of plasma.[11]

Plasma was also desirable for crushing injuries, burns, abdominal wounds, and heat dehydration.[12] While treating shocked and severely wounded soldiers, plasma was not as successful as whole blood. Plasma blood transfusions aided patients in their recovery from shock, but frequently they were unable to get them ready for major surgery, which may have been required for a complete recovery.[13] It was widely acknowledged throughout World War I and the time between World War I

---

[4] Jordan J.A. War on Two Fronts: Race, Citizenship, and the Segregation of the blood supply during World War II. Penn History Review. 2018; 24(2), article 3, p. 32–70. https://repository.upenn.edu/entities/publication/c995dc51-efaa-40c1-a234-94e2caf4e3b5. Accessed 12 March 2022.

[5] Blood transfusion service [video] 1941.

[6] Lbid.

[7] LeBlanc, 2016, p. 4.

[8] National World War II museum New Orleans. Fact Sheet: Blood Plasma. https://www.nationalww2museum.org/sites/default/files/2017-07/blood-plasma-fact-sheet.pdf. Accessed 24 Feb 2024.

[9] Whaler J. A World Where Blood Was Made Possible. https://pabook.libraries.psu.edu/literary-cultural-heritage-map-pa/feature-articles/world-where-blood-was-made-possible Accessed 2 March 2024.

[10] U.S. Food and Drug administration. Lyophilization of Parenteral (7/93). https://www.fda.gov/inspections-compliance-enforcement-and-criminal-investigations/inspection-guides/lyophilization-parenteral-793. Accessed 3 March 2024.

[11] Rossi, Simon, 2016, p. 8.

[12] Kendrick D. B. Blood program in World War II, Washington, D.C.: Office of the surgeon general department of the army, 1964, p. 13–391. https://collections.nlm.nih.gov/catalog/nlm:nlmuid-0014773-bk. Accessed 18 March 2022.

[13] LeBlanc, 2016, p. 4.

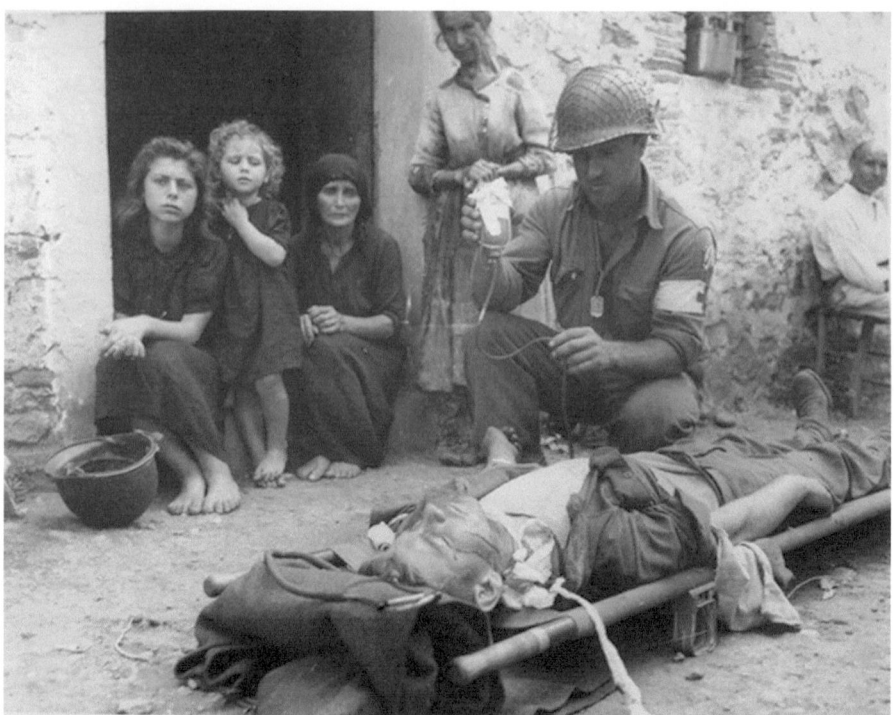

Image 13.1 Plasma transfusion. (Source: Plasma transfusion. Private Roy Humphrey of Toledo, Ohio, is being given blood plasma by Private First Class Harvey White of Minneapolis, Minnesota, after he was wounded by shrapnel, on 9 August 1943 in Sicily. From The U.S. National Archives and Records Administration. https://catalog.archives.gov/id/531161 Free to use.)

and later that hemoconcentration[14] and a decrease in blood volume were both important factors in the genesis of shock.[15] The rather general belief at the outbreak of WWII that plasma alone could compensate for the loss of whole blood in shock simply derived from the mistaken opinion that blood loss was not the primary cause of shock. Both the mortality rate and the incidence of wound infection were reduced by the use of whole blood at the time of initial wound surgery. Whole blood was a more desirable replacement fluid than plasma because both red cells and plasma had been lost. This recognition started in 1941 by the US Army and was employed in 1943, while the British army at the battlefront has used whole blood instead of plasma since 1941.[16] Nonetheless, in addition to whole blood, the US Army still continued to use blood plasma throughout the war.

---

[14] Hemoconcentration means increase in the relative number of RBC.
[15] LeBlanc, 2016, p.4.
[16] Kendrick, 1964, p. 13–391.

13.2.1 Liquid and Dried Plasma and Serum

Plasma was accumulated in WWII largely for the prevention and treatment of shock. The collected plasma was stored in a liquid state; it was also frozen and dried. In the liquid state, it retained its colloidal properties necessary for the treatment of shock, but the more labile components of plasma, the prothrombin, and fibrinogen, concerned with blood coagulation, complement, and antibodies, concerned with immunity, deteriorated with time. For an economical civilian program, therefore, liquid plasma had distinct limitations. In the frozen state, the labile components of plasma were better preserved; here the limitation was the inconvenience for storage, transport, and immediate emergency use. In the dried state, most of the labile components of plasma were preserved.[17]

The pioneer in the field of using liquid blood plasma instead of whole blood in surgery, obstetrics, and traumatic shock in 1936 was the American Alvin John Elliott.[18, 19] Plasma was separated from whole blood in bottles by passing it through filters until it became clear and sterile. After this process, it was bottled, and the contents were checked again before being shipped out of the laboratories. The serum, the liquid part of the blood after clotting, was prepared and used in an identical way. Liquid plasma and serum were easier to transport to the front than whole blood. It was not necessary to store them in the refrigerator; rough handling did not spoil them, and they had a longer shelf life than whole blood. This solved the problem of throwing away blood and shipping it overseas. The problem with the supply of blood across the sea was the shelf life of the blood, as stored blood was only usable for up to 14 days in 1941 with citrated blood.[20] The preservation of blood was prolonged in the following years with experience and with available methods for at least one more week. The US Army used different preservative solutions, such as Denstedt's solution, Rous-Turner, McGill, and Rous-Turner, mainly Alsever, and finally, in the autumn of 1944, the US Navy used acid citrate dextrose (ACD), which the US Army started to use on April 1, 1945.[21] In comparison to other preservatives, ACD had various advantages, including the need for a smaller volume and less fragile RBC that could be handled and transported better.[22] Plasma was, at this time, also stored for longer periods. Liquid plasma kept at room temperature had a safe

---

[17] Cohn, Edwin J. Blood proteins and their therapeutic value. Science. 1945; 101(2612), p. 51–56.

[18] Schmidt, P. J. The plasma wars: a history. Transfusion. 2012; 52(1), p. 2S–4S. https://pubmed.ncbi.nlm.nih.gov/22578368/.

[19] Schmidt P. J. John Elliott and the evolution of American blood banking, 1934 to 1954, Transfusion. 2000; 40(5), p. 608–612. https://pubmed.ncbi.nlm.nih.gov/10827268/ .

[20] Blood transfusion service [video] 1941.

[21] Kendrick, 1964, p. 217–227.

[22] Ruddell J. P.The effect of room temperature storage on the in vitro storage characteristics of CPDA-1 packed RBC. MS thesis. Bowling Green State University, 1996, p. 3. https://apps.dtic.mil/sti/tr/pdf/ADA318714.pdf Accessed 24 March 2024.

storage period of 2 years; frozen plasma was stored for up to 3 years,[23] while dried plasma could be stored for up to 5 years.[24]

In August 1937, the American Red Cross initially expressed interest in blood supply and donation. This new initiative was led by William DeKleine. The initiative was largely based on the blood donation work done by the British Red Cross. Blood donors at that time in the USA gave blood through direct transfusions. DeKleines initial partnership with Elliot eventually led the US Army to accept liquid plasma as a treatment by 1940.[25] Max Maurice Strumia (1896–1972) had been studying plasma as an antimicrobial agent since 1927, and he was also exploring how to change the liquid plasma pioneered by Elliot into dried plasma.[26] He developed the method of dried plasma in October 1940.[27, 28] Max Strumia had built a compact device that could shell-freeze liquid plasma and dry it in a vacuum.[29] He transfused plasma intravenously.[30] Interestingly, the use of serum intravenously has been around since 1927, when it was first used to treat serious infections, particularly those with a streptococcic origin.[31] The method of turning liquid plasma and serum into powder was a complicated process. The liquid plasma or serum was placed on a centrifuge and spun at a low temperature until it solidified. The frozen liquid was then placed in a drying chamber, which evaporated all the water. In this way, plasma or serum was turned into a powder that was bottled.[32] Dried plasma is mentioned in different sources as powder plasma, freeze-dried plasma, and dry plasma.

---

[23] Alsever J. B. Plasma Reserves for Civilian Defense, Their Distribution, Control, Preparation and Clinical Use With Special Reference to the Treatment of Infectious Diseases. American Journal of Public Health and the Nations Health. 1944; 34(2): 165–173. https://ajph.aphapublications.org/doi/pdf/10.2105/AJPH.34.2.165.

[24] Anon. The Blood Transfusion Service and Blood Banks in India. The Indian medical gazette. 1947; 82(8), p. 483–485. https://www.ncbi.nlm.nih.gov/pmc/articles/PMC5190797/?page=1.

[25] Schmidt, 2000, p. 609.

[26] Schmidt, 2012, p. 3.

[27] Blood transfusion service [video] 1941.

[28] McDonough S. J. Blood bank tanks filed for Soldiers. The Brooklyn Daily Eagle. Brooklyn, New York · Friday, October 04, 1940, p. 5. https://bklyn.newspapers.com/image/53589509/?terms=max%20strumia&match=1.

[29] Schmidt, 2012, p. 3.

[30] Strumia M.M., McGraw J.J., Reichel J. The Preparation and Preservation of Human Plasma: IV. Drying of Plasma From the Frozen State by Low Temperature Condensation in Vacuo, American Journal of Clinical Pathology. 1941;11(3), p. 175–194. https://academic.oup.com/ajcp/article-abstract/11/3/175/1757294?redirectedFrom=fulltext. Accessed 18 March 2022.

[31] Strumia M. M. Wagner J. A., Monaghan J. F. The intravenous use of serum and plasma, fresh and preserved. Annals of Surgery. 1940;111(4), p.623 https://www.ncbi.nlm.nih.gov/pmc/articles/PMC1390782/pdf/annsurg00497-0111.pdf.

[32] Blood transfusion service [video] 1941.

Besides Strumia's "The Hot Water Jacket Drier Apparatus," that achived excellent results, there were also other apparatuses and methods for drying plasma that were available by 1949.[33]

The package containing dried plasma, distilled water, and intravenous equipment was all sent to the battlefront in boxes. The plasma can, packaged under a vacuum, contained a double-ended needle, an intravenous needle, and a bottle of dried plasma. The water can, packaged under nitrogen to protect the rubber tubing, contained an intravenous set, an airway assembly, and a bottle of distilled water.[34] At the battlefront before the plasma transfusion, distilled water was added to the powder, which turned into a liquid and was immediately ready for use. Dried plasma could be stored for a long time in any climate.[35] In October 1942, the US military discussed the options to use whole blood from a universal group O blood donor instead of dried plasma. The use of whole blood started in May 1943. The blood group O was not only suggested because it is universal but also because it was also preferred to avoid the necessity for immediate cross-matching.[36] This was because the casualties that were admitted were in severe shock and in critical condition. Blood donors of any blood group were given low-titer group O blood immediately and rapidly, while the blood group O with the high titer was used for group O recipients only. The blood was sometimes transfused through two to four veins, depending on the critical condition of the patient. For grouping, blood was obtained at the first venipuncture and for cross-matching in subsequent transfusions.[37] The difference between low and high titers is that the antibody titer test shows that blood donors who have a low titer of whole blood also have low levels of anti-A and anti-B antibodies; high levels of these antibodies are able to cause transfusion reactions in patients with other blood types.[38] The abnormal results of the antibody titer may indicate immune disorders or current or past infections.[39]

In terms of the use of blood substitutes, there was never a truly urgent need for them during WWII because of the abundant whole blood donations, rapid advances in the processing of blood into plasma, and comparable advancements in the fractionation of plasma and the development of some of its derivatives, most notably serum albumin. Extensive research proved that gelatin was the safest and most effective of the agents investigated. The principal reason for the suggestion was that a 6% solution had been found to have the viscosity of whole blood at room

---

[33] Alsever J. B. Dried plasma, Chapter 18. In: DeGowin E. L., Hardin R. C., Alsever B. J. Blood transfusion. W.B. Saunders Company Philadelphia & London, 1949, p. 400–419.

[34] Kendrick, 1964, p. 700.

[35] Blood transfusion service [video] 1941.

[36] Kendrick, 1964, p. 53–391.

[37] Lbid., p. 434–689.

[38] Military Health System. Low-Titer O Whole Blood Saves Lives on the Battlefield. https://www.health.mil/News/Dvids-Articles/2023/06/23/news447762?page=1#youMayAlso. Accessed 24 Feb 2024.

[39] Luo E. K., Krause L. Antibody Titer Test, Healthline. https://www.healthline.com/health/abdomen-swollen#seeking-help Accessed 14 March 2024.

temperature and an oncotic (osmotic) pressure of 65 mm H20m, and it was not antigenic.[40, 41]

Edwin Joseph Cohn (1892–1953), an American biochemist, contributed to the development of blood fractionation techniques.[42, 43] Early clinical trials from Cohn included experimenting with bovine blood in 1941, but because of adverse reactions such as serum sickness, this program was terminated by 1943. After this, the focus was on human albumin, which was developing at the same time as the bovine program.[44] The development of serum albumin in the treatment of shock really began at the first meeting of the Subcommittee on Blood Substitutes on November 30, 1940, with the suggestion, already mentioned, of the chairman, Dr. Cannon, that "it would be in the interest of clear thinking" if protein chemists were brought into the picture. In response to the suggestion, Dr. Cohn, whose work on plasma fractionation was already outstanding, undertook his work on serum albumin. The Red Cross in 1941 had already begun to supply Dr. Cohn with 15 bloods per week.[45] The first fractionation of human plasma was carried out by Armstrong at the Harvard laboratory in August 1940. The first use of Cohn's human albumin preparation for the treatment of traumatic shock was by Charles Janeway at the Brigham Hospital in April and May 1941.[46] Purified serum albumin was used to treat shock instead of dried plasma because it was stable, reliable, transportable, and safe.[47] The fractionation process that Cohn developed and perfected was carried out in a cold room at −5 °C. Each protein fraction was precipitated in a different concentration of ethyl alcohol under specific conditions of temperature, pH, ionic strength, and protein concentration. The fluid portion was removed by centrifugation, leaving the precipitated protein as a paste. The paste was then quickly frozen and dried. The bacterial growth was inhibited because the entire process was carried out at a cold temperature and the alcohol did not denature the plasma proteins. Ten fractions (I, II, III-1,

---

[40] Kendrick, 1964, p. 373.

[41] Antigenic means being a part to or made up of antigens (= materials that trigger an immunological response in the body, particularly the production of antibodies)

[42] Blood fractionation techniques are the division of plasma proteins into fractions.

[43] Britannica, The Editors of Encyclopedia. Edwin Joseph Cohn. Encyclopedia Britannica. https://www.britannica.com/biography/Edwin-Joseph-Cohn Accessed 23 Feb 2023.

[44] Curling, Goss, Bertolini, 2012, p. 6.

[45] Kendrick, 1964, p. 336–337.

[46] Curling, Goss, Bertolini, 2012, p. 6.

[47] Creager A. N. H. Douglas M. Surgenor, Edwin J. Cohn and the Development of Protein Chemistry: With a Detailed Account of His Work on the Fractionation of Blood During and After World War II. 2003; 94(4), p.763–765. https://www.researchgate.net/publication/290622142_Douglas_M_Surgenor_Edwin_J_Cohn_and_the_Development_of_Protein_Chemistry_With_a_Detailed_Account_of_His_Work_on_the_Fractionation_of_Blood_During_and_After_World_War_II_xx434_pp_frontis_illus_index_Bo. Accessed 23 February 2023.

III-2, III-3, III-0, IV-1, IV-4, V, and VI) altogether were gained with this process by 1945.[48, 49]

Content of Cohn's Ten-Plasma Fractions:
- **I** (majority of fibrinogen and antihemophilic globulin).
- **II** (gamma globulin by subfractionation of II plus III).
- **III-1** (other antibodies: typhoid, isoagglutinin, and anti-Rh).
- **III-2** (prothrombin that was converted to thrombin for the preparation of fibrin products and one of the components of complement).
- **III-3** (plasminogen, the predecessor of plasmin, and fibrinolytic enzyme).
- **III-0** (rich in lipoproteins that were cholesterol, carotene, and vitamin A). This fraction also included beta-globulin.
- **IV-1** (lipoprotein and alpha-globulin).
- **IV-4** (enzymes and hormones such as hypertensinogen and thyrotropin).
- **V** (albumin).
- **VI** (salts, minor amounts of protein, and small organic molecules).[50]

WWII marked the beginning of blood components and derivative therapy. The credit goes to Elliott and Strumia for the separation of plasma from the whole blood.[51] The acknowledgment also goes to Edwin Joseph Cohn and his associates, who invented the cold ethanol method of plasma fractionation, which marked the beginning of component and derivative therapy. Their efforts led to the development of albumin, globulin, and fibrinogen for use in medicine.[52] To summarize, the Cohn process was an ongoing process from the separation of human albumin from 1941 to the year 1945, when it was possible to gain ten fractions.

13.2.1.1 Development of Cryoprecipitate

In the years following WWII, clotting factor concentrates were developed for the treatment of hemophilia and other hemorrhagic illnesses.[53] An American biomedical researcher, Dr. Judith Graham Pool (June 1, 1919 to July 13, 1975), noted in 1964 that the "gelatinous sludge" at the bottom of previously frozen plasma containers was highly concentrated in factor VIII (FVIII, or antihemophilic factor). She employed a technique currently used in blood banks to separate cryoprecipitate from plasma by utilizing the "last-to-thaw" feature of FVIII. Dr. Pool showed how cryoprecipitate blood transfusion could increase FVIII levels in patients with hemophilia A. The treatment of patients with hemophilia A was transformed by cryoprecipitate, greatly extending their life expectancy. Furthermore, Dr. Pool's work laid

---

[48] Alsever J.B. Plasma derivatives. Preparation and administration of the whole blood derivatives and plasma substitutes—plasma derivatives, part VII. In: DeGowin E. L., Hardin R. C., Alsever B. J. Blood transfusion. W.B. Saunders Company Philadelphia & London, 1949, p. 446.

[49] Cohn, Edwin J. The separation of blood into fractions of therapeutic value. Annals of Internal Medicine, 1947; 26 (3), p. 351. https://www.acpjournals.org/doi/abs/10.7326/0003-4819-26-3-341.

[50] Alsever, 1949, p. 446.

[51] Carmichael, Lin, Evangelista, Holcomb, 2021, p. 1.

[52] Rossi, Simon, 2016, p. 7.

[53] Lbid.

the groundwork for the creation of contemporary hemophilia medicines, ushering in a new age of hemophilia treatment.[54] Preparing a cryo requires the use of blood donor plasma. The plasma is initially frozen and then slowly thaws. The precipitate or insoluble fraction of the plasma is left behind while the liquid portion drains away. When the precipitate has a volume large enough for blood transfusion, it is collected and combined with donations from other blood donors. It can be stored for a full year. Many blood-clotting proteins are present in cryo, including fibrinogen, factor VIII, factor XIII, and Von Willebrand factor. Those whose own blood does not clot sufficiently can use cryotherapy to halt or control bleeding. The group of patients includes those with severe but uncommon hereditary illnesses such as Von Willebrand Disease (VWD) and hemophilia A. The essential clotting protein fibrinogen can also be obtained through cryotherapy for patients who are unable to produce enough of it on their own.[55] VWD was originally identified by Erik Adolf von Willebrand, who in early 1924 investigated a large family suffering from a bleeding disorder that seemed to differ from hemophilia. By the end of the 1960s, VWD was accepted as a combined deficiency of factor VIII (FVIII) and another plasma factor responsible for normal platelet adhesion.[56]

13.2.2 Plasma for Britain

The British Red Cross requested assistance from the US National Red Cross on July 14, 1940, to supply them with liquid blood plasma because the Third Reich had bombed them and left many wounded. In August 1940, the *"Plasma for Britain"* initiative got underway. The Red Cross was in charge of locating blood donors and setting up the shipments, while the Blood Transfusion Society of New York was in charge of processing the plasma. Almost 14,000 blood donors participated. Dr. Charles Drew (1904–1955) oversaw the effort.[57] Dr. Drew had important work regarding setting the criteria for production, developing standard techniques, and ensuring the safety of the final product.[58] Eight hospitals provided plasma, which was then examined, pooled, diluted, and packaged for delivery to Britain.[59] Special apparatus was developed in laboratories to prepare plasma for large-scale needs.[60] For this program, liquid plasma was chosen instead of dried plasma because of the

---

[54] Swenson E., Hollenhorst MA. Dr. Judith Graham Pool and the development of cryoprecipitate, Transfusion. 2021; 61 (6), p. 1676–1677. https://pubmed.ncbi.nlm.nih.gov/33894065/.

[55] American Red Cross. What Is Cryoprecipitate? Why Is It Important? https://www.redcrossblood.org/donate-blood/dlp/cryoprecipitate.html Accessed 21 April 2022.

[56] Favaloro EJ, Diagnosing von Willebrand disease: a short history of laboratory milestones and innovations, plus current status, challenges, and solutions, Semin Thromb Hemost. 2014; 40(5), p. 551–570. https://pubmed.ncbi.nlm.nih.gov/24978322/.

[57] Strumia, McGraw, Reichel, 1941, p. 175–194.

[58] Kendrick, 1964, p. 13–15.

[59] Strumia, McGraw, Reichel, 1941, p. 175–194.

[60] Blood transfusion service [video] 1941.

tight schedule, the operation of installing equipment for drying plasma was expensive, and the functionality of the equipment was not satisfying. Plasma was separated from whole blood using centrifugation or sedimentation techniques. It was diluted with equal parts of a sterile physiologic salt solution to lessen viscosity. Six bottles holding 1000 cc of the completed product were supplied per carton. Strict bacteriologic and toxicity controls were established before any amount of plasma was sent overseas. Dr. Frank L. Meleney supervised controls that were carried out both in the laboratories of the participating hospitals and in a central laboratory. When plasma reached the UK, it was mandatory to take samples from each carton for bacteriological controls before being sent to the casualties in need. Unfortunately, certain pools of plasma that were within 3–7 days examined after their collection and processing and that were considered to be without bacteria were later identified as being contaminated.[61] Bacterial contamination of plasma was also a common occurrence during transport across the sea.[62] However, eventually the Brits stopped using their plasma out of concern for bacterial contamination, and the program to deliver plasma to Britain was terminated in January 1941. Despite the program's suspension, the US military made the decision to keep using blood plasma in the conflict with newly developed dried plasma at the time.[63, 64] Because of its link to hepatitis epidemics, the USA discontinued using frozen and dried plasma after WWII.[65, 66] The hepatitis epidemics derived from pool plasma, and at that time, blood donor screening was not completely sufficient to ensure the safety of plasma, particularly when blood donors were paid.[67] Since then, security testing has completely improved, and dried plasma is now used by the US military again, as of 2012, as well as a few other armies across the world.[68]

13.2.3 Race Segregation of Blood Products

There was also controversy regarding race. In 1941, it was mostly forbidden for African Americans to donate blood or plasma. Because of the pressure from the general public, on January 21, 1942, the American Red Cross, in agreement with the Navy and Army, allowed African Americans to donate blood or plasma. The donated

---

[61] Kendrick, 1964, p. 13–15.
[62] Strumia, McGraw, Reichel, 1941, p.175–194.
[63] Schmidt, 2012, p. 3
[64] Schmidt, 2000, p. 609–610.
[65] Schmidt, 2012, p. 3
[66] Schmidt, 2000, p. 610.
[67] Lee L., Moore E. E., Hansen K. C., Silliman C. C., Chandler J. G., & Banerjee A. It's not your grandfather's field plasma. Surgery, 2013; 153(6), 857–860. https://www.ncbi.nlm.nih.gov/pmc/articles/PMC4065714/.
[68] Galvan S. U.S., France Armies Join Forces to Expand Freeze-Dried Plasma. https://mrdc.health.mil/index.cfm/media/articles/2014/armies_join_forces_to_expand_freeze-dried_plasma. Accessed 18 March 2022.

components from white and black people were processed and labeled separately. Also, blood transfusions were carried out in this matter.[69] The Red Cross did not stop requiring the separation of blood from so-called "Negro" populations until 1950. It was not until the latter half of the 1960s and the beginning of the 1970s that southern states like Louisiana and Arkansas abolished analogous regulations.[70]

13.3 The Soviet Union

When the Soviet Union entered WWII in Moscow, roughly 2000 people donated blood every day. To entice blood donors, they employed every propaganda strategy at their disposal. Almost 95% of blood donors were women, compared to 50% in the USA. This was due to the fact that the majority of men were on the frontlines fighting. The amount of blood drawn varied between 225 and 450 mL. After 4–6 weeks of the initial blood donation, a second donation was permitted, but only if the blood count readings were normal. Some blood donors have contributed for 12–15 years without experiencing any negative health effects, thanks to these safeguards. Bottles with isothermal boxes that could be used in both cold and warm weather were used to convey the blood to the battlefield by plane. Blood was also put into 200-cc ampoules. For the majority of battlefield blood transfusions, the Soviets employed group O blood and significant amounts of type-specific, unpooled plasma. The institute developed a technique for drying plasma that ensured its solubility without turbidity or precipitation, as well as one that allowed the preservation of blood for 3–4 weeks without losing any of its biological features. Even while blood transfusions were administered up to the regimental medical aid station (battalion aid station), they were most frequently utilized at the level of the medical-sanitary battalion service (collecting station). Hemorrhage with shock in their casualties from the war was the main symptom, especially in wounds on the limbs and abdomen. Their experiences showed that quick and large blood transfusions between 1000 and 1500 cc in volume work well in dealing with shock.[71]

13.4 The Third Reich

The Germans had a civilian blood donation program in 1940. Only Aryans were allowed to donate blood. They were paid 10 marks for the first 100 cc and 5 marks for each additional 100 cc. In Berlin, there was a laboratory for blood transfusion, which oversaw the military operation. But their supply of blood was insufficient,

---

[69] Guglielmo T. A."Red Cross, Double Cross:"Race and America s World War II-Era Blood donor Service, The Journal of American History. 2010; 97(1), p. 63–90. Available at: https://academic.oup.com/jah/article-abstract/97/1/63/719496 [Accessed 18 March 2022].
[70] Guglielmo T. A. When the Red Cross didn't accept black blood. https://www.chicagoreporter.com/when-the-red-cross-didnt-accept-black-blood/ [Accessed 18 March 2022].
[71] Kendrick, 1964, p. 21–23.

and containers and technical equipment were in short supply. Medical professionals, nursing sisters, office assistants, and men who had just minor injuries were among the blood donors. Attempts were always made to rule out tuberculosis, malaria, and syphilis in blood donors, but serologic tests were rarely useful, and it was always necessary to accept the blood donor's assurance that he had not had the disease. The blood groups listed in the troops' pay books were frequently wrong, necessitating fresh determinations before each blood transfusion. A test injection of 10 cm of blood was conducted if this was not achievable. In Germany, preserved blood usage occurred mostly between 1940 and 1942. Medical professionals lost interest in it as a result of the numerous adverse reactions. Individuals who claimed positive results were typically in advantageous positions, particularly in the realm of transportation. Other medical personnel have never witnessed the field use of preserved blood without experiencing deleterious shivers. Although commanders who used captured US plasma stocks were enthused about it, plasma and serum were rarely used.[72] In the German-occupied territories, it was banned for Jews to donate their blood to Aryans.[73]

During WWII, new methods and techniques were required for saving lives and improving the safety of blood transfusions. Plasma was very important in treating shock and severe hemorrhage. During the period of this war, there were experts, mostly from the USA, who made great achievements. Developmental fractionation techniques for human plasma were introduced. The discovery was also important for later use in civilian medicine. But none of this would be possible without the generosity of altruistic blood donors. Even immediately after this horrible war, blood transfusion centers all around the world had to develop strategies to recruit more blood donors to meet the daily requirements of supplies of blood for hospitals.

References

1. Alsever JB, Plasma derivatives. Preparation and administration of the whole blood derivatives and plasma substitutes—plasma derivatives, part VII. In: Degowin EL, Hardin RC, Alsever BJ, editors. Blood transfusion. Philadelphia & London: W.B. Saunders Company; 1949. p. 446.
2. Alsever JB. Plasma reserves for civilian defense, their distribution, control, preparation and clinical use with special reference to the treatment of infectious diseases. Am J Public Health Nations Health. 1944;34(2):165–73. https://doi.org/10.2105/AJPH.34.2.165.
3. Alsever JB. Dried plasma, chapter 18. In: DeGowin EL, Hardin RC, Alsever BJ, editors. Blood transfusion. Philadelphia & London: W.B. Saunders Company; 1949. p. 400–19.
4. Anon. The blood transfusion service and blood banks in India. Indian Med Gazette. 1947;82(8):483–5. https://www.ncbi.nlm.nih.gov/pmc/articles/PMC5190797/?page=1.
5. American Red Cross. What Is Cryoprecipitate? Why Is It Important? https://www.redcrossblood.org/donate-blood/dlp/cryoprecipitate.html. Accessed 21 Apr 2022.
6. Britannica, The Editors of Encyclopedia. Edwin Joseph Cohn. Encyclopedia Britannica. https://www.britannica.com/biography/Edwin-Joseph-Cohn. Accessed 23 Feb 2023.

---

[72] I.bid.

[73] Heier H.E. Blood, ideology, science and the birth of the ISBT, VOXS. 2018; 15(29, p. 207–211). https://onlinelibrary.wiley.com/doi/full/10.1111/voxs.12539.

7. Creager ANH, Douglas M, Surgenor EJ. Cohn and the development of protein chemistry: with a detailed account of his work on the fractionation of blood during and after world war II. Isis. 2003;94(4):763–5. https://www.researchgate.net/publication/290622142_Douglas_M_Surgenor_Edwin_J_Cohn_and_the_Development_of_Protein_Chemistry_With_a_Detailed_Account_of_His_Work_on_the_Fractionation_of_Blood_During_and_After_World_War_II_xx434_pp_frontis_illus_index_Bo Accessed 23 February 2023.
8. Cohn EJ. Blood proteins and their therapeutic value. Science. 1945;101(2612):51–6.
9. Cohn EJ. The separation of blood into fractions of therapeutic value. Ann Intern Med. 1947;26(3):351. https://doi.org/10.7326/0003-4819-26-3-341.
10. Favaloro EJ. Diagnosing von Willebrand disease: a short history of laboratory milestones and innovations, plus current status, challenges, and solutions. Semin Thromb Hemost. 2014;40(5):551–70. https://pubmed.ncbi.nlm.nih.gov/24978322/.
11. Guglielmo TA. Red cross, double cross: race and America s world war II-era blood donor service. J Am Hist. 2010;97(1):63–90. https://academic.oup.com/jah/article-abstract/97/1/63/719496. Accessed 18 Mar 2022.
12. Guglielmo T.A. When the red cross didn't accept black blood. https://www.chicagoreporter.com/when-the-red-cross-didnt-accept-black-blood/. Accessed 18 Mar 2022.
13. Galvan S. U.S., France Armies Join Forces to Expand Freeze-Dried Plasma. https://mrdc.health.mil/index.cfm/media/articles/2014/armies_join_forces_to_expand_freeze-dried_plasma. Accessed 18 Mar 2022.
14. Heier HE. Blood, ideology, science and the birth of the ISBT. VOXS. 2018;15(29):207–11. https://doi.org/10.1111/voxs.12539.
15. Jordan JA. War on two fronts: race, citizenship, and the segregation of the blood supply during world war II. Penn History Rev. 2018;24(2):32–70. https://repository.upenn.edu/entities/publication/c995dc51-efaa-40c1-a234-94e2caf4e3b5. Accessed 12 Mar 2022.
16. Kendrick DB. Blood program in world war II. Washington, D.C, Office of the Surgeon General Department of the Army; 1964. p. 13–391. https://collections.nlm.nih.gov/catalog/nlm:nlmuid-0014773-bk. Accessed 18 Mar 2022.
17. Lee L, Moore EE, Hansen KC, Silliman CC, Chandler JG, Banerjee A. It's not your grandfather's field plasma. Surgery. 2013;153(6):857–60. https://www.ncbi.nlm.nih.gov/pmc/articles/PMC4065714/.
18. Luo E.K, Krause L. Antibody Titer Test, Healthline. https://www.healthline.com/health/abdomen-swollen#seeking-help. Accessed 14 Mar 2024.
19. McDonough SJ. Blood bank tanks filed for Soldiers. Brooklyn, New York: The Brooklyn Daily Eagle; 1940. p. 5. https://bklyn.newspapers.com/image/53589509/?terms=max%20strumia&match=1.
20. Military Health System. Low-Titer O Whole Blood Saves Lives on the Battlefield. https://www.health.mil/News/Dvids-Articles/2023/06/23/news447762?page=1#youMayAlso. Accessed 24 Feb 2024.
21. National World War II museum New Orleans. Fact Sheet: Blood Plasma. https://www.nationalww2museum.org/sites/default/files/2017-07/blood-plasma-fact-sheet.pdf. Accessed 24 Feb 2024.
22. Ruddell J.P. The effect of room temperature storage on the in vitro storage characteristics of CPDA-1 packed RBC. MS thesis. Bowling Green State University, 1996, p. 3. https://apps.dtic.mil/sti/tr/pdf/ADA318714.pdf. Accessed 24 Mar 2024.
23. Strumia MM, McGraw JJ, Reichel J. The preparation and preservation of human plasma: IV. Drying of plasma from the frozen state by low temperature condensation in Vacuo. Am J Clin Pathol. 1941;11(3):175–94. https://academic.oup.com/ajcp/article-abstract/11/3/175/1757294?redirectedFrom=fulltext. Accessed 18 Mar 2022.
24. Schmidt PJ. John Elliott and the evolution of American blood banking, 1934 to 1954. Transfusion. 2000;40(5):608–12. https://pubmed.ncbi.nlm.nih.gov/10827268/.
25. Schmidt PJ. The plasma wars: a history. Transfusion. 2012;52(1):2S–4S. https://pubmed.ncbi.nlm.nih.gov/22578368/.

26. Swenson E, Hollenhorst MA. Dr. Judith Graham Pool and the development of cryoprecipitate. Transfusion. 2021;61(6):1676–7. https://pubmed.ncbi.nlm.nih.gov/33894065/.
27. U.S. Food and Drug administration. Lyophilization of Parenteral (7/93). https://www.fda.gov/inspections-compliance-enforcement-and-criminal-investigations/inspection-guides/lyophilization-parenteral-793. Accessed 3 Mar 2024.
28. Whaler J. A World where blood was made possible. https://pabook.libraries.psu.edu/literary-cultural-heritage-map-pa/feature-articles/world-where-blood-was-made-possible. Accessed 2 Mar 2024.
29. Strumia MM, Wagner JA, Monaghan JF. The intravenous use of serum and plasma, fresh and preserved. Ann Surg. 1940;111(4):623. https://www.ncbi.nlm.nih.gov/pmc/articles/PMC1390782/pdf/annsurg00497-0111.pdf.

Image Source

Plasma transfusion. Private Roy Humphrey of Toledo, Ohio, is being given blood plasma by Private First Class Harvey White of Minneapolis, Minnesota, after he was wounded by shrapnel, on 9 August 1943 in Sicily. From The U.S. National Archives and Records Administration. https://catalog.archives.gov/id/531161. Free to use.

Equipment and Technology for Collection of Whole Blood and Blood Components

14

Contents

14.1 Equipment and Material for Whole Blood Collection.................................. 175
14.2 Equipment and Material Standards... 181
    14.2.1 Plastic Bags in Transfusion Medicine.. 184
    14.2.2 Whole Blood and Apheresis Technology....................................... 188
References.. 200

14.1 Equipment and Material for Whole Blood Collection

The early beginnings of collecting, storing, and administering blood from WWI eventually led to the development of different equipment, materials, and methods for clinical use.

In the beginning, blood was stored in glass vessels of different shapes and closed in different ways.[1] In the first flasks, the preserved blood was stoppered with cotton wool. This allowed oxygen to freely enter the blood mixture. Blood flasks developed later were partly filled and sealed with gas-tight stoppers. This allowed a small gaseous exchange to occur between the trapped air and the blood mixture. Blood was also preserved in ampoules that were entirely sealed to prevent the entry of any air. The first person to document this intriguing finding with the usage of ampoules was

---

[1] Grozdanić V., Fišer-Herman M., Maher V. Pribor za transfuziju krvi, krvnih derivate I zamenika krvne plazme-chapter. V. In: Polak A., Dinić B., Papo I., Fišer- Herman M., Lah P., Stefanović S., Vuletin V., editors. Transfuzija krvi. Beograd: Savezni Zavod za Zdravstvenu Zaštitu; 1966, p. 193–205.

© The Author(s), under exclusive license to Springer Nature Switzerland AG 2024
Z. Kvržić, *History of Blood Donation and Transfusion Medicine*,
https://doi.org/10.1007/978-3-031-68715-0_14

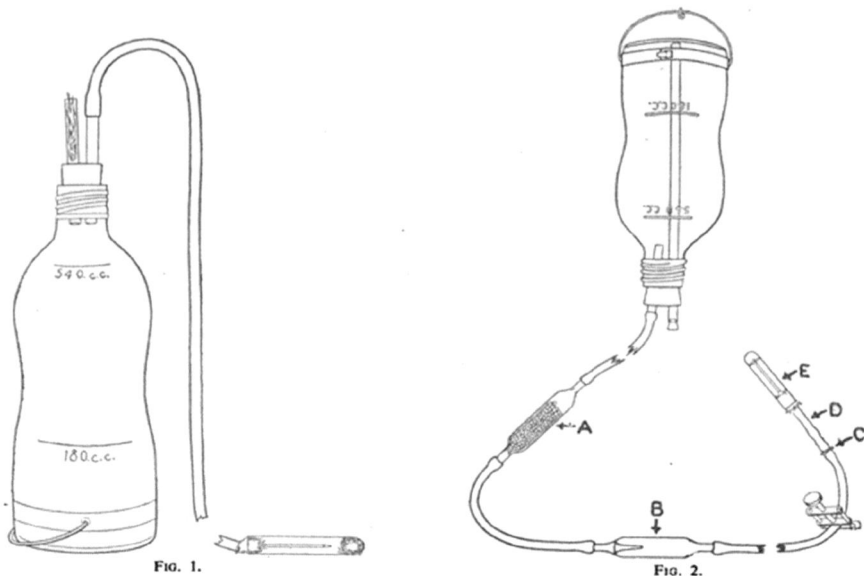

Image 14.1 The MRC bottle for blood donation and blood transfusion 1939. (Source: Vaughan J. M. The MRC bottle for blood donation and blood transfusion Vaughan J.M. Blood Transfusion Outfit. British Medical Journal, 1939, 2(4117), p. 1084. https://www.ncbi.nlm.nih.gov/pmc/articles/PMC2178860/pdf/brmedj04174-0013.pdf Accessed March 3, 2024. Permission for usage of this image was granted by the copyright holder, BMJ, on March 7, 2024)

Gnoinski in 1938.[2] The ampoules that were used were also made from glass.[3] In 1939, the Directors of the London Depots, in collaboration with the Medical Research Council (MRC), decided to standardize transfusion equipment. The MRC's standard transfusion kit included a modified milk bottle that was slightly curved to make it easier to hold. The bottle was fitted with an aluminum screw cap, which was lined with a rubber membrane, and at the bottom of the bottle, there was a metal strap and a loop to hang the bottle. The collection and administration assemblies were made of rubber tubing fitted with metal needles. Filters made of glass wool, glass beads, or knitted cotton were incorporated into the administration set or the neck of the bottle. The whole set was sterilized and the needles were sharpened after every use. The same equipment was used with minor modifications for almost three decades, and the MRC bottle was adopted for use in other countries (Image 14.1).[4] The bottle was

---

[2] DeGowin E.L. Storage and preservation of whole blood, chapter 13. In: DeGowin E. L., Hardin R. C., Alsever B. J. Blood transfusion. W.B. Saunders Company Philadelphia & London, 1949, p. 315.

[3] Grozdanić, Fišer-Herman, Maher, 1966, p. 193.

[4] Gunson H. H, Dodsworth H. From the 'MRC Blood Transfusion Outfit' to blood components chapter 4, In: Anstee D.J., Barbara J. A. J., Lincoln P. J., McClelland D. B. L., Voak D., editors. Fifty Years of Blood transfusion. Oxford: Blackwell Science. Blood transfusion Medicine. 1996, 6 (1), p. 25. https://www.infectedbloodinquiry.org.uk/evidence/nhbt0000028-fifty-years-blood-transfusion-01-jan-1996. Accessed 3 March 2024.

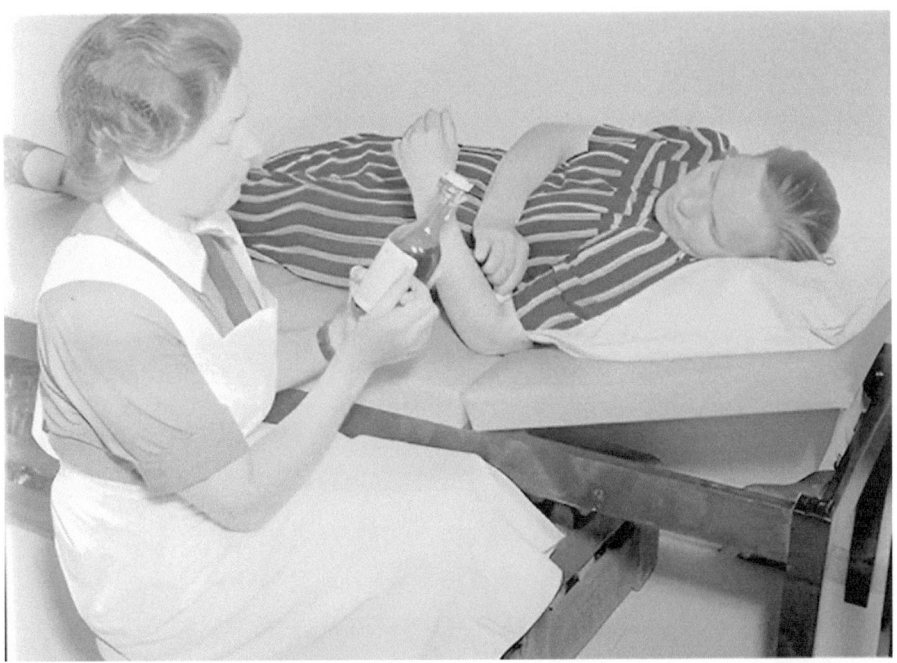

Image 14.2 Soda bottle with blood after the blood donation Finland 1941. (Source: Soda bottle with blood after the blood donation, Finland 1941. Finnish Armed Forces photograph SA-kuva. Creative Commons CC BY 4.0. http://sa-kuva.fi/neo# Accessed 9 March 2024)

marked at 180 cc and 540 cc for measuring the anticoagulant solution and blood. It was essential to mix the blood and anticoagulant in a gentle rotation throughout the time of collection.[5]

Despite the MRC bottle being used in several countries, it has to be noted that there were also other manufacturers of bottles from different countries with different dimensions and collection volumes that were used for decades in many different countries.

For comparison, the standard bottle for collection and blood transfusion in Finland in the 1940s was a soda bottle with a flip top (Image 14.2). The bottles were also known as Vichy bottles. The set includes a needle, a rubber bulb syringe, and a metal cannula that branches into two detachable rubber tubes. By pressing the bulb, the citrate blood in the bottle was pumped into the patient's vein via the tube and the needle.[6] Other similar bulb apparatuses worked on the same principle.

---

[5] Vaughan J.M. Blood Transfusion Outfit. British Medical Journal. 1939; 2(4117), p. 1084. https://www.ncbi.nlm.nih.gov/pmc/articles/PMC2178860/pdf/brmedj04174-0013.pdf.

[6] Hakkarainen S. A life-saving soda bottle, Helsinki University Museum. https://blogs.helsinki.fi/hum-object-of-the-month/2023/01/25/a-life-saving-soda-bottle/ Accessed 4 March 2024.

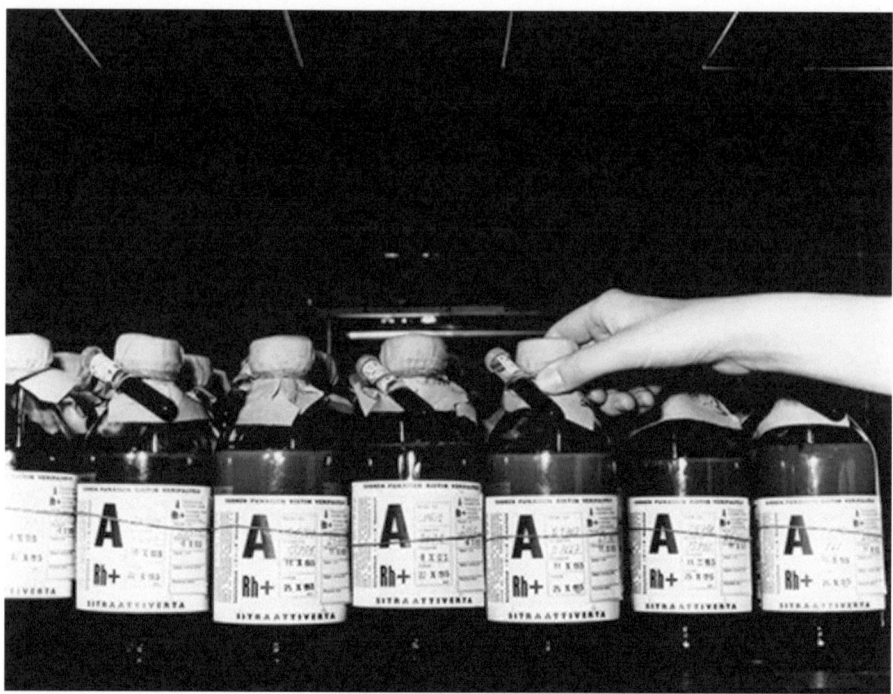

Image 14.3 Glass bottles containing blood, Finland 1960s. (Source: Finnish Red Cross Blood Service. History of Blood Service. Glass bottles containing blood, Finland, 1960s. https://www.veripalvelu.fi/en/history/ Accessed March 10, 2024. Permission for the use of this photograph was granted by Mr. Willy Toiviainen, Director of HR and Communications at the Finnish Red Cross Blood Service, on March 4, 2024)

However, in Finland, by the end of the 1940s, instead of soda bottles, they were already using a different-shaped model of a glass bottle in compliance with a Nordic standard, containing a citrate solution to prevent clotting of the blood (Image 14.3).[7]

Glass bottles had ground glass stoppers with a narrow or wide opening, and glass bottles with a wide neck closed with a rubber plate and an aluminum screw were used. Ampoules and bottles with glass stoppers had to be opened; that is, the cap had to be changed and accessories attached at the time of blood collection or transfusion. During this handling, there was a great possibility of contamination, and therefore, in order to prevent the development of possibly introduced microorganisms, bacteriostatic agents were added to the stabilizers. However, since 1950, many countries have switched to the so-called "closed system," namely, glass bottles closed with rubber stoppers or tiles were used to ensure this, which were tightened against the neck of the bottle using metal or bakelite closures. When donating blood or giving blood transfusion, the rubber was pierced with a needle, through

---

[7] Finnish Red Cross Blood Service. History of Blood Service. https://www.veripalvelu.fi/en/history/. Accessed 10 March 2024.

14.1 Equipment and Material for Whole Blood Collection

Image 14.4 Baxter Transfusovac set, USA 1938. (Source: Science Museum Group. Baxter Transfusovac set 1938. Creative Commons Attribution 4.0 license. https://collection.sciencemuseumgroup.org.uk/objects/co8692510/baxter-transfuso-vac-set-blood-taking-set Accessed March 10, 2024)

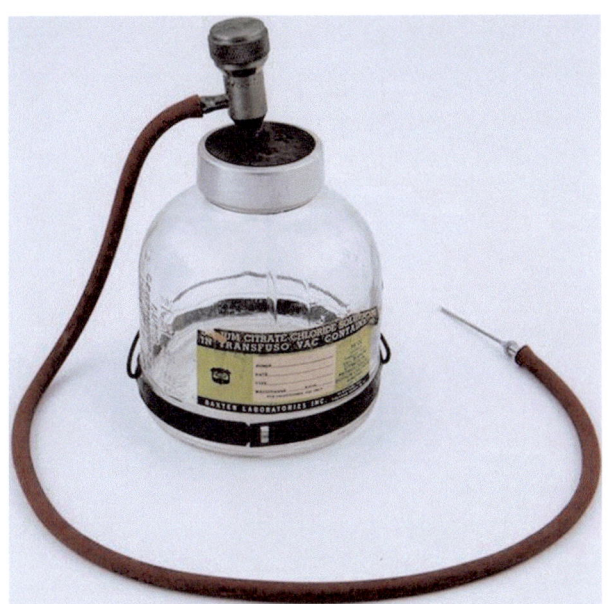

which the blood flowed into or out of the bottle. Along with this, many accessories were used that ensured that blood did not come into contact with air at any time during collection, storage, and donation.[8]

In the USA, the most popular blood donation set was Baxter Transfusovac (image 14.4). This set was used throughout World War II. Transfusovac bottles containing sodium citrate were more satisfactory from the standpoints of sterility as well as efficiency. The final contents of each flask were 500 cc. of blood, 70 cc. of citrate solution, and 5 cc. of 50 percent glucose solution, which were added before the flask was topped.[9] The Transfusovac bottle replaced the open beaker and the milk bottle in hospital practice by 1940.[10]

Also interesting facts, judging by the photographs of different countries at different time periods. In some countries, both the staff and the blood donors were dressed in their normal clothes or uniforms (Image 14.5). In other countries, only the staff wore protective clothes, and in other countries, both the staff and the blood donors wore protective clothes to prevent blood stains on their clothes and, especially, to ensure aseptic conditions for preventing the possible contamination of the glass bottle with blood. The protective uniforms included accessories as in an operating room (surgical hat, mask, gloves, etc.) (image 14.6). This also depended on which type of bottle was used (open or closed system), but this was not always the case. These sorts of protective uniforms were obsolete when plastic bags completely replaced the use of glass bottles, and that ensured a complete sterile closed system.

---

[8] Grozdanić, Fišer-Herman, Maher, 1966, p. 193.
[9] Kendrick, 1949, p. 589.
[10] Schmidt, 2012, p. 2.

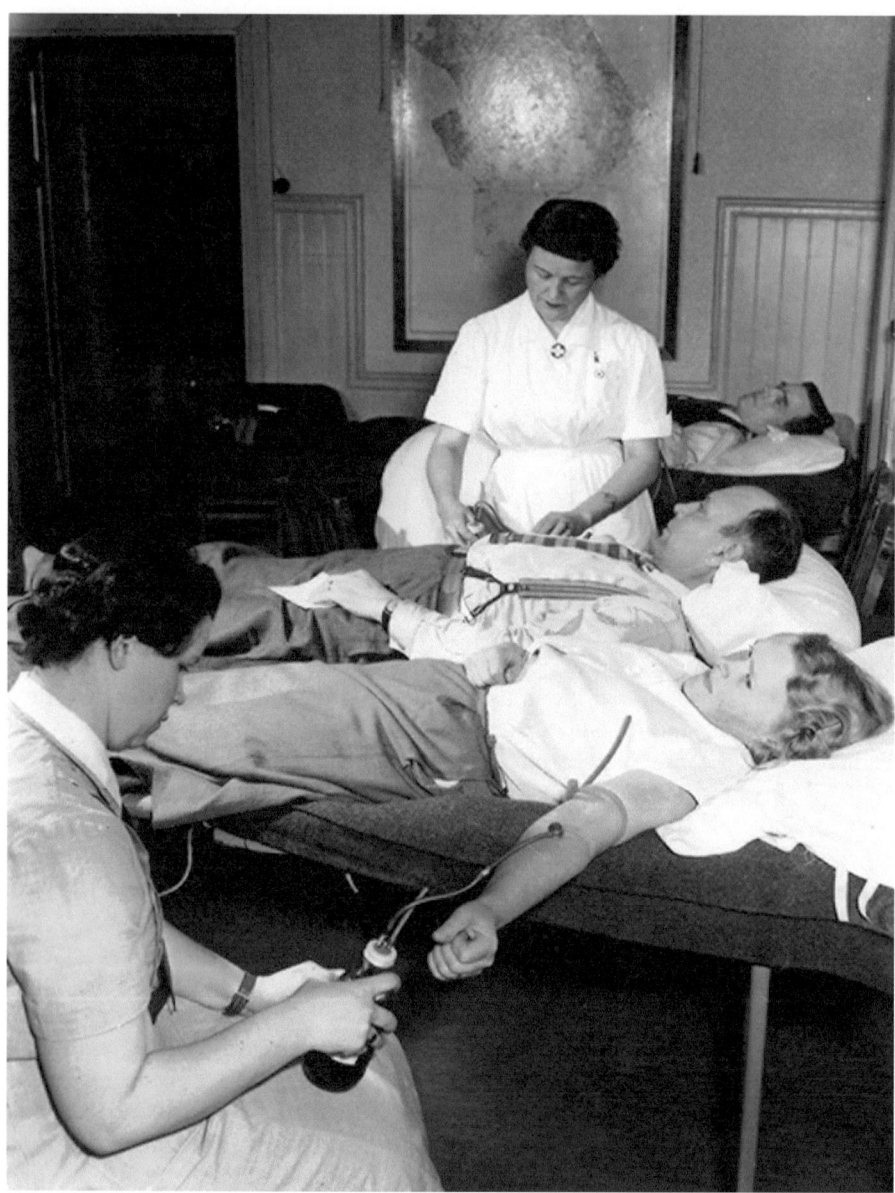

Image 14.5 Nurses drawing blood from blood donors in Sipoo Southern Finland 1955. (Source: Finnish Red Cross Blood Service. Nurses drawing blood from blood donors in sipoo, southern Finland 1955. https://www.veripalvelu.fi/en/history/ Accessed March 10, 2024. Permission for the use of this photograph was granted by Mr. Willy Toiviainen, Director of HR and Communications at the Finnish Red Cross Blood Service, on March 7, 2024)

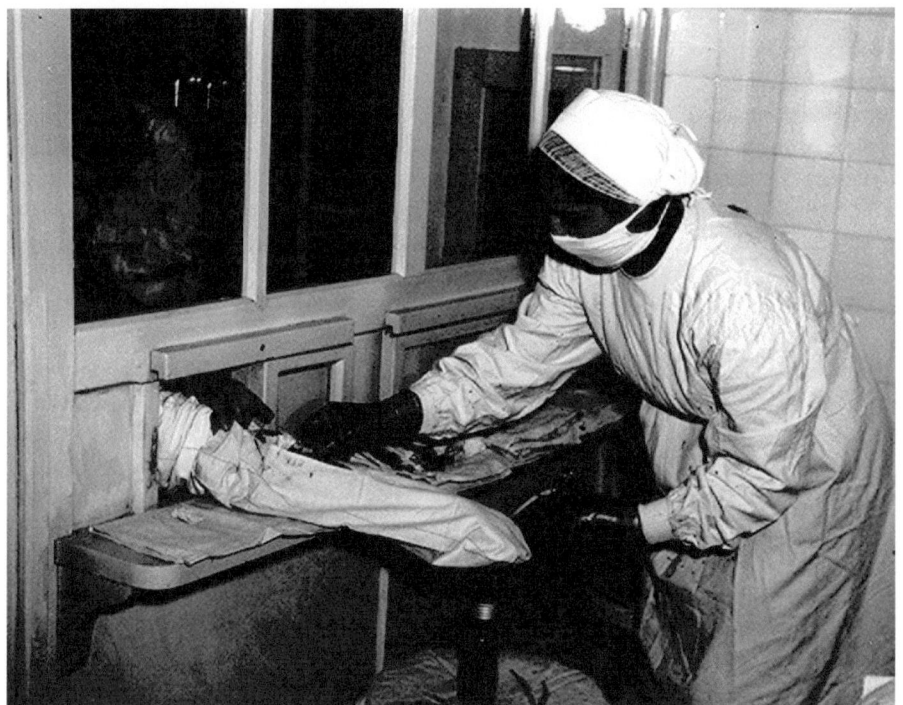

Image 14.6 Nurse drawing blood from blood donor at hospital blood transfusion department in city of Maribor 1956. (Source: Nurse drawing blood from blood donor at hospital blood transfusion department in city of Maribor 1956. From Večer https://vecer.com/ Slovenia, Public domain)

14.2 Equipment and Material Standards

The USA standards in 1949 for equipment were that all equipment had to be completely clean, pyrogen-free, and sterile.[11] Today's FDA standards have strict requirements regarding the equipment used in the collection, processing, compatibility testing, storage, and distribution of blood and blood components.[12] Strict standards are applied in Europe as well as in other parts of the world where there are strict mandatory regulations set up.

---

[11] Alsever J. B. Liquid plasma, chapter 16. In: DeGowin E. L., Hardin R. C., Alsever B. J. Blood transfusion. W.B. Saunders Company Philadelphia & London, 1949, p. 362–394.

[12] FDA. Part 606—current good manufacturing practice for blood and blood components. https://www.ecfr.gov/current/title-21/chapter-I/subchapter-F/part-606 Accessed 10 March 2024.

In the USA, there are also, as in Europe, medical device regulations. These regulations are commonly referred to as general controls applying to all sorts of medical devices. The Food, Drug, and Cosmetics Act (FDCA) Medical Device Amendments, which was enacted on May 28, 1976, contained the fundamental rules known as general controls. In order to guarantee the safety and efficacy of devices, they give the FDA the tools necessary for regulation. All medical devices are subject to general restrictions under the FDCA. They cover topics like adulteration, misbranding, premarket notification, device registration and listing, prohibited devices, records and reporting, and good manufacturing practices.[13]

Blood can be obtained and used in clinical settings using a variety of quality management systems (QMSs). While some focus more on management issues and ensure a quality environment and culture, which are essential for the consistency and dependability of the operational processes, others are "process-oriented and operations-oriented." "Good Manufacturing Practice (GMP) and Good Hospital Practice (GHP) are the most suitable QS for a blood establishment and a hospital, respectively." The FDCA Amendments of 1962 included the prototype system, which was developed in the United States and subsequently put into use for the production of human pharmaceuticals in 1963. Blood and blood derivatives were included in the Biologics Act by the US Congress in 1970, and the FDA released GMP guidelines in 1975. The first GMP regulations were established in Europe gradually, and in 1992, the EU passed a directive titled "GMP for Proprietary Medicinal Products for Human and Veterinary Use." Blood products ought to be generated in compliance with pharmaceutical principles since they serve a medicinal purpose. Aseptic conditions must be maintained during the collection and processing of human blood or plasma. In the pharmaceutical sector, raw materials must be processed into sterile or aseptic final products, typically in large batch quantities. There are various methods, like the European Foundation for Quality Management (EFQM) and the ISO 9001 series, to handle such "operations-oriented QS."[14] At the fourth International Congress of the International Society of Blood Transfusion held in Lisbon in 1951, the following resolution was adopted: "Owing to the urgent need of interchangeability of transfusion equipment, the IVth International Congress of Blood Transfusion held in Lisbon in July 1951 recommends: *that the transfusion equipment used by the various national services should, as much as is possible, be prepared in such a way that the bottle or the transfusion equipment of each country may be used indifferently with the corresponding transfusion equipment of the other countries.*" The suggestion that standardization work should be carried out on an

---

[13] Mintz P.D., Weinstein M.J. Chapter 7 - Global perspective on ensuring blood and blood product safety and availability. In: Simon TL, McCullough J., Snyder E. L., Solheim BG, Strauss RG., editors. Rossi's Principles of Transfusion Medicine, fifth Edition. USA: Wiley Blackwell. 2016, p. 73.

[14] Sibinga S., Hasan F. Quality management or the need for a quality culture in transfusion medicine. Global Journal of Transfusion Medicine. 2020; 5(1)1, p. 10–11. file:///C:/Users/zdrav/Downloads/Quality_management_or_the_need_for_a_quality_cultu.pdf

14.2 Equipment and Material Standards

international scale was first discussed at a meeting of the Committee of the International Standardization Organization (ISO) on Laboratory Glassware in 1950, when it was proposed to the ISO Council that a new technical committee of ISO be formed for this purpose. The ISO Council adopted the recommendation made by its Technical Committee on Laboratory Glassware, and accordingly, a technical committee, ISO/TC 76: Transfusion Equipment for Medical Use, was prepared in 1951. The first meeting of ISO/TC 76 was held in London at the British Standards Institution from March 3–5, 1952. The essential resolutions were made regarding containers, closure, piercing needles, needle mounts, tubing, filters, and drip counters. By 1955, there were 26 countries worldwide that were members of the ISO/TC/76. [15] World Health Organization (WHO) in 1981 and 1984 laid down the standardization requirements for the blood group reagents that the manufacturers had to comply with.[16] The introduction of ISO 9001:2000 (International Organization for Standardization) that specified requirements for a quality management system was also important for the entire chain of professional fields in transfusion medicine. These included quality management and change control, personnel and organization, and premises. Including mobile sites, equipment and materials, documentation, blood donation, processing, storage and distribution, quality monitoring, quality control and laboratory testing, contract management, deviations, complaints, adverse events and reactions, recall, corrective, and preventive actions, self-inspection, audits, and improvement.[17] The current issue of this directive is ISO 9001:2015. [18] The Medicines Control Agency (MCA), which was in charge of regulating medicines in the UK, and the Medical Devices Agency (MDA), which was in charge of medical device regulation, merged to form the Medicines and Healthcare Products Regulatory Agency (MHRA) in April 2003.[19] Directive 89/381/EEC from 1989 relating to proprietary medicinal products and laying down special provisions for medicinal products derived from human blood or human plasma was a great contribution to establishing legal provisions for plasma derivates. After this new directive in 1996, for blood safety and self-sufficiency, the European Council

---

[15] Tovey G. H. Section IV Organization, C- Travaux des organisms internationaux. International Standardization of Transfusion Equipment of Medical Use. In: Berroche L., Eyquem A., Julliard J., Mailloux M., Maupin B., Moullec J. Perrot H., Saint-Paul M., Sam Lewi, editors. Immuno-hématologie: techniques sérologiques = Immuno-hematology. Drépanocytose thalassémie [u.a.]. Ve Congrès International de Transfusion Sanguine. Paris: Croutzet; 1955, p. 1100–1105.

[16] Wagstaff W. Quality assurance of transfusion centre derived blood products, chapter 1. In: Cash J. D., editor. Progress in transfusion medicine, volume 22. London: Churchill Livingstone; 1987, p. 10.

[17] Faber J.C., Boulton F., Rouger P. Comments on the EU Blood Directive 2002/98/CE, chapter 2. In: Rouger P., Hossenlopp C., editors. Blood Transfusion in Europe. The White Book 2005. Paris: Elsevier; 2005, p. 44–45.

[18] ISO. ISO 9001:2015, Quality management systems Requirements. https://www.iso.org/standard/62085.html. Accessed 1 April 2024.

[19] Breckenridge A. The changing scene of the regulation of medicines in the UK. Paper from The Use of Medicines: Regulation & Clinical Pharmacology in the twenty-first Century Symposium - December 2003. British journal of clinical pharmacology. 2004;58 (8), p. 571–574. https://www.ncbi.nlm.nih.gov/pmc/articles/PMC1884637/.

adopted Resolution 96/C374/01. After this, in 1998, the European Commission issued Council Recommendation 98/463/EEC on the suitability of blood and plasma donors and the screening of donated blood in the European Community. In 1999, the Treaty of Amsterdam, Article 152, 4(a), invited the European Parliament and the Council to adopt measures that set high standards for the quality and safety of organs and substances of human origin, including blood and blood derivatives. Based on the basis of this article, a proposal for a European Blood Directive was submitted by the European Commission in December 2000, and on January 27, 2003, the Directive 2002/98/EC was adopted and published in the Official Journal of the European Union. On February 8, 2003, the Directive of the European Parliament and of the Council setting standards of quality and safety for the collection, testing, processing, storage, and distribution of human blood and blood components and amending Directive 2001/83/EC was born.[20] By 2010, there were also several European (EU) guidelines for blood banking. These were the already mentioned general standards for the quality and safety of human blood and blood components (EU Directive 2002/98/EC), then there were the technical standards (Directive 2004/33/EC), quality systems (2005/62/EC), and traceability (2005/61/EC). Today in Europe, materials, reagents, and equipment must meet the requirements of Regulation (EU) medical devices and Regulation (EU) 2017/746 (repealing Directive 98/79/EC) of the European Parliament and of the Council for in vitro diagnostic medical devices, or comply with equivalent standards in the case of collection in third countries (Directive 2005/62/EC, Annex 4.3). These requirements include general requirements, data processing systems, qualification and validation, process validation, validation of test methods, change control, and control of equipment and materials.[21]

14.2.1 Plastic Bags in Transfusion Medicine

The idea of using plastic equipment for the blood container was first discussed at the Symposium on Blood Preservation held under the auspices of the Committee on Blood and Blood Derivatives, National Research Council, on December 2, 1949. Carl Walter (1905–1992), who was a surgeon, inventor, and professor, introduced the criteria for the blood bag as follows: 1. simple, one-piece equipment that would permit hermetic sealing during processing, storage, and transportation of the blood and that could be employed with a bacteriologically safe technique; 2. a slow rate of collection, causing minimal physiological disturbance to the donor; 3. the elimination of air vents, both during collection (by venous pressure and gravity) and during administration; 4. transparency; 5. non-wettability; 6. compressibility, to permit positive pressure infusion; 7. stability to sterilizing temperatures (121 °C for 30 min); 8. low vapor transmission; 9. good tissue tolerance. It was additionally specified, in view of the logistic difficulties, that the plastic equipment

---

[20] Faber, Boulton, Rouger, 2005, p. 38–39.
[21] EDQM GUIDE, 2023, p. 57–82.

14.2 Equipment and Material Standards

recommended must be light-weight, unbreakable, collapsible, and sized to accommodate the volume of liquid it was intended to contain. Also, it had to be inexpensive enough to warrant discarding after a single use.[22] The early research of Carl W. Walter in search for the appropriate plastic film and tubing began in fall of 1947.[23]

Dr. Walter's studies had been carried out with equipment fabricated from elastic thermoplastic vinylite resin that incorporated an ion-exchange column of sulfonated polystyrene copolymer. Blood was collected in this apparatus, essentially as in regular collecting bottles. After the bag had been filled by gravity, the tourniquet was released, and a spring clip was placed across the tube distal to the exchange column. Samples for testing were collected in pilot tubes before the needle was removed from the vein. The tube was sealed or knotted close to the bag, and the bag of blood, after being hermetically sealed, was refrigerated. The transfusion could be given by suspending the bag from a gravity pole by the grommet provided, or the blood could be squeezed into the recipient's vein by placing the bag under his shoulder or buttock. If rapid transfusion was desired, the intra-arterial technique was used, or the operator could stand on the bag. Although it took slightly longer to collect the blood than when bottles were used, the quality and yield of the blood collected were equal, if not superior, to the quality and yield of the blood collected in bottles. Moreover, blood collected in plastic bags practically never had to be discarded because of hemolysis. The bags did not require refrigeration before the blood was collected. A plastic bag containing 500 cc. of blood occupies only half the space of a bottle holding the same amount, and it was used in the Korean War.[24] Walter designed this model in 1950 together with his colleague William Parry Murphy Jr. (1923–2023), who was a medical doctor and inventor.[25] Walter in 1950, regarding the material for equipment, additionally stated that the equipment fabricated of a polyvinyl chloride resin base material, for example, a polyvinyl chloride acetate copolymer, has been found to meet all the requirements.[26] Walter and Murphy Jr. introduced a collapsible bag in 1952 containing 75 mL of ACD solution A. The bag contained a plastic donor tube and a needle. The bag was sterilized with saturated steam.[27] Newly developed poly-

---

[22] Wandell, F. A. (1968). Plastic in Blood Transfusion—Plastic Containers—Development of Criteria. In International Society of Blood Transfusion, 11th Congress, Karger Publishers. 1966; Part 3 (Vol. 29,) p. 978–988. https://karger.com/books/book/416/chapter-abstract/5569976/Plastic-in-Blood-Transfusion-Plastic-Containers?redirectedFrom=fulltext.

[23] Walter Car.l W. Invention and development of the blood bag. Vox Sanguinis. 1984; 47 (6), p. 318–319. https://www.semanticscholar.org/paper/Invention-and-Development-of-the-Blood-Bag-Walter/a467ad1e71abe108b5dc581fb73fae9664c338aa.

[24] Kendrick, 1964, p. 758–759.

[25] AABB. in memoriam: william p. murphy, jr., md. https://www.aabb.org/news-resources/news/article/2023/12/06/in-memoriam%2D%2Dwilliam-p.-murphy%2D%2Djr.%2D%2Dmd Accessed 10 March 2024.

[26] Walter C. W. Apparatus for collecting, storing, and dispensing whole blood. https://patents.google.com/patent/US2702034A/en?q=(blood)&q=(bag)&q=(container)&q=(needle)&q=(collection)&before=priority:19530430&scholar Accessed 17 March 2024.

[27] Carmen R. The selection of plastic materials for blood bags. Transfusion medicine reviews. 1993; 7(:1), p. 1–10. https://europepmc.org/article/med/8431654.

vinyl chloride (PVC) plastic multiple-bag collection systems in the early 1980s made it easy and safe to prepare blood components with virtually no risk of air embolism or contamination, sometimes a problem with glass containers. The red cell concentrate was prepared and stored in the primary bag of the collection system, and depending on the number of integrally attached transfer packs, a platelet concentrate, fresh frozen plasma, cryoprecipitate, or cryoprecipitate-poor fresh frozen plasma were prepared.[28] Since the innovation of plastic bags, many manufacturers have gradually produced blood bags of different types. Also important to mention regarding the structure of the material that vinylite, a copolymer of vinyl chloride and vinyl acetate, differs slightly from PVC homopolymer in terms of composition.

By the late 1950s, the largest hospitals in the USA and Canada were using plastic equipment, at least for some of their transfusion requirements. It took quite some time for plastic bags to be distributed from the USA across the world and manufactured elsewhere. There were several reasons for this, including some as follows: In the UK, the plastic bag set could be used only once in comparison with rubber sets, which could be used up to four times. There was also a concern that the staff who sharpened needles and assembled rubber sets for glass bottles would lose their jobs. There was also concern regarding the manufacturing of plastic bags since there was only one factory in the UK, which was opened there in 1960. The main issue was the price, since plastic bags cost more than glass bottles with rubber sets. By 1962, plastic sets were still in the minority, up until July 1975, when plastic bags replaced glass bottles.[29] For comparison, in 1976, plastic blood bags were mostly used in the USA and Europe, but in Japan, they still used glass bottles.[30] Plastic bags in Finland were used for the first time in 1957. They gradually replaced glass bottles in the 1960s. At the same time, component therapy was introduced.[31] Despite initial concerns, it was proven that the plastic bags for transfusion medicine were better than the glass bottles. Handling and storing the heavy, delicate bottles required extreme caution. For reuse, they also needed to be cleaned and sterilized. Blood components could be transported and kept considerably more conveniently. The process of separating platelets, plasma, and cryoprecipitate using glass bottles proved difficult, inconsistent, and prone to bacterial contamination.[32] The inadequate sterility of glass bottles lead to bacterial contamination, and the presence of air bubbles lead to

---

[28] Valeri C. R. New developments in red blood cell preservation using liquid and freezing procedures. J Clin Lab Auto, 1982; 2, p. 6. https://apps.dtic.mil/sti/tr/pdf/ADA140442.pdf Accessed 24 March 2024.

[29] Gunson, Dodsworth, 1996, p. 27–28.

[30] Sasakawa S.; Tokunaga E. Physical and chemical changes of ACD-preserved blood: a comparison of blood in glass bottles and plastic bags. Vox Sanguinis. 1976; 31 (4), p. 199–200. https://karger.com/vox/article-abstract/31/3/199/311820/Physical-and-Chemical-Changes-of-ACD-Preserved.

[31] Finnish Red Cross Blood Service, 2024.

[32] The Royal College of Pathologists. Object 47: Plastic blood bag. https://www.rcpath.org/static/1c305fd3-6e4e-4427-802aa646720ec6e8/47-Plastic-Blood-Bag.pdf Accessed 10 March 2024.

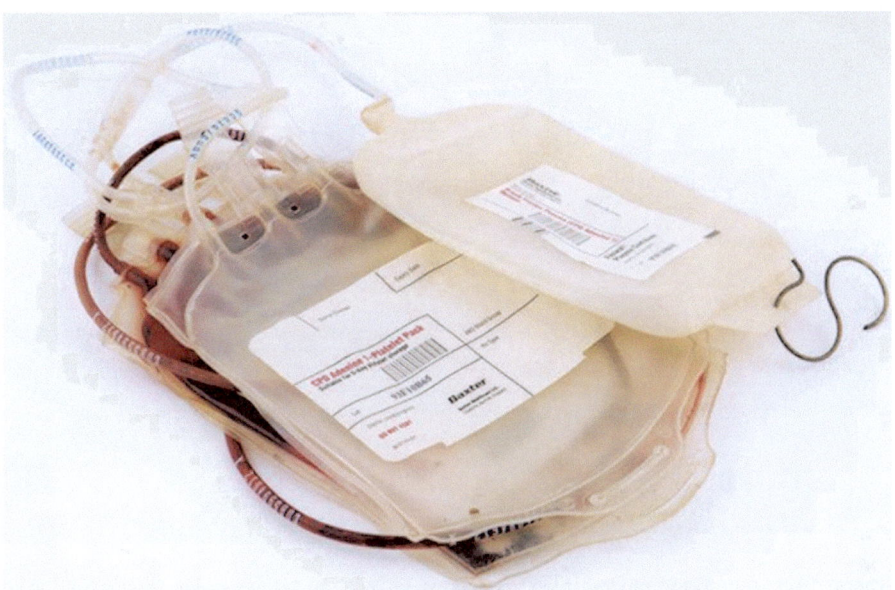

Image 14.7 Fenwal triple blood pack for storage of whole blood used in transfusions, by Baxter healthcare ltd, Thetford, Norfolk, supplied by South Thames blood transfusion service 1993–1994. (Source: Science Museum Group. Fenwal triple blood pack for storage of whole blood used in transfusions, by Baxter Healthcare Ltd., Thetford, Norfolk, supplied by South Thames Blood Transfusion Service, 1993–1994. Creative Commons Attribution 4.0 license. https://collection.sciencemuseumgroup.org.uk/objects/co143636/fenwal-triple-blood-pack-for-storage-of-whole-blood-used-in-transfusions-medical-equipment. Accessed 10 March 2024)

severe complications during blood transfusion.[33] In 1957, platelet concentrates were recognized for reducing mortality from hemorrhage in cancer patients.[34]

With the plastic blood bag, component therapy was easier and, most importantly, safer (Image 14.7). Eventually, double bags were made for the preparation of platelet concentrates, with platelet-poor plasma being put back onto the packed cells. This led to the production of triple-and quadruple-bag systems for the collection of plasma for fractionation and the preparation of cryoprecipitate.[35] The plastic bag systems also have a sample bag, from which the blood samples are taken into tubes for further testing.

Today, blood bags must comply with the requirements of the relevant regulations (such as EU directives, the European Pharmacopoeia, and ISO standards). Polyvinylchloride (PVC) with an adequate plasticizer is satisfactory for red blood

---

[33] Jegrelius institute for applied green chemistry. Blood bags- history, p. 10 https://pvcfreebloodbag.eu/wp-content/uploads/2013/11/BloodBags_final_report_krcopy.pdf Accessed 10 March 2024.

[34] Ajmani, P.S. History of Blood Transfusion. In: Immunohematology and Blood banking. Springer, Singapore. 2020, p. 121.

[35] Carmen 1993, p. 1–10.

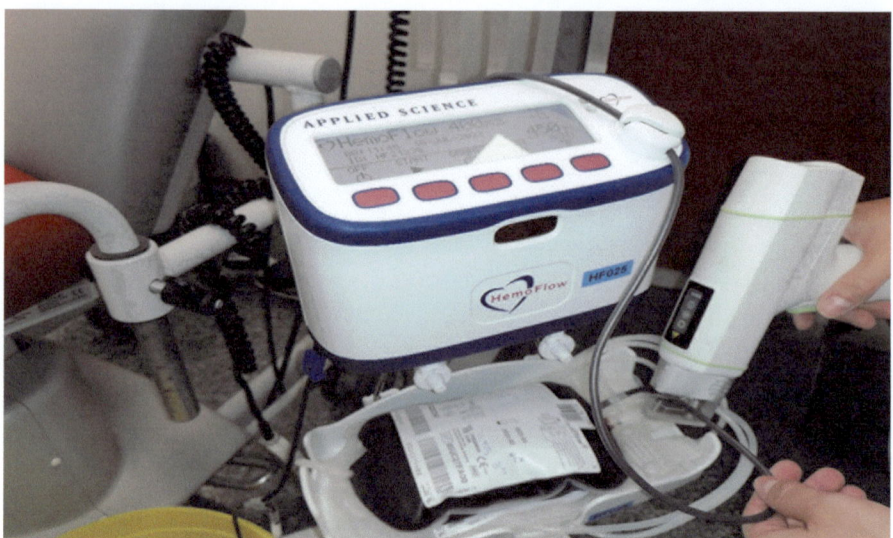

Image 14.8 Automated modern blood collection mixer with a tube sealer. (Source: Zdravko Kvržić. Automated modern blood collection mixer with a tube sealer. Permission to reuse the image from the article Zdravko Kvržić, Odvzem polne krvi pri krvodajalcu skozi različna zgodovinska obdobja (1875–2023). Utrip 31 (6), August–September, p. 17–21, was given by the Nurses and Midwives Association of Slovenia on November 29, 2023. The permission was also obtained from the V.D. director of the Blood Transfusion Center of Slovenia, Peter Kavčič, M.Sc. business and economic. Science, on November 24, 2023)

cell storage. Platelets stored between +20 °C and + 24 °C require a plastic with increased oxygen permeability, such as special polyolefins or PVC with butyryl trihexyl citrate (BTHC) plasticizer.[36]

14.2.2 Whole Blood and Apheresis Technology

For blood donation or the donation of different components and the separation of whole blood, different technologies are used. This includes automated blood collection mixers with or without sealers, automated apheresis machines, and information technology.

14.2.2.1 Blood Collection Mixers

Automated blood collection mixers, also known as blood collection scales or automatic blood collectors, are a combination of a scale and mixer devices with an adjustable or preset volume that collect whole blood (Image 14.8). The color touchscreen display enables the operator to easily monitor the procedure. During the blood donation, the removable mixing tray on which the blood bag lies mixes the

---

[36] EDQM GUIDE, 2023, p. 185.

14.2 Equipment and Material Standards

blood with the anticoagulant to prevent blood clots. The devices also weigh the amount of blood, display the precise collection volume in progress, flow rate, elapsed time, and estimated time. The devices alarm the operator if they detect any errors during the procedure, such as a change in the speed of blood flow or other technical errors. The devices also signal when a sufficient amount of whole blood has been collected. The devices automatically end the procedure by clamping the bag system tube. The blood bag is then separated from the needle system with a tube sealer. They also record and send data to the information system. Some of these devices have integrated laser barcode scanners, while others have a single-line handheld laser barcode scanner. These devices can be used to collect whole blood from blood donors, collect blood for patients for autotransfusion, or as a treatment for patients with blood dyscrasias. There are differences in the designs of these devices that are all unique in their own way.

The first models were quite different in their performance from the modern versions. The apparatus of Max Strumia for the collection and cooling of blood on April 30, 1953, was released to the public on May 8, 1958. The method for collecting blood, according to this invention, comprised withdrawing the blood from the vein of a donor at a constant controlled rate, cooling the blood continuously as it was withdrawn, mixing the cooled blood with anticoagulant solution by agitation at a constant rate, maintaining a constant low temperature during the mixing, continuously measuring the exact amount of blood collected, and stopping the withdrawal of blood when the desired amount had been withdrawn. The apparatus comprised a tank for containing a cooling liquid, which was water, brine, or other suitable coolant, and which provided a circulating line with a circulating pump. The cooling liquid was cooled with ice or by circulating a coolant through suitable heat-exchange pipes that were connected to a refrigerating system (not shown). A temperature gauge was provided to indicate the temperature of the liquid in the tank. The blood withdrawn from the donor at the normal temperature of 37 °C was delivered to the collecting bag at a temperature of about 8 °C. Lower temperatures could be obtained by using longer tubing and a larger number of coils, or by using a cooling liquid. The container was designed to accommodate a plastic collapsible blood collection bag. This device was also used for collecting the whole blood from a patient's vein.[37]

Different models of blood collection mixers gradually emerged in the 1980s. On May 19, 1981, the device of Robert W. Purdy and Don A. Arneson Sbr Lab Inc. was released in public. This device was called the "Standard Blood Ratiometer." The primary object of this device was to provide a method and apparatus for collecting blood from a donor in a controlled manner so as to minimize trauma to the blood so collected. Conventional blood collection bags from that period consisted of a donor blood transfer tube attached to a main collection bag in which anticoagulant was placed during manufacture. Also connected to the main collection bag by similar but separate tubing were one or more satellite bags similar in construction but smaller than the main collection bag. These satellite bags usually contained no

---

[37] Strumia M. M. Apparatus for the collection and cooling of blood, 1958. https://patents.google.com/patent/US2845929A/en Accessed 16 march 2024.

liquid. The satellite bags were isolated from the main bag by a tube diaphragm, which was opened when the use of the satellite bag was desired. Conventional blood collection procedures involve approximately one pint of blood (450 mL) in a plastic bag containing 63–75 mL of anticoagulant. Nearly all of the conventional anticoagulants, such as ACD, CPD, and CPD-Adenine, are highly acidic, having a pH in the range of 4.95 to 5.63. In addition, these anticoagulants contain the complexing agent citrate, which was at that time known to strip RBC of essential cations, e.g., Ca^{+2} and Mg^{+2}. The initial exposure of blood collected into the bag containing the anticoagulant caused trauma to a high percentage of the early collected cells because of the relatively hostile environment presented by the high proportion of anticoagulant. As the proportion of blood to anticoagulant increased, this tendency diminished, but the damaged early cells still remained within the collection bag. In that period, conventional blood collection procedures were also found to have an adverse effect on the stability of blood coagulation factors (particularly Factors V and VIII) in plasma and also had an adverse effect on the preservation of platelet function. This device from Sbr Lab Inc. comprised two plastic bags, one of which contained a liquid anticoagulant and the other of which served as a receiving bag for the collected blood. The collection bag was connected to a resilient means, which allowed the collection bag to descend vertically due to the weight of the blood collected. The anticoagulant bag was interconnected by a suitable tube, and the anticoagulant was injected into the collected blood at a controlled rate so as to maintain a substantially constant ratio of blood to anticoagulant. The device also allowed the blood and the anticoagulant to flow freely together at a fixed rate during the entire collection process. This improved method and apparatus removed the initial shock of the high concentration of anticoagulant. Another important aspect of the device was that the main collection bag, which was wetted with anticoagulant prior to the introduction of blood, thus precluded undesired coagulation or clotting.[38] The next interesting invention was the "Hemolator" by the inventors Ronald O. Gilcher, Allen Latham Jr., Jonathan D. Schiff, and Donald W. Schoendorfer from the Haemonetics Corporation. This device was released on May 31st, 1983. The hemolator consisted of a 500-cc flexible plastic bag that was supplied with a 75-cc anticoagulant. The bag was placed in a rigid chamber. A vacuum between the inside of the chamber and the outside of the bag was created by a vacuum pump, causing negative pressure inside the bag. Blood flowed from a donor's vein, which was under a slight positive pressure, through a needle and tube to the bag, which was under controlled negative pressure. Means were supplied for agitating the bag while the blood was being drawn, as also for automatically detecting and measuring the presence of a desired amount of fluid volume in the bag. The rate of flow of blood into the bag was determined by the adjustment of a vacuum regulator valve. During the collection of blood, the chamber was continuously pumped and maintained at a level of vacuum

---

[38] Purdy R. W., Arneson D. A. Blood collection monitoring device and method, 1981. https://patents.google.com/patent/US4267837A/en?oq=US+patent+5147330 Accessed 16 March 2024.

14.2 Equipment and Material Standards

as determined by the setting of a screw on the vacuum regulator valve.[39] On March 15, 1989, the automatic blood mixer of an inventor, Bai Yichang Zhang Shuping, of the Institute of Automation of Heilongjiang Academy of Sciences, was released to the public. This device, with an attached tray, was used for many things, such as blood sampling and blood donation. During work, the mixing dish, powered by a motor, was swung up and down.[40] On October 18, 1989, the devices of Arne Kogel of Ljungberg and Kögel Ab from Sweden were released to the public. This device also had a tray that moved on an axle. The device had a weight measurement function and a control circuit, which was constructed to control at least the clamping device.[41] The device of Matsumi Toya and Yasuyuki Miyairi of Tiyoda Seisakusho KK and SB Kawasumi Laboratories Inc., released to the public on May 8, 1990, had a box-shaped casing. This device collected blood via a collapsible inflow pipe into an inflatable bag with an anticoagulant prefilled therein. The bag was placed on a weighing platform coupled to a load cell, which produced an electric voltage signal representative of the weight of the blood being collected in the bag. The load cell was mounted on a swing cradle capable of oscillation about a horizontal axis, so that the bag was shaken during blood collection to intimately intermingle the collected blood and the anticoagulant. When a predetermined amount of blood was collected, as ascertained from the voltage output of the load cell, a controller actuated a collection stop mechanism, thereby causing the same to tightly grip and collapse the inflow pipe.[42] By 1992, there were several models with a tray on the market. Some models included a bag-carrying surface that was caused to rock forward and backward with the aid of a crank device that rotated about an axle that extended perpendicularly to the bag-carrying surface. It was also known to provide such cradles with a weight-measuring device that functioned to measure the amount of blood that had flowed into the bag and to produce an alarm signal when blood flowed too quickly or too slowly into the bag.[43] Since then, commercial producers have developed a variety of models.

14.2.2.2 Apheresis Technology

The term *"apheresis"* is the Greek word for "to separate." Automated apheresis machines of different kinds allow the collection of specific blood components during the apheresis process. The remaining components are returned to the donor's bloodstream. The collected blood components are used to treat patients. The blood

---

[39] Gilcher R.O., Latham A., Schiff J.D., Schoendorfer D. V. Blood donation unit, 1983. https://patents.google.com/patent/US4385630A/en Accessed 16 march 2024.
[40] Shuping B. Y. Z. Automatic blood mixer, 1989. https://patents.google.com/patent/CN2034039U/en. Accessed 16 March 2024.
[41] Kögel A. Blood Rock, 1989. https://patents.google.com/patent/SE8903440D0/en?q=(~patent%2fUS5147330A). Accessed 16 March 2024.
[42] Toya M., Miyairi Y. Apparatus for collecting constant amounts of blood from individual donors, 1990. https://patents.google.com/patent/US4923449A/en. Accessed 16 March 2024.
[43] Kögel A. Blood cradle, 1992. https://patents.google.com/patent/US5147330A/en?oq=US+patent+5147330. Accessed 16 march 2024.

components can be obtained from blood donors or from patients. There are different types of apheresis procedures that are different in the duration of collection, type of collected blood components, and intention. Because the whole blood is returned to the donor, the apheresis procedure can be performed more frequently.

Apheresis, also known as pheresis or hemapheresis procedures, can be divided into two categories: cytapheresis, where the cellular elements are removed, and plasmapheresis, where plasma is removed. There are different types of cytapheresis, as well as plasmapheresis. Cytapheresis includes leukocytapheresis, adsorptive cytapheresis, extracorporeal photopheresis, plateletpheresis, thrombocytapheresis, erythrocytapheresis, and red cell exchange. Plasmapheresis includes plasmapheresis, therapeutic plasma exchange, double-filtration plasmapheresis, rheopheresis, immunoadsorption, and lipid apheresis. The means by which the separation of blood components is performed is by centrifugation, membrane filtration, or a combination. Centrifugation uses centrifugal force and blood component-specific gravity to separate the elements in the blood. Membrane filtration separates elements based on size. Blood is anticoagulated prior to extensive contact with the tubing.[44] There are also two types of flows for the apheresis procedure. One is continuous, and the other is discontinuous flow centrifugation. In continuous flow, blood components are simultaneously removed, processed, and reinfused. Continuous flow systems require two sites of vascular access or a central apheresis line with two lumens, but they have the advantage of more rapid procedures and higher hemodynamic stability. The discontinuous flow centrifugation involves the processing of small volumes of blood in cycles (a cycle consists of blood withdrawal, processing, and reinfusion). Compared to continuous flow devices, the use of discontinuous flow has the benefit of single-site venous access; nevertheless, the procedure takes longer and results in greater fluctuations in extracorporeal blood volume and hemodynamics.[45]

In 1877, Swedish engineer and inventor Karl Gustaf Patrik de Laval (1845–1913) invented the earliest continuous flow centrifugation device with his hand-cranked cream separator.[46] The idea for plasmapheresis came in 1914 from an American biochemist and pharmacologist named John Jacob Abel (1857–1913). In 1914, he and his colleagues Rowntree and Turner published a paper titled "*Plasma removal with corpuscle return (plasmaphaeresis*) (image 14.9)." They experimented on dogs, from which they took plasma and returned the rest of the blood. They named

---

[44] Burgstaler E. A. Winters J. L. Apheresis: principles and technology of hemapheresis, chapter 32. In: Simon TL, McCullough J., Snyder E. L., Solheim BG, Strauss RG., editors. Rossi's Principles of Transfusion Medicine, fifth Edition. USA: Wiley Blackwell. 2016, p. 1–14.

[45] Canadian Blood Services: Chapter 14, therapeutic apheresis. https://professionaleducation.blood.ca/en/transfusion/clinical-guide/therapeutic-apheresis Accessed 19 March 2024.

[46] Corbin F., Cullis H.M., Freireich E.J., Ito J., Kellogg R.M., Lathman Jr. A., McLeod B.C. Development of apheresis instrumentation- chapter 1.In McLeod B.C., Price T.H., Weinstein R.,editors. Apheresis principles and practice second Edition. Maryland USA: American Association of Blood Banks (AABB); 2003, p. 2.

14.2 Equipment and Material Standards

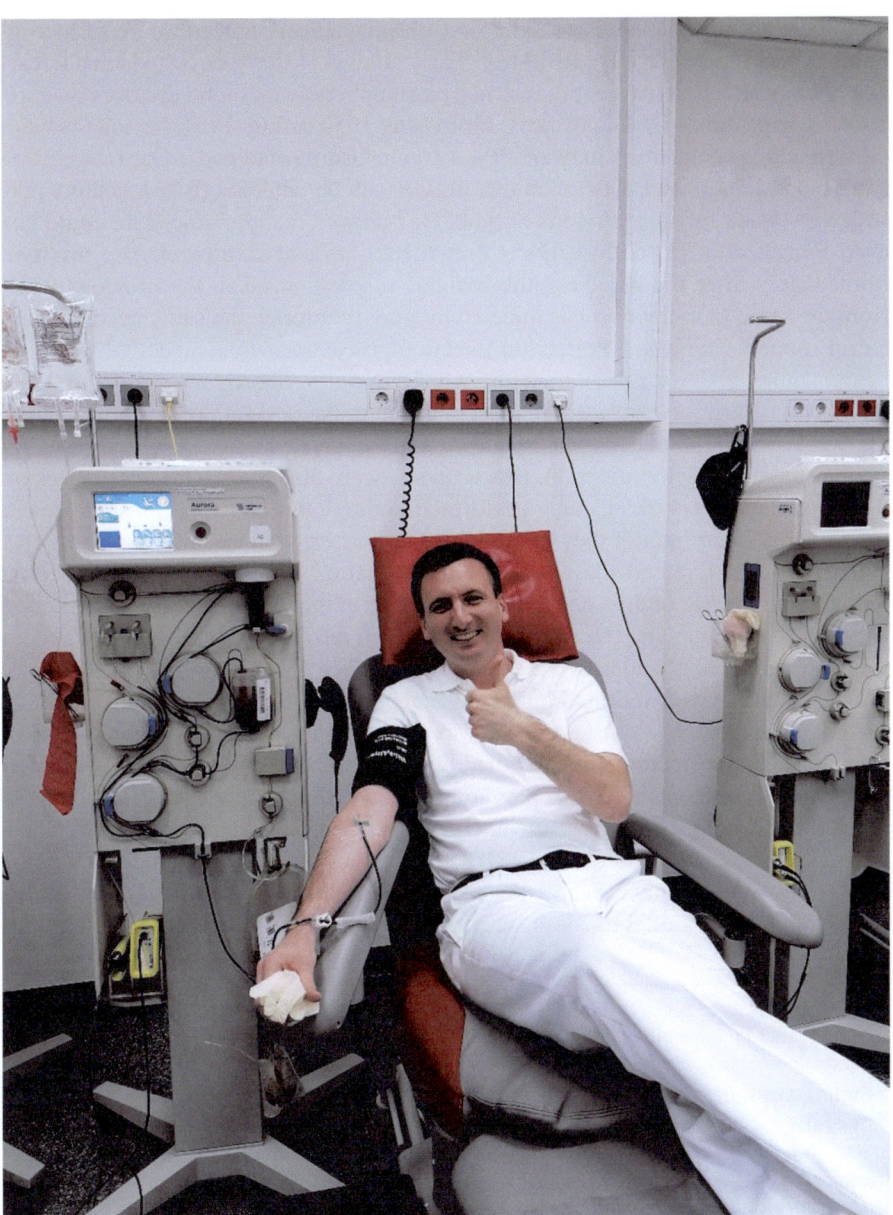

Image 14.9 Modern plasmapheresis. (Source: Zdravko Kvržić. Modern plasmapheresis procedure by Zdravko Kvržić. Permission to use the image was obtained from the V.D. director of the Blood Transfusion Center of Slovenia, Peter Kavčič, M.Sc. business and economic. Science, on November 24, 2023)

the procedure plasmapheresis.[47] The first plasmapheresis procedure performed in humans was reported by Tui in 1944.[48] Early studies of therapeutic plasmapheresis began in 1951.[49] Extensive studies to use plasmapheresis on blood donors was done by Dr. Josep Antoni Grifols I Lucas. From May 1950 to July 1951, he and his team performed plasmapheresis in over 320 cases. Dr. Grifols obtained 200 mL of plasma from blood donors and concluded that plasma can be obtained from a healthy person every week for short periods of time. He believed that the procedure could last even longer. 400 mL of blood was drawn into an acid-citrate-dextrose mixture. Immediately after the bleeding, the red-cell suspension taken the previous week from the same blood donor was injected by gravity through the same needle, using a drip counter. The whole collection-injection process was thus made with a single venipuncture, and as a rule, it took about 8–10 minutes. Shortly after collection, the blood was centrifuged and kept in this condition in the refrigerator until the following week, when the plasma was removed and the packed cells were suspended in citrate-saline, ready for injection. Blood donors were bled for plasma every week on the same day. Every week, they performed hemoglobin and total plasma protein estimations. Every month they carried out the Wassermann and Meinicke tests for syphilis and determined the albumin-globulin ratio.[50] The Grifols-Lucas method required the storage of the donor's blood. Storage of the blood increased the interval between withdrawal and return of the red cells to the donor, amplified the chances for misidentification, and added the risks of shortened red cell survival and bacterial growth. These considerations limited the acceptance of the procedure, even though special equipment was not needed. It was revived with the use of a constant-flow centrifuge (Cohn fractionator) and the elimination of red cell storage.[51] Cohn was the pioneer of the mechanical separation of blood into components. His work was built on the principles of the de Laval cream separator.[52] Cohn separator based on a dairy centrifuge was invented in 1951. Tullis further improved it, which included a swiftly revolving conical vessel that separated cells from plasma.[53] Despite the Cohn fractionator's effectiveness for plasmapheresis, the price and complexity of

---

[47] Abel J.J., Rowntree L.G., Turner B.B. Plasma removal with return of corpuscles (plasmaphaeresis). Journal of Pharmacology and Experimental Therapeutics July 1. 1914; 5 (8) 625–641. https://jpet.aspetjournals.org/content/5/6/625.short.

[48] Curling, Goss, Bertolini, 2012, p. 4.

[49] Biancalana A. Exsanguinação e transfusão de glóbulos (plasmaferese) no tratamento do edema agudo do pulmão [Withdrawal of blood and transfusion of erythrocytes (plasmapheresis) in the treatment of acute pulmonary edema]. Arq Cir Clin Exp. May-Jun 1951; 14 (4):156–61. Undetermined Language. https://pubmed.ncbi.nlm.nih.gov/14895430/.

[50] Grifols-Lucas J.A. Use of plasmapheresis in blood donors. British medical journal.1952; 1(4763), p. 854. https://www.ncbi.nlm.nih.gov/pmc/articles/PMC2023259/.

[51] Kliman A., Lesses M.F. Plasmapheresis as a Form of Blood Donation, Transfusion. 1964; 4 (8), p. 469–472. https://onlinelibrary.wiley.com/doi/abs/10.1111/j.1537-2995.1964.tb02907.x.

[52] Summerfield D. D. Burgstaler E. A. Donor Apheresis Separators and Their Development. In: Vassallo R.R., editor. Apheresis: principles and practice fourth edition, volume 2. Maryland USA: American Association of Blood Banks (AABB). 2021, p. 2–11.

[53] Curling, Goss, Bertolini, 2012, p. 4.

14.2 Equipment and Material Standards

the apparatus severely restricted its use. To avoid this, the relevant features of the Cohn fractionator were replicated by use of modified plastic equipment and regular blood bank centrifuges. In the Cohn separator, whole blood slowly filled the rotating separating chamber, and the separation of the red cells, buffy coat with the white cells and platelets, and plasma was based on density. When the equilibrium state was reached, the red cells and plasma could be drawn off. In 1952, Cohn and Allen Latham Jr. together invented the ADL Cohn blood fractionator for plasmapheresis. With this device albumin was further purified, and it was also used for freezing and deglycerolizing RBC. [54] Getting huge quantities of various blood components from a single blood donor is effective when using an automated blood cell separator. As an illustration, one of these devices was developed by Dr. Allen "Jack" Latham from a design by Dr. Edwin Joseph Cohn. His device is commonly known as a Latham bowl from 1971. With it the components were separated using differential centrifugation.[55] This type of centrifugation is a separation method where the components of a cell are separated on the basis of their density in a centrifuge according to the centrifugal force they experience.[56] With the Latham bowl, which is still today used in certain machines, RBC and plasma, for instance, are given back to the blood donor, but platelets, which are big and can be divided into a different layer, are not returned. The Latham bowl can be used repeatedly. It is conically-shaped, held in a chuck which is attached to a spindle and powered by a motor. The bowl has a rotor portion where blood components are separated and a stator portion with an input and output port.[57] By 1957, autotransfusion of the sedimented red cells was demonstrated to be a practical way to keep men's hemoglobin levels normal after blood withdrawal. Between 1957 and 1959, evidence was gathered to support the usefulness of plasmapheresis using a single venipuncture, the safety of chronic plasma withdrawal, and the benefits of a large plasma pool from carefully chosen blood donors.[58] The prototypes of continuous flow blood cell separators were developed in the 1960s.[59] Through the use of plasmapheresis and the recruitment of compensated blood donors by commercial processors, plasma collection was increased in the United States in the late 1950s.[60] In 1956, products made from blood plasma were developed to treat diseases such as chicken pox. In 1960, A. Solomon and J. L. Fahey reported the first therapeutic plasmapheresis procedure.[61] Plasmapheresis in the USA had established itself as a common method of blood donation and a significant

---

[54] Summerfield, Burgstaler, 2021, p. 2–11.

[55] NIH, Object record, Haemonetics Blood Cell Separator Bowl, Model 30. https://onih.pastperfectonline.com/webobject/20343EA6-60F2-4146-A111-345241338000. Accessed 20 March 2024.

[56] Royal Society of Chemistry. Differential centrifugation. https://www.rsc.org/publishing/journals/prospect/ontology.asp?id=CMO:0002015&MSI. Accessed 19 March 2024.

[57] NIH, 2024.

[58] Kliman, Lesses, 1964, p. 469–470.

[59] Millward B.L., Hoeltge G.A. The historical development of automated hemapheresis. J. Clin. Apher. 1982;1 (1), p. 25–32. https://pubmed.ncbi.nlm.nih.gov/6765453/

[60] Curling, Goss, Bertolini, 2012, p. 4.

[61] Ajmani, 2020, p. 121.

source of plasma by the year 1964. Plasma was then collected in plastic containers. Different techniques and tools were used for collection, but they all had one thing in common: a safe return of RBC to the blood donor as soon as possible after donation to prevent the risks of blood storage, particularly misidentification, bacterial growth, and reduced red blood cell survival. The blood donor is required to be in good nutritional condition, have a normal serum protein level, and meet other standards for blood donors.[62] In Europe, collecting plasma for fractionation began in 1950. The first company in Europe to introduce widespread plasmapheresis centers in both Austria and Germany was Immuno AG, formed in 1953, which commenced plasma fractionation in Vienna in 1954, opening the first center in 1960.[63] By the European directive the collection volume for each plasmapheresis (including anticoagulant) should never exceed 880 mL, and the donated volume (excluding anticoagulant) should not exceed 16% of the estimated TBV. In any type of apheresis procedure, the total volume of all components donated (plasma, platelets, and red cells) should not exceed 16% of the estimated TBV. Platelet apheresis must not be carried out on individuals whose platelet count is less than 150×10^9/L (Directive 2004/33/EC, Annex III)[64] Manual plasmapheresis procedures, as they were carried out by Grifols and others in similar circumstances, are no longer in use.

Single-blood donor platelet collection, which started in the 1960s, was done manually with manual centrifugation prior to the invention of automatic cell separators. As an example, four serial whole blood collections made up the collection. The buffy coat was removed from the centrifuged blood after each collection cycle, and the RBC and plasma fractions were given back to the blood donor.[65] Manual centrifugation resulted in low yields and was labor-and time-intensive.[66] It was also exhausting for the blood donor, who had to undergo this procedure for several hours.[67] An interesting case was reported in 1965 of the separation and collection of leukocytes. An instrument had been designed to process large volumes of blood on a continuous flow basis. The instrument collected venous blood, separated leukocytes in a centrifuge, and reinjected the red cells, plasma, and platelets.[68] This is one of the earliest cases where the centrifuge was used as a cell separator.[69] The first automated cell separator with a fully closed tubing system was the Fenwal CS3000. Cullis and his team of seven co-workers completed the Fenwal CS3000 in 1972. In

---

[62] Kilman, Lesses, 1964, p. 469.

[63] Curling, Goss, Bertolini, 2012, p. 4.

[64] EDQM GUIDE, 2023, p. 158–159.

[65] Summerfield, Burgstaler, 2021, 2–11.

[66] NIH, 2024.

[67] Summerfield, Burgstaler, 2021, p. 3.

[68] Emil J. Freireich, George Judson, Robert H. Levin; Separation and Collection of Leukocytes. Cancer Res 1 October. 1965; 25 (9_Part_1), p. 1516–1520. https://aacrjournals.org/cancerres/article/25/9_Part_1/1516/475783/Separation-and-Collection-of-Leukocytes.

[69] Vogt A. The Italian Consensus Conferences on low density lipoprotein-cholesterol apheresis. Blood transfusion = Trasfusione del sangue. 2017; 15 (1), 1–3. https://www.ncbi.nlm.nih.gov/pmc/articles/PMC5269421/#b3-blt-15-001.

14.2 Equipment and Material Standards

1979, the Fenwal CS3000 started to be utilized in clinical practice and was made available internationally.[70] The CS3000 was for decades used for collecting platelets and granulocytes. Significant quantities of granulocytes could be collected from a donor by the early 1970s.[71] Also in 1970s Granulocyte transfusions in patients with transient bone marrow aplasia were introduced.[72] Automated single-donor plateletpheresis was available by 1973, and by 1975 it had moved into general use.[73] By the 1970s, apheresis was being used to produce blood components and remove materials from blood that could not be dialyzed, such as hazardous chemicals and antibodies.[74] Today's automated cell separators for apheresis procedures allow blood donors to donate individual blood components regularly, relatively quickly, reliably, and, above all, safely.

14.2.2.3 Information Technology

Today, it is unimaginable to be in the healthcare system without information technology (IT), which offers a wide range of activities for users, whether employees, patients, or other healthcare clients.

The history of IT can be divided into pre-mechanical, mechanical, electromechanical, and electronic eras that began in the early 1940s.[75] The early beginnings of electronic IT in the healthcare system began to appear in the 1960s, with not only serious discussions but also the introduction of electronic health records. The use of computers in the healthcare system began in the early 1980s.[76] IT technology in modern times is developing rapidly with the high demands of the healthcare profession. IT technology in transfusion medicine was present before the electronic era in the form of documentation, which was, of course, constantly developing and expanding. Today, extensive automated and computerized high-tech IT activities are used in transfusion medicine.

The history of barcodes dates to before World War II, with a mention in a 1934 patent by John Kermode, Douglass Young, and Harry Sparkes. Assigned to Westinghouse Electric Co., LLC, the patent was for a machine that sorted cards and recorded data and utilized "photo-electric cells or other light-responsive means in accordance with the marks on the cards or records." But the first actual barcode prototype was designed in 1949 by Bernard Silver and Joseph Woodland, a pair of graduate students from the Drexel Institute of Technology in Philadelphia. The institute was contacted by a nearby grocery store regarding the development of an automated system for scanning product information. After accepting the challenge,

---

[70] Corbin, Cullis, Freireich, Ito, Kellogg, Lathman, 2003, p. 15–16.
[71] Summerfield, Burgstaler, 2021, p. 6.
[72] Högman, 1992, p. 142.
[73] Summerfield, Burgstaler, 2021, p. 6.
[74] Högman, 1992, p. 142.
[75] Open book project. History Of Information Technology. https://openbookproject.net/courses/intro2ict/history/history.html Accessed 19 March 2024.
[76] Net Health. Electronic Health Records: A Comprehensive History of EHR Systems. https://www.nethealth.com/blog/the-history-of-electronic-health-records-ehrs/ Accessed 19 March 2024.

the two students started developing a technique that made use of UV-light ink patterns. They created something that functioned, but they soon abandoned their initial concept due to the ink's instability and high cost. Woodland carried on solving the issue by using some stock market profits. Woodland, in the 1950s, sold the patent to the Radio Corporation of America (RCA). The RCA started to use their system in 1967. George Laurer designed the 10-digit barcode that is the UPC barcode of today, and it started to be widely used in 1974. The barcode business expanded throughout the 1980s.[77] The barcode has gone through various iterations and advancements, including the 2D barcode and the QR code. Barcodes in the healthcare system are often used to identify patients, medications, and medical equipment, which can help reduce errors and improve patient safety.[78] There are many different types of codabars. The Codabar Barcode system is the most adaptable. It is an excellent option for companies that mostly rely on complicated data structures because it can encode digits 0 through 9. The Codabar Barcode, also known as Ames Code, USD-4, Codeabar, or NW-7, is a linear barcode symbology that encodes a few special characters and numeric digits. Codabar Barcode was primarily intended for retail and package labeling when it was developed by Monarch Marking Systems in the early 1970s. Accurate reading, even in high-speed scanning environments, is one of its distinctive features. In the healthcare industry, Codabar Barcode is widely used for medical recordkeeping, tracking of specimens, patient identification, and many other important tasks. These applications benefit greatly from its capacity to encode numerical information. [79] Regarding the use of barcodes in transfusion medicine, it was the Committee for Commonality in Blood Banking Automation (CCBBA), established in 1974 and operating under the American Blood Commission since 1975, that first gave consideration to the important factors that would determine the criteria for the construction of a barcode for use in blood transfusion. In 1977, they recommended a standard label design and the allocation of numeric codes for blood groups and blood products. By 1987, a number of countries had adopted the recommendations of the CCBBA. In Scandinavia in the 1980s, they used an OCR-B system, which was not so efficient. In 1979, the ISBT established a working party on automation and data processing. By 1981, the computerization of donor files had been well researched. In 1983, in the USA, great work was done to standardize barcodes in health care services. By 1984, it was recognized that the labels used in blood transfusion were printed to specification and were subjected to exacting quality control. These specifications were included in the same-year Guidelines for the Uniform Labeling of Blood and Blood Components. In 1985, the ISBT issued the Guide to Barcodes in Blood

---

[77] Goldberg A. A History of Barcodes & Barcoding Technology. Labtag blog. https://blog.labtag.com/a-history-of-barcoding-technology/. Accessed 19 March 2024.

[78] Viziotix. The History of Barcodes. https://www.viziotix.com/2023/04/03/history-of-the-barcode-bl/. Accessed 19 March 2024.

[79] QodeNext. Codabar Barcode—Everything You Need to Know. https://www.qodenext.com/blog/codabar-barcode-everything-you-need-to-know/. Accessed 20 Apr 2024.

14.2 Equipment and Material Standards

Collection and Transfusion.[80] Today's barcodes are essential in healthcare and in transfusion medicine.

The physics of the separation in a spinning bowl in the centrifuge and the optimization of the separation process were not well understood until 1992, when Hein Smit Sibinga, a Dutch graduate student in mechanical engineering at Enschede Technical University in the Netherlands, created software and a computer imaging program based on artificial intelligence algorithms. About the year 2000, with ever-expanding databases, processing, and testing, artificial intelligence (AI) began to quietly seep into the expanding area of transfusion medicine.[81]

Another important aspect of IT in transfusion medicine is found in hemovigilance. The Latin word "vigilans" (watchful) and the Greek word "hema" (blood) are the origins of the word hemovigilance. Hemovigilance is the process of identifying and evaluating any adverse effects of blood transfusion in order to identify the underlying cause, stop the impact from happening again, and ultimately increase the safety of the procedure. Hemovigilance plays a significant role in the blood transfusion quality system. It includes techniques like warning systems, complaint inquiry, traceability systems, notification systems, and practice audits for detecting mistakes, unfavorable events, and reactions. In order to gather and evaluate data on unanticipated or undesirable effects resulting from the therapeutic use of labile blood products and to prevent their occurrence and recurrence, hemovigilance is defined as "a set of surveillance procedures covering the whole transfusion chain from the collection of blood and its components to the follow-up of its recipients."[82] Blood Transfusion Committees installed monitoring systems and a national hemovigilance system in France in 1994, marking the beginning of the groundbreaking work on hemovigilance in that country. Later, in 1995, a resolution was released by the European Council with the aim of enhancing public confidence in a safe supply of blood. Legal authorities soon took control of the hemovigilance system. The United Kingdom's Serious Hazards of Transfusion (SHOT), Canada's Transfusion Transmitted Injuries Surveillance System (TTISS), the Netherlands' Transfusion Reactions in Patients (TRIP), Japan, Russia, Switzerland, and the United States of America are just a few of the nations whose well-established hemovigilance systems have provided data that shed light on a variety of strategies that can be used to increase blood safety. Currently operating on a global level is the International Hemovigilance Network (IHN), which developed from the European Hemovigilance Network (EHN—founded in 1998). IHN's mission is to create and uphold a global framework for hemovigilance in blood transfusion and transfusion medicine, as

---

[80] Gunson H. H. Machine readable labels, chapter 5. In: Cash J. D., editor. Progress in transfusion medicine, volume 22. London: Churchill Livingstone;1987, p. 59–65.

[81] Cees Th., Sibinga S. Transfusion Medicine: From AB0 to AI (Artificial Intelligence) In: Linwood SL, editor. Digital Health [Internet]. Brisbane (AU): Exon Publications; 2022 Apr 29. Chapter 8. https://www.ncbi.nlm.nih.gov/books/NBK580623/ Accessed 19 March 2024.

[82] De Vries R.R., Faber J.C., Strengers P.F.W.; Board of the International Haemovigilance Network. Haemovigilance: an effective tool for improving transfusion practice. Vox Sang. 2011;100 (1) p. 60–7. https://pubmed.ncbi.nlm.nih.gov/21175656/.

well as for the safety of blood and blood components. A standard definition for a hemovigilance system was proposed by the IHN in 2011 in collaboration with the International Society of Blood Transfusion (ISBT) working party on hemovigilance.[83] SHOT started to operate in the UK in 1996.[84] TTISS started to operate in 2001[85], and TRIP started to operate in 2003.[86] The Blood Safety Directive of the European Union (EU) established a legal obligation to notify the appropriate competent authority of any major adverse reactions or events that take place within EU Member States. The UK Competent Authority is the Medicines and Healthcare Products Regulatory Agency (MHRA), which has been recognized by the Department of Health. In order to make reporting easier, the MHRA created the SABRE (Serious Adverse Blood Reactions and Events) online reporting system in 2005.[87]

IT technology in transfusion medicine consists of sophisticated and diverse high-tech technologies and equipment with complete traceability for the entire chain of transfusion medicine, ranging from the donation, processing, testing, storing, delivering, and blood transfusion itself.

References

1. Alsever JB. Liquid plasma, chapter 16. In: DeGowin EL, Hardin RC, Alsever BJ, editors. Blood transfusion. Philadelphia & London: W.B. Saunders Company; 1949. p. 362–94.
2. Abel JJ, Rowntree LG, Turner BB. Plasma removal with return of corpuscles (plasmaphaeresis). J Pharmacol Exp Ther. 1914;5(6):625–41. https://jpet.aspetjournals.org/content/5/6/625.short.
3. AABB. in memoriam: william p. murphy, jr., md. https://www.aabb.org/news-resources/news/article/2023/12/06/in-memoriam%2D%2Dwilliam-p.-murphy%2D%2Djr.%2D%2Dmd. Accessed 10 Mar 2024.
4. Ajmani PS. History of blood transfusion. In: Immunohematology and blood banking. Singapore: Springer; 2020. p. 121.
5. Bolton-Maggs PHB, Cohen H. Serious hazards of transfusion (SHOT) haemovigilance and progress is improving transfusion safety. Br J Haematol. 2013;163(3):303. https://pubmed.ncbi.nlm.nih.gov/24032719/.

---

[83] Jain A., Kaur R. Hemovigilance and blood safety. Asian journal of transfusion science. 2012; 6 (2), p. 137. https://www.ncbi.nlm.nih.gov/pmc/articles/PMC3439750/.

[84] Bolton-Maggs, P. H. B., Cohen H. Serious Hazards of Transfusion (SHOT) haemovigilance and progress is improving transfusion safety. British journal of haematology. 2013; 163 (4), p. 303. https://pubmed.ncbi.nlm.nih.gov/24032719/.

[85] Government of Canada. Transfusion Transmitted Injuries Surveillance System 2011–2015 Summary Report. https://www.canada.ca/en/public-health/services/publications/drugs-health-products/transfusion-transmitted-injuries-surveillance-system-ttiss-2011-2015-summary-results.html Accesssed 20 March 2024.

[86] TRIP.TRIP annual report 2009 Hemovigilance, p. 2. https://www.notifylibrary.org/sites/default/files/TRIP%20hemovigilance%202009.pdf Accessed 20 March 2024.

[87] Joint UK Blood Transfusion and Tissue Transplantation Services Professional Advisory Committee (JPAC). Section 5 Haemovigilance. https://www.transfusionguidelines.org/document-library/documents/section-5-haemovigilance. Accessed 20 March 2024.

References

6. Breckenridge A. The changing scene of the regulation of medicines in the UK. Paper from the use of medicines: Regulation & Clinical Pharmacology in the twenty-first century symposium—December 2003. Br J Clin Pharmacol. 2004;58(6):571–4. https://www.ncbi.nlm.nih.gov/pmc/articles/PMC1884637/.
7. Burgstaler EA, Winters JL. Apheresis: principles and technology of hemapheresis. In: Simon TL, McCullough J, Snyder EL, Solheim BG, Strauss RG, editors. Rossi's principles of transfusion medicine. 5th ed. New York: Wiley Blackwell; 2016. p. 1–14.
8. Biancalana A. Exsanguinação e transfusão de glóbulos (plasmaferese) no tratamento do edema Agudo do pulmão [withdrawal of blood and transfusion of erythrocytes (plasmapheresis) in the treatment of acute pulmonary edema]. Arq Cir Clin Exp. May-Jun. 1951;14(3):156–61. Undetermined Language. https://pubmed.ncbi.nlm.nih.gov/14895430/.
9. Cees T, Sibinga S. Transfusion medicine: from AB0 to AI (Artificial Intelligence). In: Linwood SL, editor. Digital Health [Internet]. Brisbane, AU: Exon Publications; 2022. https://wwwncbinlmnihgov/books/NBK580623/. Accessed 19 Mar 2024.
10. Carmen R. The selection of plastic materials for blood bags. Transfus Med Rev. 1993;7(1):1–10. https://europepmc.org/article/med/8431654.
11. Canadian Blood Services, therapeutic apheresis. https://professionaleducation.blood.ca/en/transfusion/clinical-guide/therapeutic-apheresis. Accessed 19 Mar 2024.
12. Corbin F, Cullis HM, Freireich EJ, Ito J, Kellogg RM, Lathman A Jr, McLeod BC. Development of apheresis instrumentation. In: McLeod BC, Price TH, Weinstein R, editors. Apheresis principles and practice. 2nd ed. Maryland: American Association of Blood Banks (AABB); 2003. p. 2.
13. DeGowin EL. Storage and preservation of whole blood. In: DeGowin EL, Hardin RC, Alsever BJ, editors. Blood transfusion. Philadelphia & London: W.B. Saunders Company; 1949. p. 315.
14. De Vries RR, Faber JC, Strengers PFW, Board of the International Haemovigilance Network. Haemovigilance: an effective tool for improving transfusion practice. Vox Sang. 2011;100(1):60–7. https://pubmed.ncbi.nlm.nih.gov/21175656/
15. Freireich EJ, Judson G, Levin RH. Separation and collection of leukocytes. Cancer Res. 1965;25(9_Part_1):1516–20. https://aacrjournals.org/cancerres/article/25/9_Part_1/1516/475783/Separation-and-Collection-of-Leukocytes.
16. Finnish Red Cross Blood Service. History of Blood Service.https://www.veripalvelu.fi/en/history/. Accessed 10 Mar 2024.
17. FDA. Part 606—current good manufacturing practice for blood and blood components. https://www.ecfr.gov/current/title-21/chapter-I/subchapter-F/part-606. Accessed 10 Mar 2024.
18. Faber JC, Boulton F, Rouger P. Comments on the EU blood directive 2002/98/CE, chapter 2. In: Rouger P, Hossenlopp C, editors. Blood transfusion in Europe. The white book 2005. Paris: Elsevier; 2005. p. 38–45.
19. Grozdanić V, Fišer-Herman M, Maher V. Pribor za transfuziju krvi, krvnih derivate I zamenika krvne plazme. In: Polak A, Dinić B, Papo I, Fišer- HM, Lah P, Stefanović S, Vuletin V, editors. Transfuzija krvi. Beograd: Savezni Zavod za Zdravstvenu Zaštitu; 1966. p. 193–205.
20. Gunson HH, Dodsworth H. From the 'MRC Blood Transfusion Outfit' to blood components. In: Anstee DJ, Barbara JAJ, Lincoln PJ, McClelland DBL, Voak D, editors. Fifty Years of Blood transfusion. Blood transfusion Medicine, vol. 6. Oxford: Blackwell Science; 1996. p. 25. https://www.infectedbloodinquiry.org.uk/sites/default/files/2023-06-09%20Oral%20Evidence%20Docs%20-%20Row%202701-2900%20%20copy/2023-06-09%20Oral%20Evidence%20Docs%20-%20Row%202701-2900%20%20copy/NHBT0000028%20-%20Fifty%20Years%20of%20Blood%20Transfusion%20-%2001%20Jan%201996.pdf. Accessed 3 Mar 2024.
21. Gilcher RO, Latham A, Schiff JD, Schoendorfer D. Blood donation unit. 1983. https://patents.google.com/patent/US4385630A/en. Accessed 16 Mar 2024.
22. Grifols-Lucas JA. Use of plasmapheresis in blood donors. Br Med J. 1952;1(4763):854. https://www.ncbi.nlm.nih.gov/pmc/articles/PMC2023259/.
23. Goldberg A. A history of barcodes & barcoding technology. Labtag blog https://blog.labtag.com/a-history-of-barcoding-technology/. Accessed 19 Mar 2024.

24. Gunson HH. Machine readable labels. In: Cash JD, editor. Progress in transfusion medicine, vol. 22. London: Churchill Livingstone; 1987. p. 59–65.
25. Government of Canada. Transfusion Transmitted Injuries Surveillance System 2011–2015 Summary Report. https://www.canada.ca/en/public-health/services/publications/drugs-health-products/transfusion-transmitted-injuries-surveillance-system-ttiss-2011-2015-summary-results.html. Accessed 20 Mar 2024.
26. ISO. ISO 9001:2015, Quality management systems Requirements. https://www.iso.org/standard/62085.html. Accessed 1 Apr 2024.
27. Jegrelius institute for applied green chemistry. Blood bags-history, p. 10. https://pvcfree-bloodbag.eu/wp-content/uploads/2013/11/BloodBags_final_report_krcopy.pdf. Accessed 10 Mar 2024.
28. Jain A, Kaur R. Hemovigilance and blood safety. Asian J Trans Scie. 2012;6(2):137. https://www.ncbi.nlm.nih.gov/pmc/articles/PMC3439750/.
29. Joint UK Blood Transfusion and Tissue Transplantation Services Professional Advisory Committee (JPAC). Section 5 Haemovigilance. https://www.transfusionguidelines.org/document-library/documents/section-5-haemovigilance. Accessed 20 Mar 2024.
30. Kliman A, Lesses MF. Plasmapheresis as a form of blood donation. Transfusion. 1964;4(6):469–72. https://doi.org/10.1111/j.1537-2995.1964.tb02907.x.
31. Kögel A. Blood rock. 1989. https://patents.google.com/patent/SE8903440D0/en?q=(~patent%2fUS5147330A). Accessed 16 Mar 2024.
32. Kögel A. Blood cradle. 1992. https://patents.google.com/patent/US5147330A/en?oq=US+patent+5147330. Accessed 16 Mar 2024.
33. Hakkarainen S. A life-saving soda bottle, Helsinki University Museum. https://blogs.helsinki.fi/hum-object-of-the-month/2023/01/25/a-life-saving-soda-bottle/. Accessed 4 Mar 2024.
34. Mintz PD, Weinstein MJ. Global perspective on ensuring blood and blood product safety and availability. In: Simon TL, McCullough J, Snyder EL, Solheim BG, Strauss RG, editors. Rossi's principles of transfusion medicine. 5th ed. New York: Wiley Blackwell; 2016. p. 73.
35. Millward BL, Hoeltge GA. The historical development of automated hemapheresis. J Clin Apher. 1982;1(1):25–32. https://pubmed.ncbi.nlm.nih.gov/6765453/.
36. Net Health. Electronic health records: a comprehensive history of EHR systems. https://www.nethealth.com/blog/the-history-of-electronic-health-records-ehrs/. Accessed 19 Mar 2024.
37. NIH Object record, haemonetics blood cell separator bowl, model 30. https://onih.pastperfectonline.com/webobject/20343EA6-60F2-4146-A111-345241338000. Accessed 20 Mar 2024.
38. Open book project. History of information technology. https://openbookproject.net/courses/intro2ict/history/history.html. Accessed 19 Mar 2024.
39. Purdy RW, Arneson DA. Blood collection monitoring device and method. 1981. https://patents.google.com/patent/US4267837A/en?oq=US+patent+5147330. Accessed 16 Mar 2024.
40. QodeNext. Codabar Barcode—Everything You Need to Know. https://www.qodenext.com/blog/codabar-barcode-everything-you-need-to-know/ Accessed 20 Apr 2024.
41. Royal Society of Chemistry. Differential centrifugation. https://www.rsc.org/publishing/journals/prospect/ontology.asp?id=CMO:0002015&MSI. Accessed 19 Mar 2024.
42. Summerfield DD, Burgstaler EA. Donor apheresis separators and their development. In: Vassallo RR, editor. Apheresis: principles and practice, vol. 2. 4th ed. Maryland: American Association of Blood Banks (AABB); 2021. p. 2–11.
43. Sibinga S, Hasan F. Quality management or the need for a quality culture in transfusion medicine. Global journal of. Transfus Med. 2020;5(1):10–1. file:///C:/Users/zdrav/Downloads/Quality_management_or_the_need_for_a_quality_cultu.pdf.
44. Sasakawa S, Tokunaga E. Physical and chemical changes of ACD-preserved blood: a comparison of blood in glass bottles and plastic bags. Vox Sang. 1976;31(3):199–200. https://karger.com/vox/article-abstract/31/3/199/311820/Physical-and-Chemical-Changes-of-ACD-Preserved.
45. Strumia M.M. Apparatus for the collection and cooling of blood. 1958. https://patents.google.com/patent/US2845929A/en%20Accessed%2016%20march%202024. Accessed 16 Mar 2024.

46. Shuping BYZ. Automatic blood mixer. 1989. https://patents.google.com/patent/CN2034039U/en. Accessed 16 Mar 2024.
47. Tovey GH. Section IV Organisation, C-Travaux des organisms internationaux. International standardization of transfusion equipment of medical use. In: Berroche L, Eyquem A, Julliard J, Mailloux M, Maupin B, Moullec J, Perrot H, Saint-Paul M, Lewi S, editors. Immuno-hématologie: techniques sérologiques = Immuno-hematology. Drépanocytose thalassémie [u.a.]. Ve Congrès International de Transfusion Sanguine. Paris: Croutzet; 1955. p. 1100–5.
48. The Royal College of Pathologists. Object 47: Plastic blood bag. https://www.rcpath.org/static/1c305fd3-6e4e-4427-802aa646720ec6e8/47-Plastic-Blood-Bag.pdf. Accessed 10 Mar 2024.
49. Toya M, Miyairi Y. Apparatus for collecting constant amounts of blood from individual donors. 1990. https://patents.google.com/patent/US4923449A/en
50. TRIP.TRIP annual report 2009 Hemovigilance, p 2 https://wwwnotifylibraryorg/sites/default/files/TRIP%20hemovigilance%202009pdf. Accessed 20 Mar 2024.
51. Vaughan JM. Blood transfusion outfit. Br Med J. 1939;2(4117):1084. https://www.ncbi.nlm.nih.gov/pmc/articles/PMC2178860/pdf/brmedj04174-0013.pdf.
52. Viziotix. The History of Barcodes. https://www.viziotix.com/2023/04/03/history-of-the-barcode-bl/. Accessed 19 Mar 2024.
53. Valeri CR. New developments in red blood cell preservation using liquid and freezing procedures. J Clin Lab Auto. 1982;2:6. https://apps.dtic.mil/sti/tr/pdf/ADA140442.pdf. Accessed 24 March 2024.
54. Vogt A. The Italian Consensus Conferences on low density lipoprotein-cholesterol apheresis. Blood transfusion = Trasfusione del sangue. 2017;15(1):1–3. https://www.ncbi.nlm.nih.gov/pmc/articles/PMC5269421/#b3-blt-15-001.
55. Wagstaff W. Quality assurance of transfusion center derived blood products, chapter 1. In: Cash JD, editor. Progress in transfusion medicine, vol. 22. London: Churchill Livingstone; 1987. p. 10.
56. Wandell FA. Plastic in blood transfusion—plastic containers—development of criteria. In: International Society of Blood Transfusion, 11th congress, vol. 29. Karger Publishers; 1968. p. 978–88. https://karger.com/books/book/416/chapter-abstract/5569976/Plastic-in-Blood-Transfusion-Plastic-Containers?redirectedFrom=fulltext.
57. Walter Car W. Invention and development of the blood bag. Vox Sang. 1984;47(4):318–9. https://www.semanticscholar.org/paper/Invention-and-Development-of-the-Blood-Bag-Walter/a467ad1e71abe108b5dc581fb73fae9664c338aa
58. Walter C.W. Apparatus for collecting, storing, and dispensing whole blood. https://patents.google.com/patent/US2702034A/en?q=(blood)&q=(bag)&q=(container)&q=(needle)&q=(collection)&before=priority:19530430&scholar. Accessed 17 Mar 2024.

Image Source

Vaughan JM. The MRC bottle for blood donation and blood transfusion Vaughan J.M. Blood Transfusion Outfit. Br Med J. 1939;2(4117):1084. https://www.ncbi.nlm.nih.gov/pmc/articles/PMC2178860/pdf/brmedj04174-0013.pdf. Accessed March 3, 2024. Permission for usage of this image was granted by the copyright holder, BMJ, on March 7, 2024

Soda bottle with blood after the blood donation, Finland 1941. Finnish Armed Forces photograph -SA-kuva. Creative Commons CC BY 4.0. http://sa-kuva.fi/neo#. Accessed 9 Mar 2024.

Finnish Red Cross Blood Service. History of Blood Service. Glass bottles containing blood, Finland 1960s. https://www.veripalvelu.fi/en/history/ Accessed 10 Mar 2024. Permission for the use of this photograph was granted by Mr. Willy Toiviainen, Director of HR and Communications at the Finnish Red Cross Blood Service, on March 4, 2024.

Science Museum Group. Baxter Transfusovac set, 1938. Creative Commons Attribution 4.0 license. https://collection.sciencemuseumgroup.org.uk/objects/co8692510/baxter-transfusovac-set-blood-taking-set. Accessed 10 Mar 2024.

Finnish Red Cross Blood Service. Nurses drawing blood from blood donors in Sipoo, Southern Finland 1955. https://www.veripalvelu.fi/en/history/. Accessed 10 Mar 2024. Permission for the use of this photograph was granted by Mr. Willy Toiviainen, Director of HR and Communications at the Finnish Red Cross Blood Service, on March 4, 2024.

Nurse drawing blood from blood donor at hospital blood transfusion department in city of Maribor, 1956. From Večer https://vecer.com/ Slovenia, Public domain.

Science Museum Group. Fenwal triple blood pack for storage of whole blood used in transfusions, by Baxter Healthcare Ltd., Thetford, Norfolk, supplied by South Thames Blood Transfusion Service, 1993–1994. Creative Commons Attribution 4.0 license. https://collection.sciencemuseumgroup.org.uk/objects/co143636/fenwal-triple-blood-pack-for-storage-of-whole-blood-used-in-transfusions-medical-equipment Accessed 10 Mar 2024.

Kvržić Z. Automated modern blood collection mixer with a tube sealer. Permission to reuse the image from the article Zdravko Kvržić, Odvzem polne krvi pri krvodajalcu skozi različna zgodovinska obdobja (1875–2023). Utrip. 2023;31(6):17–21. was given by the Nurses and Midwives Association of Slovenia on November 29, 2023. The permission was also obtained from the V.D. director of the Blood Transfusion Center of Slovenia, Peter Kavčič, M.Sc. business and economic. Science, on November 24, 2023.

Kvržić Z. Modern plasmapheresis donation by Zdravko Kvržić. Permission to use the image was obtained from the V.D. director of the Blood Transfusion Center of Slovenia, Peter Kavčič, M.Sc. business and economic. Science, on November 24, 2023.

Anticoagulants and Additive Solutions 15

Contents

15.1 Important Facts About Anticoagulants and Additive Solutions.......................... 205
    15.1.1 Some Important Events for Storing Red Blood Cells.......................... 208
References.......................... 210

15.1 Important Facts About Anticoagulants and Additive Solutions

Anticoagulants are used to prevent clotting during the blood donation procedure.[1] Additive solutions are used to maintain the shelf life of the donated blood products.[2] The early experiments with preventing blood from clotting by using different substances until the introduction of the anticoagulant sodium citrate in 1914 proved to be insufficient.

Rous and Turner in 1916 were the first to report the successful storage of blood, but in a small way.[3, 4] During the 1930s, the definition of the major carbohydrate pathway of the red blood cell, including the generation of ATP (adenosine

---

[1] Australian Red Cross Lifeblood. Additives and anticoagulants. https://www.lifeblood.com.au/health-professionals/products/additives-anticoagulants Accessed 22 March 2024.
[2] Lbid.
[3] Rajashekharaiah V., Ravikumar S., Krishnegowda M., Hsieh C. Storage lesions in blood components. Oxidants and Antioxidants in Medical Science, ScopeMed Publishing. 2015; 4 (4), p. 13. https://www.ejmoams.com/ejmoams-articles/storage-lesions-in-blood-components.pdf Accessed 24 March 2024.
[4] Whitby L. 1949, p. 457.

© The Author(s), under exclusive license to Springer Nature Switzerland AG 2024
Z. Kvržić, *History of Blood Donation and Transfusion Medicine*, https://doi.org/10.1007/978-3-031-68715-0_15

triphosphate) by oxidation of glucose to lactate, provided a rational biochemical basis for studies in red cell preservation.[5] By 1949, the anticoagulants that were in use were trisodium citrate, also known as sodium citrate, disodium citrate, and heparin. Among them, trisodium citrate was the most commonly employed for the blood transfusion of fresh blood. This solution was only an anticoagulant, not a blood preservative. The difference between stored and preserved blood was first pointed out by Muether and Andrews in 1941.[6] Stored blood was citrated blood, which has been kept for hours or days at temperatures between 2° and 8 °C and to which nothing has been added to inhibit deterioration of the erythrocytes. In preserved blood, some additional substances were added to prevent the erythrocytes from breaking down.[7] Disodium monohydric citrate was introduced in 1943 by Loutit and Mollison as an anticoagulant in blood preservative mixtures. While heparin was available as an anticoagulant for intravenous application.[8] J.F. Loutit and Patrick L. Mollison made the storage of red cells possible in 1943 by introducing the acid citrate-dextrose ACD, which was both an anticoagulant and preservative solution.[9] The introduction of an ACD solution for the preservation of blood for transfusion was a great achievement.[10] Additionally, ACD significantly lowers the anticoagulant volume, enables larger blood transfusion volumes, and allows for longer-term storage.[11]

By 1949, there were several mixtures containing dextrose, sodium citrate, and citric acid. The term ACD did not refer to any particular formula. Some of the different variations of ACD were composition of solution 2, composition of solution 8, and composition of an American solution. They all contained trisodium citrate, citric acid, anhydrous dextrose, and water. But they differed in the quantity of each composition. Besides the ACD solutions, different preservative mixtures were also used, such as Rous-Turner solution, modified Rous-Turner solution, buffered Rous-Turner solution, dextrose-saline-citrate solution, McGill solution I, McGill solution II, Medical Research Council (British) solution, British Army Blood Transfusion Service Solution, disodium-citrate-dextrose solution, and citrated blood.[12] Today the ACD solution A (ACD-A) is meant to be used in extracorporeal blood collection, apheresis, and processing as well as an anticoagulant and preservative for

---

[5] Dawson, R. B. Preservation of RBC for transfusion. Human Pathology. 1983; 14 (4), p.213. https://www.sciencedirect.com/science/article/abs/pii/S0046817783800197.

[6] DeGowin, 1949, p. 302–337.

[7] Kendrick, 1964, p. 217–227.

[8] DeGowin, 1949, p. 302–337.

[9] Högman, 1992, p. 139–144.

[10] De verdier C., Killander J. Storage of human RBC. I. The effect of acd solution on breakdown of glucose. Acta physiol scand. Mar-apr. 1962; 54 (4, 5), p. 346–353. https://pubmed.ncbi.nlm.nih.gov/13925397/.

[11] Cannas, Thomas, 2015, p. 206–207.

[12] DeGowin, 1949, p. 334–335.

15.1 Important Facts About Anticoagulants and Additive Solutions

human blood.[13, 14] There is also 4% sodium citrate that is used as an anticoagulant for plasmapheresis procedures.[15]

Since citrate-phosphate-dextrose (CPD) was less acidic than ACD, it replaced ACD's place in 1957. With both the ACD and CPD, the storage of RBC was 21 days. The FDA gave its approval for adenine to be added to CPD in August 1978. Citrate-phosphate-dextrose-adenine, or CPDA-1, is formed when adenine raises the amount of adenosine diphosphate, which drives glycolysis toward the synthesis of ATP (adenosine triphosphate).[16] CPDA-1 prolonged the storage of RBC to 35 days. Adenine's role in the enhanced production of adenosine triphosphate has been pointed out as the cause of the shelf life extensions.[17] When CPDA-1 was approved, it became widely used, and in many blood banks, it replaced citrate-phosphate-dextrose (CPD) as the anticoagulant-preservative solution of choice.[18] Since the 1970s, blood and blood products intended to sustain red blood cells (RBCs) have been treated less often with citrate-phosphate-double dextrose (CP2D), an anticoagulant with a higher osmolarity and greater dextrose content than CPD. The anticoagulated whole blood containing CP2D has the same 21-day shelf life as CPD. Although there is a greater likelihood of diminished hemostatic capacity due to a later-growing storage lesion, CPD is still the recommended option for whole blood; however, the 35-day shelf life of CPDA-1 is advantageous for waste reduction and logistical reasons.[19] A red blood cell storage lesion (RSL) is a complex physiologic condition. It refers to a decline in RBC quality marked by abnormalities that are both reversible and irreversible, as well as fatal and sub-lethal.[20] Today whole blood is collected into plastic bags containing a buffered, sodium-citrate anticoagulant solution. Typically citrate, phosphate, dextrose (CPD) or CPDA-1. They both contain citric acid, sodium citrate, monosodium phosphate, and dextrose in

---

[13] Cepham Life Sciences, Inc. Acid Citrate Dextrose (ACD) Solution A. https://www.cephamls.com/acid-citrate-dextrose-acd-solution-a/ Accessed 24 March 2024.

[14] Fisher scientific. BD Vacutainer™ Glass ACD Solution Tube with Yellow Closure. https://www.fishersci.se/shop/products/vacutainer-glass-acd-solution-tube-yellow-closure/p-8579010. Accessed 24 March 2023.

[15] Australian Red Cross Lifeblood. Additives and anticoagulants. https://www.lifeblood.com.au/health-professionals/products/additives-anticoagulants Accessed 22 March 2024.

[16] Ruddell, 1996, p. 4

[17] Meledeo M. A., Peltier G. C., McIntosh C. S., Bynum J. A., Cap A. P. Optimizing whole blood storage: hemostatic function of 35-day stored product in CPD, CP2D, and CPDA-1 anticoagulants. Transfusion. 2019; 59(S2), 1549–1559. https://www.researchgate.net/publication/332405259_Optimizing_whole_blood_storage_hemostatic_function_of_35-day_stored_product_in_CPD_CP2D_and_CPDA-1_anticoagulants.

[18] Sohmer P., Moore G., Beutler E., Peck C. In vivo viability of RBC stored in CPDA-2. Transfusion. 1982; 22 (7), p. 479. https://pubmed.ncbi.nlm.nih.gov/7147326/.

[19] Lbid.

[20] Antonelou, M. H., Seghatchian, J. Insights into red blood cell storage lesion: Toward a new appreciation. Transfusion and Apheresis Science. 2016; 55 (4), p. 292. https://www.sciencedirect.com/science/article/abs/pii/S1473050216301628.

different concentrations. Except that CPD does not contain adenine.[21] There is also a platelet additive solution (PAS).[22]

15.1.1 Some Important Events for Storing Red Blood Cells

Rapoport's studies published in 1947 in a special issue indicated that a maintained red cell viability was dependent on a reasonably well-maintained erythrocyte adenosine triphosphate (ATP) concentration. This finding was later confirmed and extended by others and had great importance for the improvement of storage conditions for red cells. In 1950, A. Smith, J. Lovelock, J. Farrant, H. Meryman, H. Sloviter, R. Valeri, and others showed that long-term storage of red cells as well as some other blood cells can be applied using suitable cryoprotectants. In 1955, C. Finch, E. Simon, H. Yoshikawa, M. Nakao, and others showed that purines and purine nucleosides improve the storage of red cells at 4 °C. In 1965, C. de Verdier, C. Hogman, G. Bartlett, and others proved that ACD-adenine can be used routinely for RBC storage. In 1975, C. Hogman, A. Lovric, and others introduced additive systems for the storage of red cells (SAG, SAG-M, and Circle-Pack).[23] Phosphate inclusion in the 1950s and adenine inclusion in the 1970s opened the door for the development and widespread use of additive solutions in the 1980s, considerably extending shelf life and enhancing RBC storage quality.[24] Two formulations (CPDA-2 and CPDA-3) with twice the amount of adenine as present in CPDA-1 were being actively investigated in the early 1980s, with particular emphasis on red blood cell preservation.[25] The modified CPD-adenine anticoagulants CPDA-2 and CPDA-3 were developed to improve red blood cell storage. It was predicted from the adenosine 5′-triphosphate (ATP) concentrations that whole blood drawn from CPDA-2 and CPDA-3 could be stored for 56 days.[26] Anticoagulant Citrate Phosphate Double Dextrose (CP2D) in Additive Solution 3 (AS-3) was approved by the FDA in 2002.[27] The development of red blood cell storage solutions has subsequently

---

[21] Davis W., Frantz A., Brennan M., Scher C. S. Blood Component Therapy: The History, Efficacy, and Adverse Effects in Clinical Practice, chapter 6. In: Liu H., Kaye A.D., Jahr J. S., editors. Blood Substitutes and Oxygen Biotherapeutics. Cham: Switzerland: Springer; 2022, p. 61–62.

[22] Australian Red Cross Lifeblood. Additives and anticoagulants. https://www.lifeblood.com.au/health-professionals/products/additives-anticoagulants Accessed 22 March 2024.

[23] Högman, 1992, p. 139–144.

[24] Ajmani, 2020, p. 119–123.

[25] Wong, S., & Rock, G. The effect of adenine on platelet storage. Transfusion. 1982; 22 (5), p. 283–287. https://onlinelibrary.wiley.com/doi/abs/10.1046/j.1537-2995.1982.22482251208.x.

[26] Moore, G., Ledford, M., Unruh, K., & Brummell, M. (1981). Red cell storage for 56 days in modified DPD-adenine. An in vitro evaluation. Transfusion. 1981; 21 (7), p. 699–701. https://pubmed.ncbi.nlm.nih.gov/7314217/.

[27] U.S. Food and drug administration. Anticoagulant Citrate Phosphate Double Dextrose (CP2D) & Additive Solution 3 (AS-3). https://www.fda.gov/vaccines-blood-biologics/approved-blood-products/anticoagulant-citrate-phosphate-double-dextrose-cp2d-additive-solution-3-3 Accessed 24 March 2024.

15.1 Important Facts About Anticoagulants and Additive Solutions

progressed slowly and incrementally. Because the developmental cycle typically lasts a decade and industry and regulatory bodies seemed to be able to address just one issue at a time, progress has been made gradually. Adenine in the 1970s, heat sterilization in the 1940s, phosphate in the 1950s,[28] plastic bags in the 1950s,[29] additive solutions in the 1980s, and leucoreduction in the 1990s are some examples of these cycles.[30]

The first red blood cell additive solution was developed in the late 1970s by scientists in Europe and named saline-adenine-glucose (SAG). Soon after, in 1981, the same researchers added mannitol to help maintain red blood cell membranes and reduce hemolysis, allowing RBCs to be refrigerated for up to 6 weeks. SAG-M, a modified form of SAG, is still the most commonly utilized RBC additive. Some countries only allow the use of their SAG-M-RBC components for a maximum of 5 weeks at a time, even though SAG-M can be stored for up to 6 weeks. Because SAG-M lacks an FDA license, it is not used in the United States. This has led to the development and commercialization of a number of additives, which are basically variations of SAG/SAG-M and include AS-1, AS-3, AS-5, MAP, and PAGGSM.[31] AS-3 comprises citrate, phosphate, and an adenine-glucose salt solution as its base.[32] The current generation of additive solutions allows the conservation of RBC for up to 42 days at 1–6 °C.[33] There were also studies of different solutions for the preservation of RBC in the 1970s and 1980s. Some of these studies included the usage of Bicarbonate-Adenine-Glucose-Phosphate-Mannitol (BAGPM) solution and Citrate-Phosphate-Dextrose-Adenine-Sodium Ascorbate (CPD-Ad-NaA) in 1973,[34] the usage of citrate-dextrose-sucrose-adenine-guanosine solution (CDS-AG) in 1983, etc.[35] In modern times, there are also other solutions, on which some studies in 2000 were conducted that showed the possibility of the storage of RBC for more than 42 days. These included the use of a hypotonic

---

[28] Hess, J. R. An update on solutions for red cell storage. Vox Sanguinis.2006; 91 (1), p.13. https://onlinelibrary.wiley.com/doi/full/10.1111/j.1423-0410.2006.00778.x.

[29] AABB, 2024.

[30] Hess, 2006, p.13.

[31] Sparrow R.L. Time to revisit red blood cell additive solutions and storage conditions: a role for "omics" analyses, Blood Transfus.2012; 10 (2), p. 7–11. https://www.ncbi.nlm.nih.gov/pmc/articles/PMC3418618/.

[32] D'Amici G.M., Mirasole C., D'Alessandro A., Yoshida T., Dumont LJ., Zolla L. Red blood cell storage in SAG-M and AS3: a comparison through the membrane two-dimensional electrophoresis proteome. Blood Transfus. 2012;10 (2), p. 46–54. https://www.ncbi.nlm.nih.gov/pmc/articles/PMC3418620/.

[33] García-Roa, M., Del Carmen Vicente-Ayuso, M., Bobes, A. M., Pedraza, A. C., González-Fernández, A., Martín, M. P., Sáez, I., Seghatchian, J., & Gutiérrez, L. Red blood cell storage time and transfusion: current practice, concerns and future perspectives. Blood transfusion = Trasfusione del sangue. 2017;15 (4), p.222–231. https://www.ncbi.nlm.nih.gov/pmc/articles/PMC5448828/.

[34] Wood L.A., Beutler E. The Effect of Periodic Mixing on the Preservation of 2,3-Diphosphoglycerate (2,3-DPG) Levels in Stored Blood. Blood. 1973; 42 (1), p. 17–25. https://www.sciencedirect.com/science/article/pii/S0006497120692412.

[35] Strauss D. CDS-AG medium for red blood cell preservation. Biomed Biochim Acta. 1983;42 (14, 16): S332–6. https://pubmed.ncbi.nlm.nih.gov/6675714/.

experimental additive solution (EAS) for storing RBC for up to 10 weeks.[36,][37] Research conducted in 2014 on AS-7 indicated that, compared to AS-1, which loses membrane integrity after 42 days, AS-7 can maintain RBC membrane integrity for up to 56 days.[38]

Today's licensed anticoagulants and preservative solutions enable the highest possible quality of blood components.

References

1. Australian Red Cross Lifeblood. Additives and anticoagulants. https://www.lifeblood.com.au/health-professionals/products/additives-anticoagulants. Accessed 22 Mar 2024.
2. Antonelou MH, Seghatchian J. Insights into red blood cell storage lesion: toward a new appreciation. Transfus Apher Sci. 2016;55(3):292. https://www.sciencedirect.com/science/article/abs/pii/S1473050216301628.
3. Davis W, Frantz A, Brennan M, Scher CS. Blood component therapy: the history, efficacy, and adverse effects in clinical practice. In: Liu H, Kaye AD, Jahr JS, editors. Blood substitutes and oxygen biotherapeutics. Cham: Springer; 2022. p. 61–2.
4. D'Amici GM, Mirasole C, D'Alessandro A, Yoshida T, Dumont LJ, Zolla L. Red blood cell storage in SAG-M and AS3: a comparison through the membrane two-dimensional electrophoresis proteome. Blood Transfus. 2012;10(2):46–54. https://www.ncbi.nlm.nih.gov/pmc/articles/PMC3418620/.
5. Cepham Life Sciences, Inc. Acid Citrate Dextrose (ACD) Solution A. https://www.cephamls.com/acid-citrate-dextrose-acd-solution-a/ Accessed 24 Mar 2024.
6. Cancelas JA, Dumont LJ, Maes LA, Rugg N, Herschel L, Whitley PH, Zia M. Additive solution-7 reduces the red blood cell cold storage lesion. Transfusion. 2014;55(3):491–8. https://doi.org/10.1111/trf.12867.
7. Dawson RB. Preservation of RBC for transfusion. Hum Pathol. 1983;14(3):213. https://www.sciencedirect.com/science/article/abs/pii/S0046817783800197.
8. De Verdier C, Killander J. Storage of human RBC. I. The effect of acd solution on breakdown of glucose. Acta Physiol Scand. 1962;54(3–4):346–53. https://pubmed.ncbi.nlm.nih.gov/13925397/.
9. Fisher scientific. BD Vacutainer™ Glass ACD Solution Tube with Yellow Closure. https://www.fishersci.se/shop/products/vacutainer-glass-acd-solution-tube-yellow-closure/p-8579010. Accessed 24 Mar 2023.
10. García-Roa M, Del Carmen Vicente-Ayuso M, Bobes AM, Pedraza AC, González-Fernández A, Martín MP, Sáez I, Seghatchian J, Gutiérrez L. Red blood cell storage time and transfusion: current practice, concerns and future perspectives. Blood Transfusion. 2017;15(3):222–31. https://www.ncbi.nlm.nih.gov/pmc/articles/PMC5448828/.

---

[36] Hess, J. R., Rugg, N., Knapp, A. D., Gormas, J. F., Silberstein, E. B., & Greenwalt, T. J. (2000). Successful storage of RBC for 9 weeks in a new additive solution. Transfusion.2000; 40 (9), p. 1007–1011. https://onlinelibrary.wiley.com/doi/abs/10.1046/j.1537-2995.2000.40081007.x.

[37] Hess, J. R., Rugg, N., Knapp, A. D., Gormas, J. F., Silberstein, E. B., & Greenwalt, T. J. (2000). Successful storage of RBC for 10 weeks in a new additive solution. Transfusion. 2000; 40 (9), 1012–1016. https://onlinelibrary.wiley.com/doi/abs/10.1046/j.1537-2995.2000.40081012.x.

[38] Cancelas, J. A., Dumont, L. J., Maes, L. A., Rugg, N., Herschel, L., Whitley, P. H., Zia, M. Additive solution-7 reduces the red blood cell cold storage lesion. Transfusion. 2014; 55 (4) p. 491–498. https://onlinelibrary.wiley.com/doi/full/10.1111/trf.12867.

11. Hess JR, Rugg N, Knapp AD, Gormas JF, Silberstein EB, Greenwalt TJ. Successful storage of RBC for 9 weeks in a new additive solution. Transfusion. 2000;40(8):1007–11. https://doi.org/10.1046/j.1537-2995.2000.40081007.x.
12. Hess JR, Rugg N, Knapp AD, Gormas JF, Silberstein EB, Greenwalt TJ. Successful storage of RBC for 10 weeks in a new additive solution. Transfusion. 2000;40(8):1012–6. https://doi.org/10.1046/j.1537-2995.2000.40081012.x.
13. Hess JR. An update on solutions for red cell storage. Vox Sang. 2006;91(1):13. https://doi.org/10.1111/j.1423-0410.2006.00778.x.
14. Meledeo MA, Peltier GC, McIntosh CS, Bynum JA, Cap AP. Optimizing whole blood storage: hemostatic function of 35-day stored product in CPD, CP2D, and CPDA-1 anticoagulants. Transfusion. 2019;59(S2):1549–59. https://www.researchgate.net/publication/332405259_Optimizing_whole_blood_storage_hemostatic_function_of_35-day_stored_product_in_CPD_CP2D_and_CPDA-1_anticoagulants.
15. Moore G, Ledford M, Unruh K, Brummell M. Red cell storage for 56 days in modified DPD-adenine. An in vitro evaluation. Transfusion. 1981;21(6):699–701. https://pubmed.ncbi.nlm.nih.gov/7314217/.
16. Rajashekharaiah V, Ravikumar S, Krishnegowda M, Hsieh C. Storage lesions in blood components. Oxidants Antioxid Med Sci. 2015;4(3):13. https://www.ejmoams.com/ejmoams-articles/storage-lesions-in-blood-components.pdf. Accessed 24 Mar 2024.
17. Sohmer P, Moore G, Beutler E, Peck C. In vivo viability of RBC stored in CPDA-2. Transfusion. 1982;22(6):479. https://pubmed.ncbi.nlm.nih.gov/7147326/.
18. Sparrow RL. Time to revisit red blood cell additive solutions and storage conditions: a role for "omics" analyses. Blood Transfus. 2012;10(2):7–11. https://www.ncbi.nlm.nih.gov/pmc/articles/PMC3418618/.
19. Strauss D. CDS-AG medium for red blood cell preservation. Biomed Biochim Acta. 1983;42(11–12):S332–6. https://pubmed.ncbi.nlm.nih.gov/6675714/.
20. U.S. Food and drug administration. Anticoagulant Citrate Phosphate Double Dextrose (CP2D) & Additive Solution 3 (AS-3). https://www.fda.gov/vaccines-blood-biologics/approved-blood-products/anticoagulant-citrate-phosphate-double-dextrose-cp2d-additive-solution-3-3. Accessed 24 Mar 2024.
21. Wong S, Rock G. The effect of adenine on platelet storage. Transfusion. 1982;22(4):283–7. https://doi.org/10.1046/j.1537-2995.1982.22482251208.x.
22. Wood LA, Beutler E. The effect of periodic mixing on the preservation of 2,3-Diphosphoglycerate (2,3-DPG) levels in stored blood. Blood. 1973;42(1):17–25. https://www.sciencedirect.com/science/article/pii/S0006497120692412.

Processing and Storage of Blood Components

Contents

16.1 Processing of Whole Blood... 213
16.2 Storage of Blood Components... 215
References.. 216

16.1 Processing of Whole Blood

Blood transfusions are among the most widely used medical procedures in use today and are an essential, life-saving treatment for a variety of illnesses. Nonetheless, whole blood is not commonly used therapeutically in the USA and other developed nations. Instead, blood is separated into its components either before or after it is taken from a donor. This makes it possible to process and store every component of blood under optimal conditions. Blood components can be obtained directly through apheresis or from whole-blood donations. In both cases, whole blood is separated into components by a density gradient.[1] After collection, blood bags should be promptly placed into controlled-temperature storage and transported to the processing site under temperature conditions appropriate for the component that is to be prepared.[2] Each blood component must then be processed, preserved, and stored differently depending on the product being made. Whole blood is collected into plastic bags containing a buffered sodium-citrate anticoagulant solution. The resulting mixture is then separated into its components by centrifugation into RBC and platelet-rich plasma. The preservation solution is used

---

[1] Davis, Frantz, Brennan, Scher, 2022, p. 61–62.
[2] EDQM GUIDE, 2023, p. 441–442.

© The Author(s), under exclusive license to Springer Nature Switzerland AG 2024
Z. Kvržić, *History of Blood Donation and Transfusion Medicine*,
https://doi.org/10.1007/978-3-031-68715-0_16

to isolate and then re-suspend the concentrated RBC. The whole blood is also maintained at room temperature prior to the separation of platelets from the sample.[3] Blood components are therapeutic components of blood (red cells, white cells, platelets, and plasma) that can be prepared by centrifugation, filtration, and freezing using conventional methodologies in blood establishments. A blood product is any therapeutic product derived from human blood or plasma.[4] During the 1950s and 1960s, whole blood transfusion held a significant position in transfusion medicine, despite the availability of a suitable technique for preparing blood components—the closed plastic bag system. In the 1960s and 1970s, strong arguments were made supporting the superiority of blood component therapy, and these reasons were incorporated into medical education at all levels. From the 1980s on, the shift towards 100% blood component therapy gradually started. Also in this period, different technical developments improved, such as the automation of blood component production.[5] Using blood components instead of whole blood ensures that the individual blood components are stored under ideal conditions, minimizes volume overload on the recipient, and lowers the frequency of adverse reactions following transfusion. It also enables a more rational use of blood in terms of logistics, economics, and ethics.[6] Besides plastic bags, anticoagulants, and preservatives, refrigeration, component administration, infectious illness testing, high-risk blood donor screening, etc. made component therapy possible by the twentieth century.[7] Automatic cell separators for collecting single components also contributed to the expansion of component therapy. Today, in most cases, component therapy has expanded all around the world.

Whole blood can be separated by hard-spin centrifugation into layers of blood components according to their specific gravity. For the aftermath of the processing of whole blood into components, fully automated machines are used for the separation of centrifuged whole blood into components.[8] The equipment necessary for the blood processing is a blood bag centrifuge, scale, balances, plasma extractor, automated blood processing machines, pilot tube sealer, sterile connecting device,

---

[3] Davis, Frantz, Brennan, Scher, 2022, p. 61–62.

[4] EDQM GUIDE, 2023, p. 441–442.

[5] Högman, 1992, p. 143–146.

[6] Kvržić Z. Zgodovina krvodajalstva in transfuzijske medicine v Sloveniji. 50 letučinkovitega sodelovanja: pomembna prelomnica ali izjemna priložnost? [Elektronski vir]:zbornik prispevkov z recenzijo: Zbornica zdravstvene in babiške nege Slovenije – Zveza strokovnih društev medicinskih sester, babic in zdravstvenih tehnikov Slovenije, Sekcija medicinskih sester in zdravstvenih tehnikov v anesteziologiji, intenzivni terapiji in transfuziologiji: 53. strokovni seminar: Rogaška Slatina, 17. in 18. November, 2023, p. 98–104. http://www.dlib.si/?URN=URN:NBN:SI:doc-JKK4AQKL. Accessed 25 March 2024.

[7] Karim S., Hoque E. Hoque M.M., Rahman S.M., Islam K. Blood Component Therapy, AKMMC J. 2018; 9 (2), p. 142–147.

[8] Van der Meer P., Pietersz R., Hinloopen B., Dekker W., Reesink H. Automated separation of whole blood in top and bottom bags into components using the Compomat G4. Vox Sang. 1999;76(2), p. 90–99. https://pubmed.ncbi.nlm.nih.gov/10085525/.

platelet agitator, plasma snap freezer, low-temperature freezer, and laminar flow cabinet.[9] As an example of the method of centrifugation in the 1960s with a new bag, the procedure is described as follows: A four-bag closed-collection system was used in 1967, and the blood donor's blood was taken into the first bag. After that, the blood in this bag and the empty satellite bags that had been temporarily sealed off were centrifuged in a refrigerator at 4 °C. Only packed red cells remained in the first bag after the platelet-rich supernatant was expressed into the connecting bag. The bag was then sealed, detached, labeled, and refrigerated at 4 °C for a maximum of 21 days. After that, the third bag holding the clear plasma was frozen at −80 °C. It could then be used as fresh frozen plasma, treated for hemophilia and hypoproteinemia, or processed into one unit of cryoprecipitate high in antihemophilic factor (which was still the third bag) and one plasma unit (expressed into the fourth bag), which could be pooled and commercially fractionated into albumin, gamma globulin, and fibrinogen.[10] It is also important to mention that the irradiation of blood and blood components began in the 1970s.[11] The approval of the use of pathogen reduction technology was much later. First approved in Europe in 2002, and then in the U.S. by the FDA in 2014.[12]

16.2 Storage of Blood Components

Storage of whole blood and later blood components was quite different in the past than it is now. For comparison, in 1949, the equipment and methods for preparing plasma depended on which method of preparation was required. In the case of liquid plasma in commercial vacuum-type containers, the centrifuge method with vacuum bottles, the centrifuge method with reusable equipment, and citrate sedimentation methods were used.[13] For frozen plasma, certain frozen food refrigerators were used, and for rapid thawing, deep, electrically heated water baths were used.[14] For dried plasma, a tight vacuum drying chamber, a condenser, an oil pump, chemical desiccants, an aspirator condenser, a refrigerated condenser, heat that was

---

[9] Hardwick, J. Blood processing and components, section 11. VOXS, 2020; 15, p. 207. https://onlinelibrary.wiley.com/doi/pdf/10.1111/voxs.12598. Accessed 25 March 2024.

[10] Fotino M. New Collection, Processing Methods Provide Specific Blood Components: The Lab, Hospital Topics. 1967; 45 (7) p. 57–58.

[11] Moroff G., Luban N. L. C. "The irradiation of blood and blood components to prevent graft-versus-host disease: technical issues and guidelines." Transfusion Medicine Reviews. 1997; 11 (1), p. 15–26. https://clinlab.ucsf.edu/sites/g/files/tkssra1861/f/wysiwyg/TranMedRev-1997-BloodProductIrradiation.pdf.

[12] Cerus. A Brief History of Blood Safety and Pathogen Reduction Technology. https://www.cerus.com/blog/a-brief-history-of-blood-safety-and-pathogen-reduction-technology/. Accessed 22 Mar 2024.

[13] Alsever J. B. Liquid plasma, chapter 16. In: DeGowin E. L., Hardin R. C., Alsever B. J. Blood transfusion. W.B. Saunders Company Philadelphia & London, 1949, p. 362–394.

[14] Alsever J. B. Frozen plasma, chapter 17. In: DeGowin E. L., Hardin R. C., Alsever B. J. Blood transfusion. W.B. Saunders Company Philadelphia & London, 1949, p. 395–399.

supplied by conduction or infrared radiant heat, apparatus for shell freezing, apparatus for drying plasma, and a closed sterile room were all used.[15] For whole blood refrigerators with a recording thermometer, an installed temperature alarm that was activated in a laboratory or in the office of the hospital engineer when the temperature in the refrigerator was not according to standards was used.[16] By 1949, blood was stored in refrigerators at a temperature between 2 °C and 10 °C. There were four types of equipment used for refrigeration: watertight containers in which the bottles of blood were immersed in ice water, insulated chests, insulated chests with ice, and mechanical refrigerators.[17]

Today, for the storage of RBC, specifically designated blood bank refrigerators are used. For the storage of plasma, specifically blood plasma, storage freezers are used. For the storage of platelets, special incubators with integrated platelet agitators are used.

Today, the temperature of blood components is continuously monitored. Red cells are stored in a fluid state at a controlled temperature between +2 °C and +6 °C. Plasma can be stored for 36 months at −25 °C or below, or for 3 months at between −18 °C and −25 °C. Platelets are normally stored between +20 °C and +24 °C.[18] The storage of platelets at room temperature was shown to be feasible by S. Murphy and F. Gardner in 1969.[19]

References

1. Alsever JB. Liquid plasma, chapter 16. In: De Gowin EL, Hardin RC, Alsever BJ, editors. Blood transfusion. Philadelphia and London: W.B. Saunders; 1949. p. 362–94.
2. Alsever JB. Frozen plasma, chapter 17. In: De Gowin EL, Hardin RC, Alsever BJ, editors. Blood transfusion. Philadelphia and London: W.B. Saunders; 1949. p. 395–9.
3. Alsever JB. Dried plasma, chapter 18. In: De Gowin EL, Hardin RC, Alsever BJ, editors. Blood transfusion. Philadelphia and London: W.B. Saunders; 1949. p. 400–19.
4. Degowin EL. Operation of a hospital blood bank, Chapter 24. In: De Gowin EL, Hardin RC, Alsever BJ, editors. Blood transfusion. Philadelphia and London: W.B. Saunders; 1949. p. 482–3.
5. Cerus. A brief history of blood safety and pathogen reduction technology. https://www.cerus.com/blog/a-brief-history-of-blood-safety-and-pathogen-reduction-technology/. Accessed 22 Mar 2024.

---

[15] Alsever J. B. Dried plasma, chapter 18. In: DeGowin E. L., Hardin R. C., Alsever B. J. Blood transfusion. W.B. Saunders Company Philadelphia & London, 1949, p. 400–419.

[16] Degowin E. L. Operation of a hospital blood bank, chapter 24. In: DeGowin E. L., Hardin R. C., Alsever B. J. Blood transfusion. W.B. Saunders Company Philadelphia & London, 1949, p. 482–483.

[17] Hardin R. C. Transportation of whole blood, chapter 14. In: DeGowin E. L., Hardin R. C., Alsever B. J. Blood transfusion. W.B. Saunders Company Philadelphia & London, 1949, p. 344.

[18] EDQM GUIDE, 2023, p. 197–286.

[19] Murphy S., Gardner F.H. Effect of storage temperature on maintenance of platelet viability—deleterious effect of refrigerated storage. N. Engl. J. Med., May 15. 1969;280(20), p. 1094–1098. https://pubmed.ncbi.nlm.nih.gov/5778424/.

References

6. Fotino M. New collection, processing methods provide specific blood components: the lab. Hosp Top. 1967;45(7):57–8. https://pubmed.ncbi.nlm.nih.gov/6045568/.
7. Hardwick J. Blood processing and components, section 11. VOXS. 2020;15:207. https://doi.org/10.1111/voxs.12598. Accessed 25 Mar 2024.
8. Hardin RC. Transportation of whole blood, Chapter 14. In: De Gowin EL, Hardin RC, Alsever BJ, editors. Blood transfusion. Philadelphia and London: W.B. Saunders; 1949. p. 344.
9. Karim S, Hoque E, Hoque MM, Rahman SM, Islam K. Blood component therapy. AKMMC J. 2018;9(2):142–7.
10. Kvržić Z. Zgodovina krvodajalstva in transfuzijske medicine v Sloveniji. 50 letučinkovitega sodelovanja: pomembna prelomnica ali izjemna priložnost? [Elektronski vir]:zbornik prispevkov z recenzijo: Zbornica zdravstvene in babiške nege Slovenije – Zveza strokovnih društev medicinskih sester, babic in zdravstvenih tehnikov Slovenije, Sekcija medicinskih sester in zdravstvenih tehnikov v anesteziologiji, intenzivni terapiji in transfuziologiji: 53. strokovni seminar: Rogaška Slatina, 17. in 18. November, 2023, p. 98–104. http://www.dlib.si/?URN=URN:NBN:SI:doc-JKK4AQKL. Accessed 25 March 2024.
11. Moroff G, Luban NLC. The irradiation of blood and blood components to prevent graft-versus-host disease: technical issues and guidelines. Transfus Med Rev. 1997;11(1):15–26. https://clinlab.ucsf.edu/sites/g/files/tkssra1861/f/wysiwyg/TranMedRev-1997-BloodProductIrradiation.pdf.
12. Murphy S, Gardner FH. Effect of storage temperature on maintenance of platelet viability—deleterious effect of refrigerated storage. N Engl J Med. 1969;280(20):1094–8. https://pubmed.ncbi.nlm.nih.gov/5778424/.
13. Van der Meer P, Pietersz R, Hinloopen B, Dekker W, Reesink H. Automated separation of whole blood in top and bottom bags into components using the Compomat G4. Vox Sang. 1999;76(2):90–9. https://pubmed.ncbi.nlm.nih.gov/10085525/.

Blood Donor Screening 17

Contents

17.1 Syphilis... 220
17.2 Hepatitis B... 221
17.3 Hepatitis C... 222
17.4 HIV and AIDS.. 223
       17.4.1 LGBTQ+ Community and Blood Donation................................. 224
17.5 Interesting Facts About Different Tests... 226
References.. 228

Selecting voluntarily non-remunerated blood donors from low-risk populations who donate blood frequently is the first step in lowering the risk of infectious disease transmission through blood transfusions. These blood donors have a lower risk of spreading transfusion-transmissible infections than paid or family/replacement blood donors. Precise and strict screening of all given blood is necessary to guarantee the blood supply's safety. Before blood components or blood products are released for clinical or industrial use, the WHO advises that all blood donations be screened for evidence of infection. All blood donations should be mandatory for screening for syphilis, HIV, and hepatitis B and C. To guarantee the safety and compatibility of blood transfusions, the donated blood should also be tested for ABO and RhD.[1] Since the 1940s, it has been widely known that blood can spread infectious diseases.[2]

---

[1] World Health Organization (WHO). Testing of donated blood. https://www.who.int/teams/health-product-policy-and-standards/standards-and-specifications/blood-product-standardization/quality-and-safety/donation-testing. Accessed 30 Mar 2024.
[2] Högman, 1992, p. 146.

© The Author(s), under exclusive license to Springer Nature Switzerland AG 2024
Z. Kvržić, *History of Blood Donation and Transfusion Medicine*, https://doi.org/10.1007/978-3-031-68715-0_17

17.1 Syphilis

The ancient sexually transmitted infection syphilis is a treatable and preventive STI. Serious health problems may result if left untreated. Many syphilis patients either don't experience symptoms at all or are unaware of them. Oral, vaginal, and anal intercourse, pregnancy, and blood transfusions are the ways in which syphilis is spread. Pregnant women with syphilis run the risk of stillbirth, neonatal mortality, and syphilis in the newborn (congenital syphilis). Syphilis can be avoided with proper and consistent condom use during sexual intercourse. In a matter of minutes, rapid testing can provide results, enabling the commencement of treatment during the same clinic visit. It is estimated by the WHO that in 2020 about 7.1 million adults between the ages of 15 and 49 were infected with syphilis. Disproportionally affected are gay males and other men who have sex with men.[3,4] The bacterium Treponema pallidum, which causes the sexually transmitted disease syphilis, was the subject of the initial tests for antibodies.[5] Fritz Schaudinn (1871–1906) and Erich Hoffmann (1868–1954) made the discovery of Treponema pallidum in 1905. The first serologic test for the diagnosis of syphilis was created by German bacteriologist August Paul von Wassermann (1866–1925), dermatologist and venereologist Albert Neisser (1855–1916), and dermatologist and venereologist Carl Bruck (1879–1944). On May 10, 1906, they released their first article on it. Because they employed Octave Gengou (1875–1957) and Jules Bordet (1870–1961)'s concept of the complement fixation test, the Wassermann reaction is occasionally referred to as the Bordet–Wassermann reaction. Syphilis was diagnosed using the Wassermann response. It should be noted that although the Wassermann reaction is no longer in use, it was among the very first serodiagnostic tests ever employed in clinical practice.[6] Alexander Fleming (1881–1955) discovered penicillin in 1928, and from 1943, it became the main treatment for syphilis.[7] The United States' Centers for Disease Control and Prevention had already approved 11 tests in 1986; among these were flocculation tests, commonly referred to as nontreponemal testing.[8] Today's syphilis tests screen for and diagnose syphilis by looking for certain antibodies in our blood. Other tests for checking for syphilis antibodies are: rapid plasma reagin (RPR), Venereal Disease Research Laboratory (VDRL), fluorescent treponemal antibody absorption (FTA-ABS) test, agglutination assay (TP-PA), darkfield

---

[3] WHO. Syphilis. https://www.who.int/news-room/fact-sheets/detail/syphilis. Accessed 30 Mar 2024.

[4] Tampa M., Sarbu I., Matei C., Benea V., Georgescu S. R. Brief history of syphilis. Journal of medicine and life. 2014; 7 (1), p. 4–10. https://www.ncbi.nlm.nih.gov/pmc/articles/PMC3956094/.

[5] Dean C.L., Wade J., Roback J.D., Transfusion-Transmitted Infections: An Update on Product Screening, Diagnostic Techniques, and the Path Ahead. J. Clin. Microbiol.2018; 56 (7) e00352–18. https://pubmed.ncbi.nlm.nih.gov/29669792/.

[6] Bialynicki-Birula R. The 100th anniversary of Wassermann-Neisser-Bruck reaction. Clin Dermatol. 2008;26 (1), p. 79. https://pubmed.ncbi.nlm.nih.gov/18280907/.

[7] Tampa, Sarbu, Matei, Benea, Georgescu, 2014, p. 4–10.

[8] Bialynicki-Birula, 2008, p. 79.

microscopy.[9] As an interesting fact, the first case of syphilis-infected blood transfusion was reported in 1915.[10] Another notable fact is that, according to the available literature in the USA, Vanderbilt University Hospital serologically tested blood from blood donors for syphilis as early as 1928.[11] Nowadays, one of the ways of controlling the worldwide spreading of syphilis is through prevention and treatment programs.[12] Early syphilis can be cured with a single injection of long-acting benzathine penicillin G. This antibiotic can also be used for treating later stages of syphilis with more required doses.[13]

17.2 Hepatitis B

Hippocrates wrote about epidemic jaundice in the fifth century before the Common Era (BCE). It is believed that the first occurrences of serum hepatitis were those that occurred after German shipyard workers were given a smallpox vaccine containing human lymph in 1883. Following the use of infected needles and syringes, cases of serum hepatitis were often reported in the early and middle decades of the twentieth century. In 1943, Paul Beeson reported that jaundice had occurred in seven recipients of blood transfusions, emphasizing the significance of blood as a means of viral transmission. The Australia antigen, which subsequently became known as hepatitis B surface antigen (HBsAg), was initially reported in 1965. In 1969, the first screening of blood from blood donors for hepatitis B surface antigen (HBsAg) began in the USA.[14] Blood banks started testing for hepatitis B in 1971,[15] and mandatory testing was introduced in 1972.[16] In 1970, the entire hepatitis B virion, or Dane particle, was discovered. Following this, the discovery of serologic markers for HBV infection assisted in elucidating the disease's natural course. Eventually, HBV's surface protein, HBsAg, was produced in large quantities and is currently the immunogen in very successful vaccinations that prevent HBV infection. In 1981, the US received its first permission to provide the Hepatitis B (HepB)

---

[9] Medlineplus. Syphilis Tests. https://medlineplus.gov/lab-tests/syphilis-tests/ Accessed 28 Mar 2024.

[10] Kaur G., Kaur P. Syphilis testing in blood donors: an update, Blood Transfus.2015;13 (2), p. 197–204. https://www.ncbi.nlm.nih.gov/pmc/articles/PMC4385067/.

[11] Keller A. E., Leathers W.S. Serologic reactions for syphilis in blood transfusion blood donors. Venereal Disease Information. 1939; 20 (1), p. 5–8. https://www.cabdirect.org/cabdirect/abstract/19392701453.

[12] Tampa, Sarbu. Matei, Benea, Georgescu, 2014, p. 4–10.

[13] CDC. Syphilis Treatment and Care. https://www.cdc.gov/std/syphilis/treatment.htm Accessed 30 Mar 2024.

[14] Centers for disease control and prevention (CDC). Public Health Service Inter-Agency Guidelines for screening blood donors of blood, plasma, organs, tissues, and semen for evidence. https://www.cdc.gov/mmwr/preview/mmwrhtml/00043883.htm. Accessed 5 May 2022.

[15] Alexander T. S. Human Immunodeficiency Virus Diagnostic Testing: 30 Years of Evolution, Clinical and Vaccine Immunology.2016; 23 (4), p.249–253. https://journals.asm.org/doi/10.1128/CVI.00053-16.

[16] CDC, 2022.

vaccine, which was produced from plasma. Although the vaccination was safe and successful, it was not widely embraced, perhaps as a result of unfounded concerns about the spread of live HBV and other blood-borne infections. Commencing in 1986, recombinant HepB vaccines supplanted plasma-derived HepB vaccinations.[17] The vaccines are usually administered shortly after delivery; booster shots follow a few weeks later. It provides almost complete virus protection. Hepatitis B is a disease that infects the liver and is caused by the hepatitis B virus. The infection can be acute or chronic. The infected person is at high risk of dying from cirrhosis or liver cancer. In highly endemic areas, hepatitis B is most commonly spread from mother to child at birth or through exposure to infected blood, especially from an infected child to an uninfected child during the first 5 years of life.[18] Children can spread the disease to others through household contact or through scrapes or cuts.[19] In addition, exposure to contaminated blood and bodily fluids, including saliva and menstrual, vaginal, and seminal secretions, tattooing, piercing, and needlestick injuries, can all transmit hepatitis B. Reusing contaminated needles, syringes, or sharp items in medical establishments, among the general public, or among those who inject drugs can also be a cause of infection. Those who have several sexual partners and have not received vaccinations are more likely to transmit sexual diseases. Usually administered shortly after delivery, booster shots follow a few weeks later. It provides almost complete virus protection. According to WHO estimates, 1.5 million new cases of chronic hepatitis B infection occur each year, impacting 296 million people worldwide.[20]

17.3 Hepatitis C

The hepatitis C virus (HCV) was discovered in 1989. The intense research effort that took place in the 1970s and 1980s and led to the identification of HCV was mainly motivated by the urgent worries of medical professionals and epidemiologists who were becoming more aware of the connection between chronic non-A and non-B hepatitis and plasma-derived blood product therapy and transfusion[21] sharing needles or syringes, blood transfusions with unscreened blood products, and other unsafe medical procedures that can cause the infection of blood. The WHO estimates that 58 million people have chronic hepatitis C virus infection, with about 1.5

---

[17] Haber P., Schillie S. Hepatitis B. Centers for Disease Control and Prevention (CDC). Epidemiology and Prevention of Vaccine-Preventable Diseases. https://www.cdc.gov/vaccines/pubs/pinkbook/hepb.html. Accessed 30 Mar 2024.
[18] WHO. Hepatitis B. https://www.who.int/news-room/fact-sheets/detail/hepatitis-b. Accessed 30 Mar 2024.
[19] Stanford Medicine. Hepatitis B Causes. https://stanfordhealthcare.org/medical-conditions/liver-kidneys-and-urinary-system/hepatitis-b/causes.html. Accessed 30 Mar 2024.
[20] WHO, 2024.
[21] Simmonds P. The Origin of Hepatitis C Virus. Hepatitis C Virus: From Molecular Virology to Antiviral Therapy. 2013, p. 1–15. https://pubmed.ncbi.nlm.nih.gov/23463195/.

million new infections every year. Hepatitis C has effective therapies available. Curing the illness and preventing long-term liver damage are the two main objectives of treatment. Hepatitis C is treated with antiviral drugs such as daclatasvir and sofosbuvir. Some infections can be treated spontaneously by the immune system, and new infections don't always require medical attention. Chronic hepatitis C always requires treatment. Lifestyle modifications, such as abstaining from alcohol and keeping a healthy weight, may also be beneficial for those with hepatitis C. Many hepatitis C patients can be cured and live healthy lives with the right care. The WHO suggests pan-genotypic direct-acting antivirals (DAAs) as a treatment for chronic hepatitis C infection in all adults, adolescents, and children less than 3 years old.[22]

17.4 HIV and AIDS

The virus known as human immunodeficiency virus (HIV) targets the immune system of the body. AIDS, or acquired immunodeficiency syndrome, is the disease's most advanced stage. HIV attacks white blood cells in the body, weakening immunity. This increases the risk of contracting infections, certain cancers, and diseases like tuberculosis. HIV can spread through bodily fluids such as blood, breast milk, semen, and vaginal secretions from an infected individual. It cannot be transmitted by sharing meals, hugs, or kisses. Additionally, it can pass from a mother to her child. By the end of 2022, there were an anticipated 39.0 million HIV-positive individuals worldwide, of which 25.6 million were in the WHO African Region.[23] HIV targets monkeys' and apes' immune systems, and chimpanzees are the sources of HIV. A 1999 study discovered a chimpanzee SIV strain known as SIVcpz that was remarkably like HIV. The researcher subsequently found that chimpanzees hunt and consume red-capped mangabeys and larger spot-nosed monkeys, two smaller monkey species that harbor two strains of SIV that infect the chimps. It is possible that these two strains came together to generate SIVcpz, a virus that can infect humans and chimpanzees. SIVcpz most likely spread to humans when African hunters consumed sick chimpanzees or when the chimps' contaminated blood entered into the hunters' cuts or wounds. Researchers think that in 1920, in Kinshasa, the capital and largest city of the Democratic Republic of the Congo, there was the first human transmission of SIV to HIV, which subsequently sparked the global epidemic. It's possible that the virus left Kinshasa via migrants and the sex trade and traveled along infrastructure channels (roads, trains, and rivers). HIV first appeared in Haiti and the Caribbean in the 1960s after Haitian professionals returned from the colonial Democratic Republic of the Congo. After that, in 1970, the virus spread from the Caribbean to New York City and, a little later in the decade, to San Francisco.

---

[22] WHO. Hepatitis C. https://www.who.int/news-room/fact-sheets/detail/hepatitis-c. Accessed 30 Mar 2024.

[23] WHO. HIV AND AIDS. https://www.who.int/news-room/fact-sheets/detail/hiv-aids. Accessed 30 Mar 2024.

Travel from the United States abroad aided in the virus's global spread.[24] The virus HIV responsible for aids was identified on May 20, 1983.[25] Thanks to the efforts of Luc Montagnier (1932–2002), a French virologist, Robert Gallo, an American biomedical researcher, and their respective colleagues, the HIV virus was isolated, and a technique for identifying antibodies against the virus was created. It was discovered—quite surprisingly—that people who have HIV antibodies in circulation nearly always also have the virus. As was the case with the majority of other infectious diseases, no protective immunity developed. Techniques appropriate for mass screening blood donors became accessible and widely used around 1985.[26] HIV infection cannot be cured. Antiretroviral medications, which prevent the virus from multiplying in the body, are used to manage it. While HIV infection cannot be cured, current antiretroviral therapy (ART) helps a person's immune system become stronger. They can fend off various infections thanks to this.[27]

17.4.1 LGBTQ+ Community and Blood Donation

The LGBTQ+ community includes same-sex, transsex, and other sexual identities. Members of the LGBTQ+ community have always faced many challenges in the social sphere, including in the area of blood donation. The HIV virus, which caused tens of millions of deaths all around the world, has been the main reason for the deferral of the homosexual community's blood donation, mainly by men who have sex with men (MSM). If HIV is not treated, it leads to AIDS.

From October 1980 to May 1981, five males and active homosexuals were treated for *Pneumocystis carinii pneumonia*. This was the beginning of the HIV outbreak. Those were the initial AIDS cases to be identified. By 1983, there were 1000 confirmed cases in the USA, mostly of homosexual men. The same year, deferral policies were introduced.[28] The deferral policies were introduced because, at that time, there wasn't any blood test available to detect the presence of the AIDS-causing agent. HIV was identified in 1984 as the cause of AIDS.[29] In 1992, lifetime deferral guidelines were issued. Deferral policies spread across the world in the

---

[24] History. History of AIDS. What is AIDS? https://www.history.com/topics/1980s/history-of-aids. Accessed 30 Mar 2024.

[25] Institut Pasteur. 40 years of HIV discovery: the virus responsible for aids is identified on May 20, 1983. https://www.pasteur.fr/en/press-area/press-documents/40-years-after-discovery-hiv?language=fr. Accessed 30 Mar 2024.

[26] Högman, 1992, p. 146.

[27] WHO, 2024.

[28] Christopher M., Logan P. An Antiquated Perspective: Lifetime Ban for MSM Blood Donations No Longer Global Norm, DePaul J. Health Care L.2014; 16 (1), p. 21–47. https://via.library.depaul.edu/cgi/viewcontent.cgi?article=1006&context=jhcl.

[29] Wilson K., Atkinson K., Keelan J. Three decades of MSM blood donor deferral policies. What have we learned? Int J Infect Dis.2014;18, p. 1–3. https://www.ijidonline.com/action/showPdf?pii=S1201-9712%2813%2900308-1.

1980s.[30] Since then, countries all around the world have had different laws and regulations. Some are excluded from donating blood, both men and women, from the LGBTQ+ community.

AIDS did not just spread from the homosexual community but also from the heterosexual population, for example, because of prostitution and drug abuse.[31] HIV testing equipment has considerably improved since 1983. Modern serologic screening methods get close to being 100% sensitive and specific. Testing technologies excellently detect HIV, which has led to reassessing the ban on MSM and gradually lifting the ban.[32] Countries' deferral periods in 2014 ranged from 1 year to 5 years. Others didn't have a set MSM deferral policy. Regardless of sexual orientation, deferrals in these nations were based on the interval following a change in sexual partners and an evaluation of dangerous sexual activity. Also, several nations have prohibited MSM blood donors for life.[33] In the USA, an interesting change was made by the Food and Drug Administration (FDA) based on an evaluation of the available scientific evidence. In their guidance, *"Revised Recommendations for Reducing the Risk of Human Immunodeficiency Virus Transmission by Blood and Blood Products,"* released in April 2020, they changed the lifetime MSM deferral to a deferral for 3 months from the most recent sexual contact, meaning a man who has had sex with another man during the past 3 months.[34] Countries around the world that do not allow MSM to donate blood are defending their position to ensure safe and healthy blood for patients. Various organizations in countries where blood donation is still banned for MSM have condemned the ban as discriminatory. Today in the USA, other members of the LGBTQ+ community, as long as they are healthy and meet the strict medical criteria for blood donation, can donate blood at regular monthly intervals. Whether a patient receives blood from members of the LGBTQ+ community or from the heterosexual population, every blood transfusion of human blood received must be safe and healthy in order to save the patient's life.

---

[30] Christopher M, Logan, 2014, p. 24–26.

[31] Desvarieux M., Pape J.W. HIV and AIDS in Haiti: recent developments. AIDS Care. 1991;3 (3), p. 271–279. https://pubmed.ncbi.nlm.nih.gov/1932190/.

[32] Karamitros G., Kitsos N., Karamitrou I., The ban on blood donation on men who have sex with men: time to rethink and reassess an outdated policy, Pan Afr Med J., 2017;27(99), p. 1–4. https://www.ncbi.nlm.nih.gov/pmc/articles/PMC5554671/.

[33] Wilson K, Atkinson K, Keelan J., 2014, p. 2.

[34] U.S. Food and Drug administration. Revised Recommendations for Reducing the Risk of Human Immuno deficiency Virus Transmission by Blood and Blood Products. 2020, p. 6–9. https://www.fda.gov/media/92490/download. Accessed 8 May 2022.

17.5 Interesting Facts About Different Tests

The platelet immunofluorescence test was introduced to the general public in 1978, although the editors from the author Von Dem Borne and his colleagues received an article on this topic as early as 1977. The original name of this test was PSIFT.[35,36] Monoclonal antibodies directed against glycoproteins IIb/IIIa and Ib, the principal elements of platelet membranes, have been accessible since 1987. Currently, there are a minimum of four methods for identifying human platelet antigen (HPA) antibodies: the platelet immunofluorescence test (PIFT), the solid-phase assay, the monoclonal antibody immobilization of platelet antigens (MAIPA) assay, and several enzyme-linked immunosorbent assay (ELISA)-based methods. Furthermore, molecular typing can be utilized to obtain an indirect prediction of the existence of HPA antibodies.[37] In the early 1980s, early tests of blood donors for cytolomegalovirus (CMV) were introduced in the USA.[38] In 1985, screening of blood products for HIV began.[39] This was performed with an enzyme-linked immunosorbent assay (ELISA), which was the first blood-screening test to detect HIV antibodies.[40] In 1986, Japan became the first country in the world to screen blood donors for the human T-cell lymphotropic virus (HTLV).[41] There are two types of antibodies to human T-cell lymphotropic virus types 1 (anti-HTLV 1) and 2 (anti-HTLV 2).[42] Blood donor screening for antibodies to hepatitis B core antigen (anti-HBc) as a surrogate test for non-A and non-B hepatitis was introduced by some countries in

---

[35] Von dem Borne A.E., Verheugt F.W., Oosterhof F., Von Riesz E., De la Rivière A.B., Engelfriet C.P. A simple immunofluorescence test for the detection of platelet antibodies. Br J Haematol. 1978 Jun;39 (2), p.195–207. https://pubmed.ncbi.nlm.nih.gov/354684/.

[36] Hagenström H., Schlenke P., Hennig H., Kirchner H., Klüter H. Quantification of platelet-associated IgG for differential diagnosis of patients with thrombocytopenia. Thromb Haemost. 2000 84 (5), p. 779–83. https://pubmed.ncbi.nlm.nih.gov/11127855/.

[37] Dutra, V. D. F., Costa T. H., Santos L. D., Sirianni M. F. M., Aravechia M. G., Kutner J. M., Bub C. B. Platelet antibodies identification: comparison between two laboratory tests. Hematology, Transfusion and Cell Therapy. 2000; 44, p. 365–368. https://www.scielo.br/j/htct/a/mF8SSLcVWJCNGPVyjqtmDwK/.

[38] Hicks A. Cytomegalovirus and blood donation. What you need to know. https://stanfordbloodcenter.org/cytomegalovirus-and-blood-donation-what-you-need-to-know/. Accessed 28 Mar 2024.

[39] Alexander, 2016, p. 249–253.

[40] Sahni A.K., Nagendra A., Roy P., Patrikar S. Usefulness of enzyme immunoassay (EIA) for screening of anti HIV antibodies in urinary specimens: A comparative analysis. Med. J. Armed Forces India.2014; 70 (3), p. 211–214. https://www.ncbi.nlm.nih.gov/pmc/articles/PMC4213891/.

[41] Marano G., Vaglio S., Pupella S., Facco G., Catalano L., Piccinini V., Liumbruno G.M., Grazzini G. Human T-lymphotropic virus and transfusion safety: does one size fit all?,Transfusion. 2016; 56 (1), p. 249–260. https://pubmed.ncbi.nlm.nih.gov/26388300/.

[42] EDQM GUIDE, 2023, p. 337.

the mid-1980s.[43] In 1990, screening of blood donors for hepatitis C began.[44] In 1997, Germany was the first country in the world to introduce nucleic acid testing (NAT) testing of blood from blood donors for the hepatitis B virus, the hepatitis C virus, and human HIV-1.[45] NAT is a molecular method of screening blood donations to lower the danger of transfusion-transmitted illnesses (TTIs) in the recipients.[46] During the early stages of infection, NAT can detect very low levels of viral RNA or DNA.[47] Blood from blood donors can also be tested for antibodies against, for example, malaria, the West Nile virus, and Trypanosoma cruzi (the causative agent of Chagas' disease).[48] Also on Zika virus,[49] for the detection of hepatitis E virus (HEV) infection,[50] and for the presence of antibodies to the novel SARS-CoV-2 coronavirus.[51] The minimum mandatory serological blood donor screening tests of the Council of Europe are: antibody to HIV-1 (anti-HIV-1) and HIV-2 (anti-HIV-2), including outlying types (e.g., HIV-1 type O), antibody to hepatitis C virus (anti-HCV), and hepatitis B surface antigen (HBsAg).[52] Many transfusion services have introduced screening for HLA, HLA, and HNA antibodies to reduce the incidence of transfusion-related acute lung injury (TRALI).[53] Before a donation of granulocytes can be made, the granulocyte count in the blood of a donor must be elevated so that collection becomes technically feasible.[54] Other tests on blood can also be conducted.

---

[43] Riordan J. O. Antibody to hepatitis B core antigen, section 1: agents.In: Barbara J. A. J., Regan F. A. M., Contreras D. M., editors. Transfusion microbiology. Cambridge University Press. 2008, p. 25.

[44] Relias Media.Hospital Infection Control & Prevention. CDC develops notification letters for HCV testing, 1999. https://www.reliasmedia.com/articles/41057-cdc-develops-notification-letters-for-hcv-testing.

[45] Roth W. K. History and Future of Nucleic Acid Amplification Technology Blood donor Testing., Transfus.Med.Hemother.2019; 46 (2),p. 67–75. https://pubmed.ncbi.nlm.nih.gov/31191192/.

[46] Hans R., Marwaha N. Nucleic acid testing-benefits and constraints. Asian journal of transfusion science. 2014;8 (1), p. 2–3. https://www.ncbi.nlm.nih.gov/pmc/articles/PMC3943139/.

[47] Irish Blood Transfusion Service. Nucleic Acid Testing (NAT). https://healthprofessionals.giveblood.ie/clinical-services/national-donor-screening-laboratory-ndsl-/nucleic-acid-testing-nat-/. Accessed 6 Apr 2024.

[48] Fisayo T. Science in action? A critical view of UK blood donation deferral policy and men who have sex with men, Int. J. Health Plann. Mgmt.2021; 36 (4), p. 1207–1222. https://pubmed.ncbi.nlm.nih.gov/33834528/.

[49] CDC. Testing for Zika virus infection. https://www.cdc.gov/zika/laboratories/types-of-tests.html. Accessed 5 May 2022.

[50] Bi H., Yang R., Wu C., Xia J.Hepatitis E virus and blood transfusion safety. Epidemiology and infection. 2020; 148, e158. https://www.ncbi.nlm.nih.gov/pmc/articles/PMC7424600/

[51] Caliendo A. M., Hanson K. E. Patient education: Blood donation and transfusion (Beyond the Basics),Covid—19: diagnosis. Available at: https://www.uptodate.com/contents/covid-19-diagnosis?search=antibodies. Accessed 6 May 2022.

[52] EDQM GUIDE, 2023, p. 336.

[53] JPAC. Donor testing. https://www.transfusionguidelines.org/red-book/chapter-17-granulocyte-immunology/17-5-donor-testing. Accessed 30 Mar 2024.

[54] Universitätsklinikum Regensburg (UKR). Donating blood. Donating granulocytes. https://www.ukr.de/en/donate-blood/donating-granulocytes. Accessed 30 Mar 2024.

References

1. Alexander TS. Human immunodeficiency virus diagnostic testing: 30 years of evolution. Clin Vaccine Immunol. 2016;23(4):249–53. https://doi.org/10.1128/CVI.00053-16.
2. Bialynicki-Birula R. The 100th anniversary of Wassermann-Neisser-Bruck reaction. Clin Dermatol. 2008;26(1):79. https://pubmed.ncbi.nlm.nih.gov/18280907/.
3. Bi H, Yang R, Wu C, Xia J. Hepatitis E virus and blood transfusion safety. Epidemiol Infect. 2020;148:e158. https://www.ncbi.nlm.nih.gov/pmc/articles/PMC7424600/.
4. Centers for disease control and prevention (CDC). Public Health Service Inter-Agency Guidelines for screening blood donors of blood, plasma, organs, tissues, and semen for evidence. https://www.cdc.gov/mmwr/preview/mmwrhtml/00043883.htm. Accessed 5 May 2022.
5. CDC. Syphilis treatment and care. https://www.cdc.gov/std/syphilis/treatment.htm. Accessed 30 Mar 2024.
6. Christopher M, Logan P. An antiquated perspective: lifetime ban for MSM blood donations no longer global norm. DePaul J Health Care L. 2014;16(1):21–47. https://via.library.depaul.edu/cgi/viewcontent.cgi?article=1006&context=jhcl.
7. CDC. Testing for Zika virus infection. https://www.cdc.gov/zika/laboratories/types-of-tests.html. Accessed 5 May 2022.
8. Caliendo AM, Hanson KE. Patient education: blood donation and transfusion (beyond the basics), Covid-19: diagnosis. https://www.uptodate.com/contents/covid-19-diagnosis?search=antibodies. Accessed 6 May 2022.
9. Dean CL, Wade J, Roback JD. Transfusion-transmitted infections: an update on product screening, diagnostic techniques, and the path ahead. J Clin Microbiol. 2018;56(7):e00352–18. https://pubmed.ncbi.nlm.nih.gov/29669792/.
10. Desvarieux M, Pape JW. HIV and AIDS in Haiti: recent developments. AIDS Care. 1991;3(3):271–9. https://pubmed.ncbi.nlm.nih.gov/1932190/.
11. Dutra VDF, Costa T H, Santos LD, Sirianni MFM, Aravechia MG, Kutner JM, Bub CB. Platelet antibodies identification: comparison between two laboratory tests. Hematol Transfus Cell Therapy. 2000;44:365–8. https://www.scielo.br/j/htct/a/mF8SSLcVWJCNGPVyjqtmDwK/.
12. Fisayo T. Science in action? A critical view of UK blood donation deferral policy and men who have sex with men. Int J Health Plann Mgmt. 2021;36(4):1207–22. https://pubmed.ncbi.nlm.nih.gov/33834528/.
13. Haber P, Schillie S. Hepatitis B. Centers for Disease Control and Prevention (CDC). Epidemiology and prevention of vaccine-preventable diseases. https://www.cdc.gov/vaccines/pubs/pinkbook/hepb.html. Accessed 30 Mar 2024.
14. History. History of AIDS. What is AIDS? https://www.history.com/topics/1980s/history-of-aids. Accessed 30 Mar 2024.
15. Hagenström H, Schlenke P, Hennig H, Kirchner H, Klüter H. Quantification of platelet-associated IgG for differential diagnosis of patients with thrombocytopenia. Thromb Haemost. 2000;84(5):779–83. https://pubmed.ncbi.nlm.nih.gov/11127855/.
16. Hicks A. Cytomegalovirus and blood donation. What you need to know. https://stanfordbloodcenter.org/cytomegalovirus-and-blood-donation-what-you-need-to-know/. Accessed 28 Mar 2024.
17. Hans R, Marwaha N. Nucleic acid testing-benefits and constraints. Asian J Transfus Sci. 2014;8(1):2–3. https://www.ncbi.nlm.nih.gov/pmc/articles/PMC3943139.
18. Institut Pasteur. 40 years of HIV discovery: the virus responsible for aids is identified on May 20, 1983. https://www.pasteur.fr/en/press-area/press-documents/40-years-after-discovery-hiv?language=fr. Accessed 30 Mar 2024.
19. Irish Blood Transfusion Service. Nucleic Acid Testing (NAT). https://healthprofessionals.giveblood.ie/clinical-services/national-donor-screening-laboratory-ndsl-/nucleic-acid-testing-nat-/. Accessed 6 Apr 2024.
20. JPAC. Donor testing. https://www.transfusionguidelines.org/red-book/chapter-17-granulocyte-immunology/17-5-donor-testing. Accessed 30 Mar 2024.

21. Kaur G, Kaur P. Syphilis testing in blood donors: an update. Blood Transfus. 2015;13(2):197–204. https://www.ncbi.nlm.nih.gov/pmc/articles/PMC4385067/.
22. Keller AE, Leathers WS. Serologic reactions for syphilis in blood transfusion blood donors. Venereal Dis Inform. 1939;20(1):5–8. https://www.cabdirect.org/cabdirect/abstract/19392701453.
23. Karamitros G, Kitsos N, Karamitrou I. The ban on blood donation on men who have sex with men: time to rethink and reassess an outdated policy. Pan Afr Med J. 2017;27(99):1–4. https://www.ncbi.nlm.nih.gov/pmc/articles/PMC5554671/.
24. Medlineplus. Syphilis tests. https://medlineplus.gov/lab-tests/syphilis-tests/. Accessed 28 Mar 2024.
25. Marano G, Vaglio S, Pupella S, Facco G, Catalano L, Piccinini V, Liumbruno GM, Grazzini G. Human T-lymphotropic virus and transfusion safety: does one size fit all? Transfusion. 2016;56(1):249–60. https://pubmed.ncbi.nlm.nih.gov/26388300/.
26. Riordan JO. Antibody to hepatitis B core antigen, section 1: agents. In: Barbara JAJ, Regan FAM, Contreras DM, editors. Transfusion microbiology. Cambridge: Cambridge University Press; 2008. p. 25.
27. Relias Media. Hospital Infection Control & Prevention. CDC develops notification letters for HCV testing, 1999. https://www.reliasmedia.com/articles/41057-cdc-develops-notification-letters-for-hcv-testing.
28. Roth WK. History and future of nucleic acid amplification technology blood donor testing. Transfus Med Hemother. 2019;46(2):67–75. https://pubmed.ncbi.nlm.nih.gov/31191192/.
29. Stanford Medicine. Hepatitis B causes. https://stanfordhealthcare.org/medical-conditions/liver-kidneys-and-urinary-system/hepatitis-b/causes.html. Accessed 30 Mar 2024.
30. Simmonds P. The origin of Hepatitis C Virus. In: Hepatitis C virus: from molecular virology to antiviral therapy; 2013. p. 1–15. https://pubmed.ncbi.nlm.nih.gov/23463195/.
31. Sahni AK, Nagendra A, Roy P, Patrikar S. Usefulness of enzyme immunoassay (EIA) for screening of anti HIV antibodies in urinary specimens: a comparative analysis. Med J Armed Forces India. 2014;70(3):211–4. https://www.ncbi.nlm.nih.gov/pmc/articles/PMC4213891/.
32. Tampa M, Sarbu I, Matei C, Benea V, Georgescu SR. Brief history of syphilis. J Med Life. 2014;7(1):4–10. https://www.ncbi.nlm.nih.gov/pmc/articles/PMC3956094/.
33. U.S. Food and Drug Administration. Revised recommendations for reducing the risk of human immuno deficiency virus transmission by blood and blood products; 2020, p. 6–9. https://www.fda.gov/media/92490/download. Accessed 8 May 2022.
34. Universitätsklinikum Regensburg (UKR). Donating blood. Donating granulocytes. https://www.ukr.de/en/donate-blood/donating-granulocytes. Accessed 30 Mar 2024.
35. Von dem Borne AE, Verheugt FW, Oosterhof F, Von Riesz E, De la Rivière AB, Engelfriet CP. A simple immunofluorescence test for the detection of platelet antibodies. Br J Haematol. 1978;39(2):195–207. https://pubmed.ncbi.nlm.nih.gov/354684/.
36. World Health Organization (WHO). Testing of donated blood. https://www.who.int/teams/health-product-policy-and-standards/standards-and-specifications/blood-product-standardization/quality-and-safety/donation-testing. Accessed 30 Mar 2024.
37. WHO. Syphilis. https://www.who.int/news-room/fact-sheets/detail/syphilis. Accessed 30 Mar 2024.
38. WHO. Hepatitis B. https://www.who.int/news-room/fact-sheets/detail/hepatitis-b. Accessed 30 Mar 2024.
39. WHO. Hepatitis C. https://www.who.int/news-room/fact-sheets/detail/hepatitis-c. Accessed 30 Mar 2024.
40. WHO. HIV and AIDS. https://www.who.int/news-room/fact-sheets/detail/hiv-aids. Accessed 30 Mar 2024.
41. Wilson K, Atkinson K, Keelan J. Three decades of MSM blood donor deferral policies. What have we learned? Int J Infect Dis. 2014;18:1–3. https://www.ijidonline.com/action/showPdf?pii=S1201-9712%2813%2900308-1.

Blood Donors: The Past and the Present   18

Contents

18.1	Blood Donors		231
	18.1.1	Blood Donor Eligibility	233
	18.1.2	Variant Creutzfeldt-Jakob Disease (vCJD) as a Deferral for Blood Donation	235
18.2	Some Important Events for Blood Donors and for Blood Donation		237
18.3	Establishment of Different Worldwide Organizations for Promotion of Blood Donation and Blood Transfusion Medicine		238
	18.3.1	The International Federation of Red Cross and Red Crescent Societies (IFRC)	239
	18.3.2	International Society of Blood Transfusion (ISBT)	239
	18.3.3	The Association for the Advancement of Blood and Biotherapies (AABB)	240
	18.3.4	The World Health Organization (WHO)	240
	18.3.5	The International Federation of Blood Donor Organizations (IFBDO)	240
	18.3.6	The European Blood Alliance (EBA)	241
	18.3.7	The Council of Europe	241
	18.3.8	International Plasma and Fractionation Association (IPFA)	242
	18.3.9	Plasma Protein Therapeutics Association (PPTA)	242
18.4	Young Blood Donor Associations		243
18.5	Presented Cases of Altruistic Worldwide Blood Donation in Different Tragedies		244
References			245

18.1 Blood Donors

There are different types of blood donors. Family or family replacement donors, paid commercial or professional donors, and voluntary, non-remunerated, and anonymous blood donors.

Replacement donations are a common practice in many countries. In this system, the blood needed by a patient is supplied by one or more donors from within the patient's own family or community. In most cases, the patient's family is requested to donate blood, but in some countries, it is compulsory for every patient to provide a specified number of donors on admission to the hospital. Donors are not paid by the blood transfusion service or hospital blood bank, although they may sometimes be given money or another form of payment by the patient's relatives. There are different variations of this system. One is where the family donates the same quantity of blood as that given to their relative. This blood is added to the general pool in the blood bank and is then used as required. The donor is not told the identity of the recipient of the blood. A second variation is known as directed donation, where a donor specifically requests that their blood be given to a named patient, perhaps because of fears about the safety of blood from unknown donors.[1] There is also a direct donation method where granulocytes are collected from directed blood donors who are the patient's relatives or acquaintances, due to their greater motivation and willingness to agree to take growth factors.[2] The WHO strongly discourages paying for direct donations in order to prevent systemic exploitation and guarantee safe blood. For their blood donations, commercial or professional donors are compensated with money or other benefits that can be exchanged for cash. They may even have an agreement with a blood bank to provide blood for a particular price. They frequently donate blood on a regular basis. As an alternative, they can approach the families of patients and try to offer their services as substitute donors, or they might sell their blood to many blood banks.[3] This type of donation is not only dangerous for the patient but also for the blood donor themself because frequent donations can harm his health.

Voluntary, non-remunerated, and anonymous donors are people who give blood, plasma, or other blood components of their own free will and receive no money or other form of payment for it, which could be considered a substitute for money, such as time off work except that reasonably needed for the donation and travel. Their primary motivation is to help unknown recipients, not to obtain any personal benefit.[4] This is a sincere, altruistic form of donating a part of yourself to ensure the safety of both the blood donors and the patient.

---

[1] WHO. Guidelines and Principles for Safe Blood Transfusion Practice - Module 1: Safe Blood Donation. 2009, p. 11–16. https://cdn.who.int/media/docs/default-source/blood-transfusion-safety/guidelines-and-principles-for-safe-blood-transfudion-practice-module-1-.pdf?sfvrsn=afabe792_1&download=true. Accessed 1 Apr 2024.

[2] Domanovič D, Cukjati M., Zver S. Granulocyte concentrates and guidelines for their clinical use. ZdravVestn [Internet]. 2011;80(6), p. 443. https://vestnik.szd.si/index.php/ZdravVest/article/view/151.

[3] WHO, 2009, p. 11–16.

[4] WHO, 2009, p. 11–16.

18.1.1 Blood Donor Eligibility

It is necessary to establish and maintain protocols for the secure identification of donors, eligibility evaluation, and suitability interview. They must meet the criteria outlined in Directive 2004/33/EC's Annex II and Annex III (Directive 2005/62/EC, Annex 6.1.1) and occur right before each donation. Donors and each of their donations should be interconnected through effective methods. Donors are required to present identification upon arrival at the blood facility. A systematic screening procedure should be used to determine each donor's suitability. It is permitted only for healthy individuals with an acceptable medical history of donating blood or blood components. The purpose of the donor questionnaire should be to gather data about the donor's general health, medical history, and any other known or suspected risk factors. Every time a donor comes, the questionnaire should be presented to them and made in a way that makes sense to them. Once completed, the donor should sign it. To regulate the acceptance and deferral of donors, the blood establishment should have appropriate acceptance and deferral criteria in place. Confidentiality must be ensured during the donor interview (Directive 2005/62/EC, Annex 6.1.2). People who have been deferred should be provided with a detailed explanation of their deferral. In reality, it is not possible to perform a complete physical and medical examination on the donor. The donor's appearance, their responses to inquiries about their health in general, medical history, and relevant risk factors (such as risk behavior, travel history, and epidemiological factors), as well as laboratory testing, must all be trusted. Using established rules, a determination on the donor's eligibility will be made in light of this data. Referrals for conditions not covered by guidelines should go to the overseeing physician, who has the final say on the matter.[5] National regulatory authorities should therefore oversee the implementation of a standard donor questionnaire that requests information about a potential donor's medical history, demographics, and risk for infectious diseases.[6]

Different criteria for blood donor eligibility existed at different times and were always developing. For comparison, in 1934, blood donors were examined clinically, on X-rays, and serologically.[7] In 1949, the enrollment form asked questions about the history of anemia, malaria, jaundice, and tuberculosis in any form, including pleural effusion, and males were interrogated regarding any past sexually transmitted diseases. Questions were also asked regarding any serious illnesses in the recent past and if the blood donor was in good health on the day of the blood donation. Blood donors were physically examined (heart, lungs, and abdomen). A hemoglobin estimation was indicated if a potential blood donor exhibited pallor or if he reported a history of anemia. The blood sedimentation rate in the absence of a

---

[5] EDQM GUIDE, 2023, p. 92–135.
[6] WHO. Guidance on increasing supplies of plasma-derived medicinal products in low- and middle-income countries through fractionation of domestic plasma. 2021, p. 24. https://www.who.int/publications/i/item/9789240021815. Accessed 6 Apr 2024.
[7] Venčeslav A. Transfuzije krvi v letu 1934. Zdravniški vestnik, številka. 1935;7(7–8), p. 291—292. http://www.dlib.si/?URN=URN:NBN:SI:DOC-AQ6MXYDG.

physical examination was provided as a guide for general health. Even the urine was checked to see if there was a doubtful history of nephritis or cystitis. The arms in the antecubital region were inspected and graded as "excellent, good, moderate, poor." If there were problems during blood donation three times in a row, the blood donor was deferred. A sample of blood grouping was collected by venipuncture for blood grouping and a serological test for syphilis. Women in the UK were allowed to donate blood if they had menstruation and if there were no specifics.[8] However, in the USA, women were not allowed to donate blood during menstruation or pregnancy because they needed blood reserves.[9] The acceptable level of hemoglobin was 122 g/L in the USA and 130 g/L in the UK. During World War II, it was reduced in the UK to 117 g/L. Perhaps in order for more blood donors to give their blood even if they didn't have higher levels of hemoglobin.[10,11] In the USA, blood donors of both sexes, from the ages of 18 to 60, were welcomed.[12] In the UK, blood donors aged 18 to 65 donated blood. During World War II, there were few cases where blood donors over 80 years old donated blood without any harm. In 1949, minors in the United Kingdom were required to obtain permission from a parent or guardian. Men could donate blood once every 3 months, and women once every four months. Blood donors over 60 years old and vegetarians were advised to donate their blood once every six months. This was due to the slow process of blood regeneration.[13] In today's European standards, donors presenting with a medical condition or under medical treatment should be assessed to determine their eligibility. Reasons for donor deferral may include a wide range of non-infectious medical conditions, infectious diseases, and medical or surgical treatments. According to Directive 2004/33/EC, Annex III, prospective donors with severe active, chronic, or relapsing diseases must be permanently deferred. Information that test results detecting markers for viruses, such as HIV, HBV, HCV, or other relevant blood-transmissible microbiologic agents, will result in donor deferral and destruction of the collected unit (Directive 2004/33/EC, Annex II) and, when required by law, that the results should be reported to the relevant health authorities must be provided. The age limits for donation are a minimum of 18 years and a maximum of 65 years (Directive 2004/33/EC, Annex III). Hemoglobin concentration must be determined each time the donor donates whole blood or cellular components. Hemoglobin should not be lower than 125 g/L for women and 135 g/L for men (Directive 2004/33/EC, Annex III).[14] Regarding menstruation, some countries allow a woman to donate blood if she has menstruation on the day of donation, while others do not.

---

[8] Brewer, 1949, p. 333–343.

[9] Hardin R. C. The Donor and the Colelction of Blood, chap. 10. In: DeGowin E. L., Hardin R. C., Alsever B. J. Blood transfusion. W.B. Saunders Company Philadelphia & London, 1949, p. 233–237.

[10] Hardin, 1949, p. 234.

[11] Brewer, 1949, p. 335.

[12] Hardin, 1949, p. 233.

[13] Brewer, 1949, p. 335–343.

[14] EDQM GUIDE, 2023, p. 130–137.

The amount of collected blood also varied over different periods. In order to ensure the safety of a blood donor and the regeneration of blood, a controlled and standardized volume was accepted over time.

During World War I, there were cases where blood donors donated 1000 mL of blood.[15] Before the Second World War, on average, 400–600 mL of blood were donated. In 1949, the donated volume of blood in the bottle was on average 500 mL with a 5- to 10-min duration.[16,17] By 1990, the volume was limited to 450 mL plus or minus 45 mL.[18] By today's European standards, the donation of whole blood must not be collected from persons weighing less than 50 kg (Directive 2004/33/EC, Annex III). The volume of a standard donation of whole blood (excluding anticoagulants) should not exceed 500 mL and usually consists of a donation of 450 mL ± 10%. This does not include any allowance for samples taken for laboratory tests or for the retention of a donor sample. Male donors may give up to six standard donations of whole blood annually, while female donors may give up to four standard donations annually, with a minimum of an 8-week interval between standard donations. The volume of a standard donation of whole blood (including samples) should not exceed 15% of the calculated blood volume of the donor.[19]

18.1.2 Variant Creutzfeldt-Jakob Disease (vCJD) as a Deferral for Blood Donation

Both the deferral of blood donors and the production of any blood- or plasma-derived medicinal products (PDMPs) from the UK were significantly impacted by variant Creutzfeldt-Jakob disease (vCJD).

CJD, or classic Creutzfeldt-Jakob disease, is a rare illness that affects humans. It has distinctive clinical and diagnostic characteristics and is a neurodegenerative condition. This illness always has a fatal outcome and advances quickly. The "mad cow "disease is unrelated to classic CJD. Additionally, "variant CJD," another prion illness connected to bovine spongiform encephalopathy (BSE), is not the same as classic CJD.[20] BSE is a progressive and fatal neurological disease that affects cattle and is caused by an uncommon transmissible agent known as a prion. It's unclear exactly what the transmissible agent is made of. The most widely recognized explanation at the moment holds that the agent is a prion protein, a mutated version of a normal protein. The normal prion protein transforms into a pathogenic (dangerous)

---

[15] Kotwas L., Gilfillan A. C., Gerace N., Leach P. Z. Blood collection techniques. In Seminars in oncology nursing. WB Saunders.1990; 6(2), p. 109. https://www.sciencedirect.com/science/article/abs/pii/S0749208105801433.

[16] Brewer, 1949, p. 342–343.

[17] Hardin, 1949, p. 233–237.

[18] Kotwas, Gilfillan, Gerace, Leach, 1990;6(2), p. 109.

[19] EDQM GUIDE, 2023, p. 154–157.

[20] Centers for Disease Control and Prevention—CDC. Creutzfeldt-Jakob Disease, Classic (CJD). https://www.cdc.gov/prions/cjd/index.html. Accessed 28 Mar 2024.

form for unknown causes, which subsequently harms cattle's central nervous system.[21] BSE was first recognized in the United Kingdom (UK) in 1986, with clinical cases identified retrospectively in April 1985.[22] In 1989, specified bovine offal was banned from human food.[23] A prion illness known as vCJD was initially identified in the UK in 1996. There is now substantial scientific evidence that BSE agents are also to blame for the spread of vCJD in humans.[24] Both of these disorders have in common that they are always fatal brain diseases caused by a prion. A prion is a protein particle that is without DNA (nucleic acid). Many infectious disorders affecting the neurological system are thought to be caused by it. A person can contract mad cow disease by consuming contaminated cattle products, such as beef.[25]

Precautionary steps were implemented in numerous countries, including the UK, to lower the risk of vCJD transmission by blood and PDMPs. Among these, in 1999, the UK government banned the manufacturing of any blood- or plasma-derived medical products using domestic human plasma. Following this move, the UK imported the plasma required for the fractionation process necessary to produce PDMPs, and no other EU or EEA nation used UK plasma for fractionation. The United Kingdom (UK) removed its ban on using plasma collected from within the UK to make immunoglobulin products in February 2021. After conducting a risk-benefit analysis, the UK determined that the immunoglobulin products made from UK plasma had a very low and acceptable risk of variant Creutzfeldt-Jakob disease (vCJD) relative to the total risk of the disease in the general population.[26] In 1999, the FDA in the USA banned blood donors who spent more than 6 months in Britain from 1980 to 1997 from donating blood.[27] Switzerland and New Zealand issued a ban on blood donors who had spent more than 6 months in Britain during the original outbreak. From the year 2000 on, many countries accepted this ban.[28] The ban

---

[21] CDC. Bovine Spongiform Encephalopathy (BSE), or Mad Cow Disease. https://www.cdc.gov/prions/bse/index.html. Accessed 28 Mar 2024.

[22] Lanska, D. J. The Mad Cow Problem in the UK: Risk Perceptions, Risk Management, and Health Policy Development. Journal of Public Health Policy. 1998;19(2), p. 160. https://www.jstor.org/stable/3343296.

[23] Food and Agriculture Organization. Fao/WHO global forum of food safety regulators. 2002. https://www.fao.org/3/y2038e/y2038e.pdf. Accessed 3 Apr 2024.

[24] DC. Variant Creutzfeldt-Jakob disease. https://www.cdc.gov/prions/vcjd/index.html. Accessed 28 Mar 2024.

[25] Johns Hopkins Medicine Health. Mad Cow Disease (Bovine Spongiform Encephalopathy). https://www.hopkinsmedicine.org/health/conditions-and-diseases/bse-mad-cow-disease-and--vcjd. Accessed 3 Apr 2024.

[26] European Centre for Disease Prevention and Control (ECDC). Risk assessment: The risk of variant Creutzfeldt-Jakob disease transmission via blood and plasma-derived medicinal products manufactured from donations obtained in the United Kingdom. https://www.ecdc.europa.eu/en/publications-data/risk-assessment-risk-variant-creutzfeldt-jakob-disease-transmission-blood. Accessed 28 Mar 2024.

[27] Gottlieb S. FDA bans blood donation by people who have lived in UK. BMJ (Clinical research ed.). 1999; 319(7209) p. 535. https://www.ncbi.nlm.nih.gov/pmc/articles/PMC1116429/.

[28] Editorial Elsevier. Is it time to rethink UK restrictions on blood donation? EClinicalMedicine. 2019;15(1–2). https://www.thelancet.com/action/showPdf?pii=S2589-5370%2819%2930196-8.

on blood donors was introduced as a precautionary measure due to the outbreak of the disease and concerns about the risk of acquiring a human variant via blood or plasma transfusions. Today, based on an analysis of low-risk assessments, several countries, including the USA, Canada, Australia, and New Zealand, have lifted this ban from 2022 to 2024.[29] For American military members, Department of Defense civilians, and their families who were stationed at American military stations in Europe other than the United Kingdom between 1980 and 1996, the ban on deferral really started to be lifted in 2020.[30] It has to be noted that donors who have resided in the UK for a minimum of one year between 1980 and 1996 are subject to deferral in several non-UK nations; the European Medicines Agency (EMA) requires one year of residency in the UK for donors of plasma intended for fractionation. The deferrals have occasionally been expanded to cover donors from nations with a significant number of cases.[31] An interesting note is that there is no screening test for vCJD for blood donors.[32]

18.2　Some Important Events for Blood Donors and for Blood Donation

New methods for blood collection and preservation have been developed and adopted, which has boosted the number of blood donors. Blood transfusion services were established and made widely accessible in the USA, Europe, and the majority of developed nations after World War II. The development of systematic techniques for blood donation, storage, distribution, and testing for known blood-related infections were among the improvements. Blood transfusion became an element of medical education, and scholarly publications and international conferences provided a forum for the dissemination of new knowledge. For example, in the immediate postwar years, the UK National Blood Transfusion Service reported over 300,000 blood transfusions annually. From then on, the number steadily increased to over one million in 1958 and to 2.8 million blood transfusions in 2001. It's noteworthy to take into account that sub-Saharan Africa received blood transfusions later than Europe and North America. The practice started only during and after World War 2, with the exception of medical services provided to resident European and specific African groups (such as military and colonial forces or African mine laborers).[33]

---

[29] NZBlood. The madness is over. https://www.nzblood.co.nz/madcow/. Accessed 28 Mar 2024.
[30] America's Blood Centers. Updating vCJD Guidance. https://americasblood.org/advocacy/updating-vcjd- guidance/. Accessed 28 Mar 2024.
[31] EDQM GUIDE, 2023, p. 143.
[32] American Red Cross. Eligibility Reference Material. https://www.redcrossblood.org/donate-blood/how-to-donate/eligibility-requirements/eligibility-criteria-alphabetical/eligibility-reference-material.html. Accessed 28 Mar 2024.
[33] Schneider W.H., Drucker E. Blood transfusions in the early years of AIDS in sub—Saharan Africa. Am. J. Public Health.2006; 96(6), p. 984–994. https://www.ncbi.nlm.nih.gov/pmc/articles/PMC1470624/.

As the number of coronary artery bypass graft (CABG) procedures increased beginning in 1960, there was a growing need for transfusions. By the 1970s, the hazards associated with potentially infected paid donors for the blood supply were identified. Many nations have switched from compensated to unpaid volunteer blood donors in order to ensure the security of their blood supply.[34] In 1975, the Twenty-eighth World Health Assembly, in resolution WHA28.72, called for the development of national blood transfusion services based on voluntary blood donation to ensure safe, adequate, and sustainable blood supplies and to protect the health of blood donors and patients.[35] Health ministers from all over the globe overwhelmingly approved resolution WHA58.13 on commitment and support for voluntary blood donation at the World Health Assembly in May 2005.[36] To maintain adequate and safe blood supplies and equitable access to safe blood and blood products, the resolution urged nations to establish or strengthen mechanisms for the recruitment and retention of voluntary, unpaid blood donors.[37] The goal stated in the WHO Melbourne Declaration is for all nations to source 100% of their blood supply from unpaid, voluntary donors by 2020.[38] The WHO Resolution for Voluntary and Unpaid Blood Donation from 1975 has positively influenced the world to introduce and improve organized and voluntary blood donation. Unfortunately, the goal set for 2020 to achieve 100% blood supply from voluntary and non-paid blood donors hasn't been achieved. Some countries with this problem, especially developing countries, have had little or no success.

18.3 Establishment of Different Worldwide Organizations for Promotion of Blood Donation and Blood Transfusion Medicine

In today's modern world, there are several organizations that promote altruistic, anonymous, and non-remunerated blood donors, mandatory laws for ensuring safe blood and blood products, and the scientific importance of blood transfusion medicine. These organizations are among many that all work honorably aimed at their humanitarian and professional goals for saving lives (the International Federation of Red Cross and Red Crescent Societies, the International Society of Blood Transfusion, the Association for the Advancement of Blood and Biotherapies, the

---

[34] Biro G. P. Erythrocyte Transfusion: Brief History and Current Practice, chap. I. In: Liu H., Kaye A.D., Jahr J. S., editors. Blood Substitutes and Oxygen Biotherapeutics. Cham: Switzerland: Springer; 2022, p. 8.

[35] World Health Organization. Towards 100% Voluntary Blood Donation: A Global Framework for Action, Geneva: WHO, 2010, p. 15–38. https://www.ncbi.nlm.nih.gov/books/NBK305666/.

[36] World Health Organization. WHA58.13 Blood safety: proposal to establish World Blood Donor Day. 2005, p. 1–2. https://apps.who.int/gb/ebwha/pdf_files/WHA58/WHA58_13-en.pdf. Accessed 3 Apr 2024.

[37] WHO, 2010, p. 15–38.

[38] Editorial Elsevier, 2019, p. 1–2.

World Health Organization, the International Federation of Blood Donor Organizations, the European Blood Alliance, the Council of Europe, the International Plasma and Fractionation Association, the Plasma Protein Therapeutics Association, etc.).

18.3.1 The International Federation of Red Cross and Red Crescent Societies (IFRC)

The International Federation of Red Cross and Red Crescent Societies (IFRC) from Geneva, Switzerland, is a worldwide humanitarian aid organization. Following World War I, the IFRC was established in Paris in 1919. Henry Davison, the head of the American Red Cross War Committee, was the inspiration behind what we originally termed the League of Red Cross Organizations. At an international medical conference, Davison gathered the League's founding members, the Red Cross Societies of France, Great Britain, Italy, Japan, and the United States. They agreed that Red Cross volunteers could demonstrate the same compassion and knowledge in peacetime as they did in times of war. The first goal of the League was straightforward: to enhance the health of the populace in nations that had endured severe suffering during the war. Additionally, it aimed to advance the growth of new Red Cross societies all over the world and enhance current ones. It changed its name to the League of Red Cross and Red Crescent Societies in 1983 before becoming the IFRC in 1991.[39] It is the biggest network for humanitarian aid. Almost 15 million volunteers serve humanity locally in more than 192 countries through Red Cross and Red Crescent work. In order to assist vulnerable people and better their lives, the IFRC works before, during, and after catastrophes and medical emergencies.[40] The IFRC supports our 191 Red Cross and Red Crescent Societies to deliver and promote safe and sustainable blood programs around the world.[41]

18.3.2 International Society of Blood Transfusion (ISBT)

The International Society of Blood Transfusion is a scientific society that was founded in 1935. ISBT is a global community of professionals sharing knowledge to enhance transfusion practice. This is done by providing opportunities for advancing knowledge and education and advocating the welfare of blood donors and patients.[42]

---

[39] IFRC, Our history and archives. https://www.ifrc.org/who-we-are/about-ifrc/our-history-and-archives. Accessed 4 Apr 2022.
[40] IFRC. About the IFRC. https://www.ifrc.org/who-we-are/about-ifrc. Accessed 4 Apr 2022.
[41] IFRC. Our work. About blood donation. https://www.ifrc.org/our-work/health-and-care/community-health/blood-donation. Accessed 1 Apr 2024.
[42] ISBT. Advertise with us - International Society of Blood Transfusion. file:///C:/Users/zdrav/Downloads/ISBT-Media-Kit-2023-2024%20(2).pdf. Accessed 1 Apr 2024.

18.3.3 The Association for the Advancement of Blood and Biotherapies (AABB)

The Association for the Advancement of Blood and Biotherapies (AABB) was established in 1947. It is a global, non-profit organization that advocates on behalf of organizations and people working in the biotherapeutics and blood transfusion medicine industries. Bethesda, Maryland, in the United States, is home to the organization's headquarters. Through the creation and execution of standards, accreditation, and educational programs, the association collaborates to advance the field. The objective of the AABB is to improve lives by ensuring that blood transfusion medicine and biotherapies are reliable, accessible, and efficient on a global scale.[43]

18.3.4 The World Health Organization (WHO)

The World Health Organization, with its headquarters in Geneva, Switzerland, was created in 1948. WHO is a specialized agency of the United Nations with a broad mandate to act as a coordinating authority on international health issues.[44] WHO recommends that all activities related to blood collection, testing, processing, storage and distribution be coordinated at the national level through effective organization and integrated blood supply networks. The national blood system should be governed by national blood policy and legislative framework to promote uniform implementation of standards and consistency in the quality and safety of blood and blood products.[45]

18.3.5 The International Federation of Blood Donor Organizations (IFBDO)

The International Federation of Blood Donor Organizations (IFBDO) from Monaco was established on December 4, 1955, in Luxembourg.[46] This federation's mission is: To encourage routine, anonymous, voluntary, and unpaid blood donations throughout the world. To collaborate with the appropriate agencies in order to meet the demand for high-quality human blood products in every nation. To make sure that appropriate measures are taken to protect the patient's and blood donor's safety. It opposes all marketing and gain-related activities involving blood and blood

---

[43] WBMT. Member Societies of WBMT. https://www.wbmt.org/member-societies-of-%20wbmt/. Accessed 4 Apr 2022.

[44] KFF. The U.S. Government and the World Health Organization. https://www.kff.org/global-health-policy/fact-sheet/the-u-s-government-and-the-world-health-organization/. Accessed 4 Apr 2022.

[45] WHO: Blood safety and availability. 2023. https://www.who.int/news-room/fact-sheets/detail/blood-safety-and-availability. Accessed 1 Apr 2024.

[46] IFBDO. History. https://www.fiods-ifbdo.org/history-of-ifbdo/. Accessed 4 Apr 2022.

derivatives in accordance with the idea that every human body is a sacred possession. To take part in any research, study, or event pertaining to blood transfusion procedures, blood transfusion organizations, blood donor associations, or information and research in such areas. To approach national and international governmental bodies, as well as the general public, along with the country's representative group, and whenever necessary, promote voluntary, unpaid blood donation, respect for the ethics of donation, and respect for the selflessness of blood donors.[47]

18.3.6 The European Blood Alliance (EBA)

The European Blood Alliance (EBA) is an alliance of non-profit blood establishments in the European Union, the European Free Trade Area, and the United Kingdom. Its goal is to support the development and upkeep of an effective and robust collaboration between European blood, cells, and tissue services in order to improve the supply of blood and tissues for European residents in terms of availability, quality, safety, and cost effectiveness. To raise awareness among professionals and the general public about the importance of voluntary, unpaid blood and blood component donations as a vital therapeutic tool for patients and to support European blood establishments in their ongoing performance improvement based on moral and ethical standards for the benefit of patients. To make it easier for European services that deal with blood, cells, and tissues to network. Belgium, the United Kingdom, Finland, France, Ireland, Luxembourg, the Netherlands, Portugal, and Scotland were the original nine members of the EBA when it was founded in 1998. EBA currently has 25 members.[48]

18.3.7 The Council of Europe

The Council of Europe is the continent's oldest political organization, founded in 1949. The work of the Council of Europe in the blood transfusion area started in the 1950s. The committees in charge of questions related to blood transfusion are the Committee on Blood Transfusion and Immunohaematology (SP-HM) and the Committee on Quality Assurance in Blood Transfusion Services (SP-R-GS). These committees have built the program on blood transfusion around three major principles: the non-commercialization of substances of human origin by voluntary and non-remunerated donation, the goal of achieving self-sufficiency, and the protection of both the donors and the recipients.[49] Since 2007, the European Directorate for the Quality of Medicines and Health Care (EDQM), working under the European Pharmacopoeia Partial Agreement, has provided the Scientific Secretariat for these

---

[47] IFBDO. Statutes. http://www.fiods-ifbdo.org/statutes/. Accessed 4 Apr 2022.
[48] EBA. About EBA. https://europeanbloodalliance.eu/about-eba/. Accessed 4 Apr 2022.
[49] Hossenlopp C. Blood transfusion Organizations in Europe, chap. 3. In: Rouger P., Hossenlopp C., editors. Blood Transfusion in Europe. The White Book 2005. Paris: Elsevier; 2005, p. 75–84.

activities. The work of the Council of Europe in the area of blood transfusion is to ensure the protection of public health by elaborating, promoting, and actively contributing to the implementation of high safety and quality standards. The principles guiding this work are the promotion of voluntary, non-remunerated blood donation, mutual assistance, optimal use of blood and blood components, and protection of both the donor and recipient. With consideration for the ethical, legal, and organizational aspects of blood transfusion, these principles underpin the work of the Council of Europe. The ultimate aim is to ensure the quality and safety of blood and blood components and their optimal use, increase their availability, and avoid waste. The ethical and organizational impact of new scientific developments is also analyzed.[50]

18.3.8 International Plasma and Fractionation Association (IPFA)

IPFA was founded in 1990 and supports and promotes the activities of not-for-profit organizations around the globe engaged in the collection and fractionation of plasma to enable robust, safe supply of and patient access to plasma-derived medicines. Through education and collaboration with stakeholders, they advocate public health values and donor health protection.[51,52]

18.3.9 Plasma Protein Therapeutics Association (PPTA)

PPTA was founded in 1992. It works globally to advocate patient access to plasma-derived medicines, responsibly improve the availability of plasma, and advance the understanding of the plasma ecosystem. It administers standards programs that help to ensure the quality and safety of plasma collection and manufacturing, as well as protect both donors and patients.[53,54]

---

[50] Council of Europe. Background & Mission. https://www.edqm.eu/en/background-mission-blood. Accessed 1 Apr 2024.

[51] Global civil society database UIA. International Plasma and Fractionation Association (IPFA). https://uia.org/s/or/en/1100019703. Accessed 1 Apr 2024.

[52] International Plasma and Fractionation Association (IPFA). Mission and Vision. https://ipfa.nl/mission-and-vision/. Accessed 1 Apr 2024.

[53] Global civil society database UIA. Plasma Protein Therapeutics Association (PPTA). https://uia.org/s/or/en/1100020146. Accessed 1 Apr 2024.

[54] Plasma Protein Therapeutics Association (PPTA). What we do. https://www.pptaglobal.org/about-ppta. Accessed 1 Apr 2024.

18.4 Young Blood Donor Associations

The saying "the world stands on youth" is certainly true in the field of blood donation. Many countries around the world have their own programs and approaches to promoting blood donation among the young population. The young population, with the knowledge, experience, and values that they have acquired along the way, either on their own or from the more experienced older generation, is leading the world into a new day, and it is no different with blood donation. Every country needs young people to carry on the tradition of blood donation, but it is not enough for the population to be young. In spreading the tradition of blood donation, the young population must be made aware of the importance of providing safe blood for patients, but in order to provide safe blood themselves, the young population must first and foremost be healthy, which can be achieved by avoiding harmful lifestyles. By their example and behavior, they should be a source of pride for the community to be able to donate blood on a regular basis and further motivate the new and upcoming generation to whom they can pass on the "blood donor baton," to ensure sufficient and safe blood. There are two societies in the world that have achieved the almost impossible. Through their noble and humane work, they have "lit the torch of blood donation" among young people all over the world in the name of raising awareness of the importance of healthy living and safe blood donation. These two associations are the "Pledge Club 25" and the "Vampire Cup."

Pledge Club 25 was established on October 24, 1994, in Harare, Zimbabwe, by students. The purpose of this association was to promote a healthy lifestyle and safe blood in Africa, where millions of people were infected by the HIV virus. The association was aimed at young blood donors. Each new member pledged to donate whole blood at least 25 times during their lifetime. Since 2003, the Safe Blood for Africa Foundation (SBFA) and its parent organization, Safe Blood International (SBI), with the support of the WHO and the International Federation of Red Cross and Red Crescent Societies (IFRC), have played an important role in spreading the message of the 25 Club Pledge in more than 65 countries around the world (Asia/Pacific, South and Central America, Europe, and the Middle East).[55]

Most of the literature on the 25 Club incorrectly states that it was founded in 1989. In Africa, Pledge Club 25 works in a couple of countries. Countries around the world have also adopted country-specific names and approaches (*Red 25, Pledge Club 15, Target 25, Club 25 Africa, Club 25 International,* etc.) with, for example, slight differences in the way blood donation is promoted and the number of blood donations, such as unlimited blood donations up to the legal age of life, or for example, 25 donations up to the age of 25, or at least the same number of whole blood donations in a lifetime, and so on. The essence of all versions modeled on the original Club 25 pledge is that they retain the key objective of involving young people, as a lower-risk population, in voluntary and safe blood donation and in motivating

---

[55] Muchokwani E. Unlocking the potential for blood adequacy in Africa. 2018, p. 15–19. https://globalbloodfund.org/wp-content/uploads/2020/07/UNLOCKING_THE_POTENTIAL_FOR_BLOOD_ADEQUACY_IN_AFRICA.pdf. Accessed 3 Apr 2024.

young people to lead healthy lifestyles. At present, there are not as many Club 25s operating around the world as there used to be. However, in the countries where they operate, they are still undoubtedly an important program for recruiting new and young blood donors.

The Vampire Cup was first organized by the National Australian Pharmacy Students' Association (NAPSA) in 2006–2007 and is a blood donation competition between local associations. Pharmacy students can donate blood at the Australian Red Cross, a blood bank, or on a bus provided to the university campus by the Red Cross. At the end of the competition, the local associations reported the total amount of blood donated to the NAPSA Executive. The winner is announced during their national event, the NAPSA Congress. The International Pharmaceutical Student Federation (IPSF) saw great potential in this event, and, with NAPSA's approval, the Vampire Cup was launched worldwide. The Vampire Cup aims to increase public awareness of the blood donation process, increase the number of blood donations among IPSF members, encourage blood donation, host events to honor those who donate blood in the spirit of altruism, and raise awareness of the value of repeat blood donations in order to maintain a sufficient blood supply.[56]

18.5 Presented Cases of Altruistic Worldwide Blood Donation in Different Tragedies

In the world, there are always catastrophes that harm mankind. Fortunately, the blood donors are true heroes who selflessly help victims in different tragedies. These are just a few of the presented cases of humane solidarity.

In the days following the terrorist incident on September 11, 2001, the New York Blood Center received almost 36,000 units of blood per 450 mL.[57] More than 29,000 people died and another 23,000 were injured as a result of the Bam, Iran, earthquake in 2003. About 108,985 blood units were donated in total.[58] After the terrorist attack in Madrid, Spain, in 2004, in just two days, 7510 people donated blood for 1584 injured people.[59] Between December 27 and January 3, 2005, in Thailand, following the tragic tsunami that struck Southeast Asia on December 26, 2004, 20,682 units were donated in the national blood centers, while 15,510 units were donated at mobile blood donations. Around 1409 units were donated by foreigners, while 332

---

[56] International pharmaceutical students federation, Vampire Cup booklet, Netherlands: IPSF. 2018, p. 1–2.

[57] New York. Blood. https://nymag.com/news/9-11/10th-anniversary/blood-donations/. Accessed 10 Jun 2022.

[58] Abolghasemi H., Radfar M.H., Tabatabaee M., Hosseini-Divkolayee N.S., Burkle F.M. Jr. Revisiting blood transfusion preparedness: experience from the Bam earthquake response, Prehosp Disaster Med. 2008; 23 (5), p. 391–394. https://pubmed.ncbi.nlm.nih.gov/19189607/. Accessed 10 Jun 2022.

[59] Algora-Weber M. Madrid train bombings: what we have learnt from that sad event. ISBT Science Series. 2011; 6(1), p. 216–218. https://onlinelibrary.wiley.com/doi/pdf/10.1111/j.1751-2824.2011.01486.x.

of them were RhD-negative blood units. The disaster area received all the donated blood, which was then used to meet the needs of the victims.[60] More than 69,000 people died in the earthquake that happened in the province of Sichuan, China, on May 12, 2008.[61] Teachers and students from Tsinghua University lined up to donate blood for the Sichuan Province earthquake victims on May 13, 2008. More than 1000 Tsinghua students and staff members filled out the blood donation list in just one day. Around 653 of them have contributed the equivalent of 910 units (200 cc for each unit).[62] Thousands of people donated blood in April 2016 after at least 64 people were killed in a terrorist attack in Kabul, Afghanistan.[63] After the earthquake in Kathmandu, Nepal, in 2017, about 9000 people died. In the first three days, more than 600 units of blood were collected.[64,65] After the earthquake in Turkey and Syria in 2023, where over 55,000 people lost their lives, 300 donation centers across Turkey were established, and 1,506,002 people rushed to donate blood.[66]

References

1. America's Blood Centers. Updating vCJD Guidance. https://americasblood.org/advocacy/updating-vcjd-guidance/. Accessed 28 Mar 2024.
2. American Red Cross. Eligibility Reference Material. https://www.redcrossblood.org/donate-blood/how-to-donate/eligibility-requirements/eligibility-criteria-alphabetical/eligibility-reference-material.html. Accessed 28 Mar 2024.
3. Abolghasemi H, Radfar MH, Tabatabaee M, Hosseini-Divkolayee NS, Burkle FM Jr. Revisiting blood transfusion preparedness: experience from the Bam earthquake response. Prehosp Disaster Med. 2008;23(5):391–4. https://pubmed.ncbi.nlm.nih.gov/19189607/. Accessed 10 Jun 2022.
4. Algora-Weber M. Madrid train bombings: what we have learnt from that sad event. ISBT Sci Ser. 2011;6(1):216–8. https://doi.org/10.1111/j.1751-2824.2011.01486.x.

---

[60] Wiwanitkit V. Overview of the blood donation in acute post-tsunami in Thailand. Prehosp. Disaster. Med.2005; 20(5), p. 350. https://pubmed.ncbi.nlm.nih.gov/16295173/.

[61] Asian disaster reduction center (ADRC). Disaster information. China: Earthquake: 2008/05/12. https://www.adrc.asia/view_disaster_en.php?NationCode=&Lang=en&Key=1153. Accessed 10 Jun 2022.

[62] School of Economics and Management. Tsinghua University. Tsinghua SEM Students Donate Blood for Earthquake Victims. https://www.sem.tsinghua.edu.cn/en/info/1021/6605.htm. Accessed 10 Jun 2022.

[63] Tolo news. Thousands donate blood after Kabul attack. https://tolonews.com/afghanistan/thousands-donate-blood-after-kabul-attack. Accessed 10 Jun 2022.

[64] World Health Organization, Giving blood in a time of crisis. Available at: https://www.who.int/news-room/feature-stories/detail/giving-blood-in-a-time-of-crisis. Accessed 10 Jun 2022.

[65] Goba K. Why You Should Donate Blood for Mass Shooting Victims, Even If They Don't Benefit Directly, buzzfeednews. https://www.buzzfeednews.com/article/kadiagoba/blood-donation-uvalde-mass-shootings. Accessed 11 Jun 2022.

[66] British Red Cross. Türkiye (Turkey) and Syria earthquake 2023: a year on. 2024. https://www.redcross.org.uk/stories/disasters-and-emergencies/world/turkey-syria-earthquake. Accessed 3 Apr 2024.

5. Asian disaster reduction center (ADRC). Disaster information. China: Earthquake. https://www.adrc.asia/view_disaster_en.php?NationCode=&Lang=en&Key=1153. Accessed 12 May 2008.
6. Biro GP. Erythrocyte transfusion: brief history and current practice, chapter I. In: Liu H, Kaye AD, Jahr JS, editors. Blood substitutes and oxygen biotherapeutics. Cham: Springer; 2022. p. 8.
7. British Red Cross. Türkiye (Turkey) and Syria earthquake 2023: a year on. 2024. https://www.redcross.org.uk/stories/disasters-and-emergencies/world/turkey-syria-earthquake. Accessed 3 Apr 2024.
8. Council of Europe. Background & Mission. https://www.edqm.eu/en/background-mission-blood. Accessed 1 Apr 2024.
9. Centers for Disease Control and Prevention—CDC. Creutzfeldt-Jakob Disease, Classic (CJD). https://www.cdc.gov/prions/cjd/index.html. Accessed 28 Mar 2024.
10. CDC. Bovine Spongiform Encephalopathy (BSE), or Mad Cow Disease. https://www.cdc.gov/prions/bse/index.html. Accessed 28 Mar 2024.
11. CDC. Variant Creutzfeldt-Jakob disease. https://www.cdc.gov/prions/vcjd/index.html. Accessed 28 Mar 2024.
12. Domanovič D, Cukjati M, Zver S. Granulocyte concentrates and guidelines for their clinical use. ZdravVestn. 2011;80(6):443. https://vestnik.szd.si/index.php/ZdravVest/article/view/151.
13. European Center for Disease Prevention and Control (ECDC). Risk assessment: The risk of variant Creutzfeldt-Jakob disease transmission via blood and plasma-derived medicinal products manufactured from donations obtained in the United Kingdom. https://www.ecdc.europa.eu/en/publications-data/risk-assessment-risk-variant-creutzfeldt-jakob-disease-transmission-blood. Accessed 28 Mar 2024.
14. Editorial Elsevier. Is it time to rethink UK restrictions on blood donation? EClinicalMedicine. 2019;15:1. https://www.thelancet.com/journals/eclinm/article/PIIS2589-5370(19)30196-8/fulltext. Accessed 28 Mar 2024.
15. EBA. About EBA. https://europeanbloodalliance.eu/about-eba/. Accessed 4 Apr 2022.
16. Food and Agriculture Organization. FAO/WHO global forum of food safety regulators. 2002. https://www.fao.org/3/y2038e/y2038e.pdf. Accessed 3 Apr 2024.
17. Gottlieb S. FDA bans blood donation by people who have lived in UK. BMJ. 1999;319(7209):535. https://www.ncbi.nlm.nih.gov/pmc/articles/PMC1116429/.
18. Global civil society database UIA. International Plasma and Fractionation Association (IPFA). https://uia.org/s/or/en/1100019703 . Accessed 1 Apr 2024.
19. Global civil society database UIA. Plasma Protein Therapeutics Association (PPTA). https://uia.org/s/or/en/1100020146. Accessed 1 Apr 2024.
20. Goba K. Why you should donate blood for mass shooting victims, even if they don't benefit directly, buzzfeednews. https://www.buzzfeednews.com/article/kadiagoba/blood-donation-uvalde-mass-shootings. Accessed 11 Jun 2022.
21. Hardin RC. The donor and the Colelction of blood, chapter 10. In: De Gowin EL, Hardin RC, Alsever BJ, editors. Blood transfusion. Philadelphia and London: WB Saunders; 1949. p. 233–7.
22. Hossenlopp C. Blood transfusion organizations in Europe, chapter 3. In: Rouger P, Hossenlopp C, editors. Blood transfusion in Europe. The white book 2005. Paris: Elsevier; 2005. p. 75–84.
23. IFRC, Our history and archives. https://www.ifrc.org/who-we-are/about-ifrc/our-history-and-archives. Accessed 4 Apr 2022.
24. IFRC. About the IFRC. https://www.ifrc.org/who-we-are/about-ifrc. Accessed 4 Apr 2022.
25. IFRC. Our work. About blood donation. https://www.ifrc.org/our-work/health-and-care/community-health/blood-donation. Accessed 1 Apr 2024.
26. ISBT. Advertise with us - International Society of Blood Transfusion. file:///C:/Users/zdrav/Downloads/ISBT-Media-Kit-2023-2024%20(2).pdf. Accessed 1 Apr 2024.
27. IFBDO. History. https://www.fiods-ifbdo.org/history-of-ifbdo/. Accessed 4 Apr 2022.
28. International Plasma and Fractionation Association (IPFA). Mission and Vision. https://ipfa.nl/mission-and-vision/. Accessed 1 Apr 2024.

29. International Pharmaceutical Students Federation. Vampire cup booklet. The Hague: IPSF; 2018. p. 1–2.
30. Muchokwani E. Unlocking the potential for blood adequacy in Africa; 2018. p. 15–9. https://globalbloodfund.org/wp-content/uploads/2020/07/UNLOCKING_THE_POTENTIAL_FOR_BLOOD_ADEQUACY_IN_AFRICA.pdf. Accessed 3 Apr 2024.
31. New York. Blood. https://nymag.com/news/9-11/10th-anniversary/blood-donations/. Accessed 10 Jun 2022.
32. Johns Hopkins Medicine Health. Mad Cow Disease (Bovine Spongiform Encephalopathy). https://www.hopkinsmedicine.org/health/conditions-and-diseases/bse-mad-cow-disease-and-vcjd.
33. Kotwas L., Gilfillan A. C., Gerace N., Leach P. Z. Blood collection techniques. In Seminars in oncology nursing. WB Saunders,Philadelphia and London.1990; 6(2), p. 109.
34. KFF. The U.S. Government and the World Health Organization. https://www.kff.org/global-health-policy/fact-sheet/the-u-s-government-and-the-world-health-organization/. Accessed 4 Apr 2022.
35. Lanska DJ. The mad cow problem in the UK: risk perceptions, risk management, and Health policy development. J Public Health Policy. 1998;19(2):160. https://www.jstor.org/stable/3343296.
36. NZBlood. The madness is over. https://www.nzblood.co.nz/madcow/. Accessed 28 Mar 2024.
37. Plasma Protein Therapeutics Association (PPTA). What we do. https://www.pptaglobal.org/about-ppta. Accessed 1 Apr 2024.
38. School of Economics and Management. Tsinghua University. Tsinghua SEM Students Donate Blood for Earthquake Victims. https://www.sem.tsinghua.edu.cn/en/info/1021/6605.htm. Accessed 10 Jun 2022.
39. Schneider WH, Drucker E. Blood transfusions in the early years of AIDS in sub—Saharan Africa. Am J Public Health. 2006;96(6):984–94. https://www.ncbi.nlm.nih.gov/pmc/articles/PMC1470624/.
40. Tolo news. Thousands donate blood after Kabul attack. https://tolonews.com/afghanistan/thousands-donate-blood-after-kabul-attack. Accessed 10 Jun 2022.
41. Venčeslav A. Transfuzije krvi v letu 1934. Zdravniški vestnik, številka. 1935;7(7-8):291–2. http://www.dlib.si/?URN=URN:NBN:SI:DOC-AQ6MXYDG.
42. WHO. Guidelines and Principles for Safe Blood Transfusion Practice - Module 1: Safe Blood Donation. 2009, p. 11–16. https://cdn.who.int/media/docs/default-source/blood-transfusion-safety/guidelines-and-principles-for-safe-blood-transfudion-practice-module-1-.pdf?sfvrsn=afabe792_1&download=true. Accessed 1 Apr 2024.
43. World Health Organization. Towards 100% voluntary blood donation: a global framework for action. Geneva: WHO; 2010. p. 15–38. https://www.ncbi.nlm.nih.gov/books/NBK305666/.
44. World Health Organization. WHA58.13 Blood safety: proposal to establish World Blood Donor Day; 2005, p. 1–2. https://apps.who.int/gb/ebwha/pdf_files/WHA58/WHA58_13-en.pdf. Accessed 3 Apr 2024.
45. WHO: Blood safety and availability. 2023. https://www.who.int/news-room/fact-sheets/detail/blood-safety-and-availability. Accessed 1 Apr 2024.
46. World Health Organization, Giving blood in a time of crisis. https://www.who.int/news-room/feature-stories/detail/giving-blood-in-a-time-of-crisis. Accessed 10 Jun 2022.
47. WHO. Guidance on increasing supplies of plasma-derived medicinal products in low- and middle-income countries through fractionation of domestic plasma. 2021, p. 24. https://www.who.int/publications/i/item/9789240021815. Accessed 6 Apr 2024.
48. WBMT. Member Societies of WBMT. https://www.wbmt.org/member-societies-of-%20wbmt/. Accessed 4 Apr 2022.
49. Wiwanitkit V. Overview of the blood donation in acute post-tsunami in Thailand. Prehosp Disaster Med. 2005;20(5):350. https://pubmed.ncbi.nlm.nih.gov/16295173/.

Plasma Fractionation 19

Contents

19.1 Important Milestones in Plasma Fractionation.. 249
19.2 The Shortage of Plasma Products... 251
References... 253

19.1 Important Milestones in Plasma Fractionation

Plasma is a component of blood that helps regulate blood pressure, blood coagulation, the immune system, and the movement of nutrients. Millions of individuals are treated using drugs derived from plasma. Through a process known as fractionation, pharmaceutical companies produce medicine from components of plasma, such as coagulation factors (used to treat trauma and hemophilia patients), immunoglobulins (used to treat people whose immune systems are compromised due to genetics or external factors like viruses, bacteria, and chemotherapy), and albumin (a protein used to treat patients who have had burns or surgeries).[1] Plasma fractionation was developed by Cohn in the 1940s (Image 19.1).[2] The necessity to create blood serum products to aid soldiers suffering from shock and burns during World War II marked the beginning of plasma fractionation history. Dr. Edwin Joseph Cohn from Harvard

---

[1] Dooley J., Gallagher E.A. Blood Money: The Financial Implications of Plasma Sales for Individuals and Non-Bank Lenders. Federal Deposit Insurance Corporation. 2022, p. 1. https://www.fdic.gov/analysis/cfr/consumer/2022/papers/gallagher-paper.pdf. Accessed 6 Apr 2024.

[2] Bertolini J. Chapter 27. The purification of plasma proteins for therapeutic use. In: Simon TL, McCullough J., Snyder E. L., Solheim BG, Strauss RG., editors. Rossi's Principles of Transfusion Medicine, 5th Edition. USA: Wiley Blackwell. 2016, p. 303.

© The Author(s), under exclusive license to Springer Nature
Switzerland AG 2024
Z. Kvržić, *History of Blood Donation and Transfusion Medicine*,
https://doi.org/10.1007/978-3-031-68715-0_19

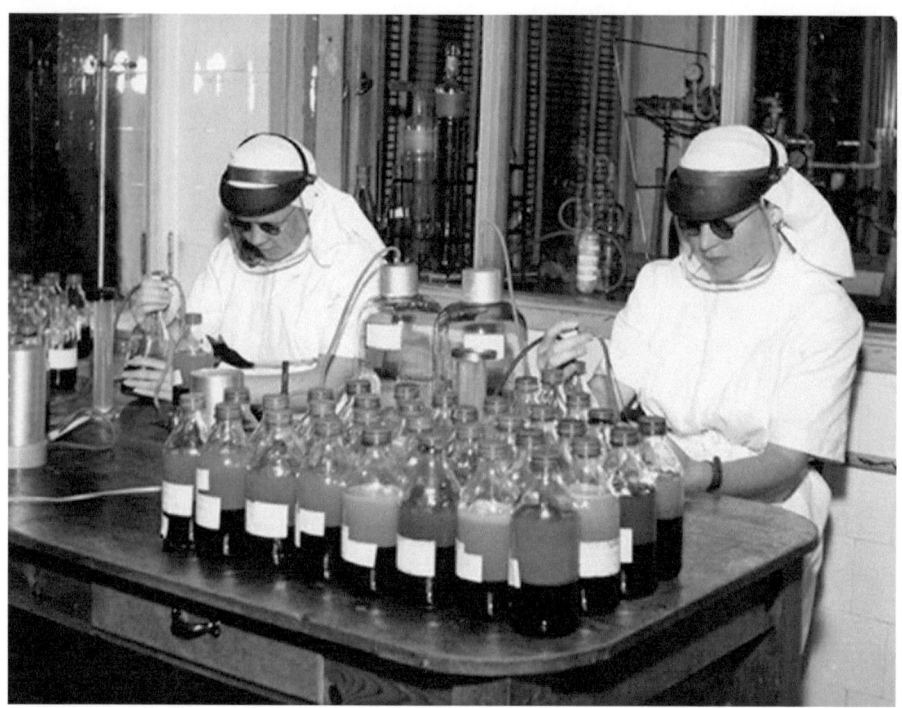

Image 19.1 Plasma Fractionation in Finland in the 1960s. (Source: Finnish Red Cross Blood Service. Plasma fractionation in the 1960s in Finland. https://www.veripalvelu.fi/en/history/. Accessed 10 Mar 2024. Permission for the use of this photograph was granted by Mr. Willy Toiviainen, Director of HR and Communications at the Finnish Red Cross Blood Service, on March 4, 2024)

University played a significant role in the process of creating a method for removing proteins from human plasma.[3] In 1944, Cohn and others introduced ethanol methods for plasma fractionation of albumin, fibrinogen, and gammaglobulin, all for clinical use. Plasma fractionation institutions were already established in the late 1940s and early 1950s. In the late 1950s, B. and M. Blomback showed that a factor VIII preparation could be obtained in a modified Cohn fraction from fresh or fresh-frozen plasma, the so-called fraction I-0. From 1975 on, the need for plasma fractionation to satisfy the need for albumin and factor VIII increased worldwide.[4] In the 1970s and 1980s, the fractionation industry grew rapidly due to self-sufficiency programs, national demands, and technological advancements that allowed for both small- and large-scale fractionation.[5] The 1980s saw examples of blood and blood

---

[3] Marketing Research Bureau. Introduction to the plasma industry. https://marketingresearchbureau.com/the-plasma-industry/. Accessed 6 Apr 2024.

[4] Högman, 1992, p. 140–144.

[5] Curling J., Goss N.; Bertolini J. The History and Development of the Plasma Protein Fractionation Industry-chapter 1. In: Bertolini J., Goss N., Curling J., editors. Production of plasma proteins for

product-borne viral transmission, specifically HIV. As a result, the plasma industry put in place stringent measures to guarantee that only donor plasma that is free of infection is used to create plasma products.[6] Plasma that was obtained from blood component production dominated the not-for-profit sector, whereas plasmapheresis production dominated the for-profit sector.[7] At the Twenty-eighth World Health Assembly in 1975, the resolution WHA28.72 was adopted. The main objective of the resolution was the worldwide establishment of nationally supported, managed, and coordinated blood systems as an essential part of the health system. The accepted resolution WHA 58.13 in 2005 at the Fifty-eighth World Health Assembly recommended the full implementation of well-organized, nationally coordinated, and sustainable blood programs with appropriate regulatory systems and stressed the essential role of voluntary, non-remunerated blood donors from low-risk populations. However, in 2010, at the sixty-third World Health Assembly, the resolution WHA63.12 on availability, safety, and quality of blood products expressed significant concerns about the unequal worldwide access to blood products, particularly PDMPs. Also emphasized was the importance of establishing reliable quality assurance systems for the whole chain of blood collection, processing, and distribution in blood establishments.[8] In addition to the WHO, the majority of regulatory bodies worldwide and the Council of Europe want to achieve self-sufficiency by establishing national blood systems that rely on voluntary, unpaid donations.[9]

19.2 The Shortage of Plasma Products

PDMPs are crucial for the prophylaxis and treatment of patients with bleeding disorders, immune deficiencies, autoimmune and inflammatory diseases and a variety of congenital deficiency disorders.[10] Currently, approximately thirty distinct protein products can be isolated from human plasma.[11] The industry for plasma products is primarily driven by immunoglobulin, albumin, and Factor VIII; however, a wide range of other plasma products are produced for rare bleeding disorders as well as other acquired and genetic diseases. These are: plasmin, von Willebrand factor, factors IX, XI, XIII, fibrinogen, antithrombin III, protein C, alpha-1-proteinase inhibitor, C-1 esterase inhibitor, and plasmin. Anti-D (Rh) IgG is also critically needed, and the market for hyperimmune medicines is growing in response to the threat of

---

therapeutic use. Hoboken, New Jersey: John Wiley & Sons, Inc.; 2013, p. 13.
[6] Marketing Research Bureau, 2024.
[7] Högman, 1992, p. 140–144.
[8] WHO, 2021, p. 1–5.
[9] Weinstein M. Regulation of plasma for fractionation in the United States. Annals of Blood. 2018; 3(1), p. 1.
[10] Strengers P. F. W. Challenges for plasma-derived medicinal products. Transfusion Medicine and Hemotherapy, 2023; 50 (2), p. 116–122. https://pubmed.ncbi.nlm.nih.gov/37066053/.
[11] WHO, 2021, p. 1–5.

bioterrorism as well as infectious diseases.[12] PDMPs are in high demand, particularly in middle- and low-income countries.[13] High-income nations can typically guarantee a sufficient supply of PDMPs, although even in these nations, there may be product shortages or financial constraints that affect the treatment of specific diseases or clinical indications.[14] The total worldwide volume of collected plasma originates from the USA. This was, by 2019, approximately 67%. Other sources come from Asia-Pacific, around 18%, of which around 75% are from China. An estimated 14% of collected plasma originates from Europe, and this continent is the largest supplier of recovered plasma. Despite making up just a modest share of the world's plasma supply, demand for PDMPs is rising quickly throughout Latin America and Africa. In high-income countries, the volume of plasma obtained from transfusion facilities has decreased in recent years, including during the SARS-CoV-2 pandemic, due to the reduced clinical use of erythrocytes following the introduction of patient blood management. A major worry and challenge for the supply of PDMPs is the imbalance in the global plasma supply and the reliance on one country or region to produce the majority of the world's plasma, even though US-sourced plasma is essential for satisfying the growing demands of other countries. Because of the SARS-CoV-2 pandemic, the worldwide volume of collected plasma has declined.[15] Donating plasma is more common than blood donation. Donors of plasmapheresis and blood are primarily non-remunerated volunteers in most European nations. In addition to the United States, Ukraine, China, and four additional European nations—Austria, Germany, the Czech Republic, and Hungary—donors of plasmapheresis receive payment for their services. A plasma donor is permitted to donate up to 25 L of plasma per year, or 33 contributions, according to the European Directorate for the Quality of Medicine (EDQM). In the United States, a plasma donor has the ability to donate up to 104 times a year, which is equivalent to twice a week and three times the recommended amount by the EDQM. In fact, the majority of nations must buy plasma products from companies that manufacture them using plasma from people who get paid for donating it, since the amount of plasma collected from each nation's altruistic donors is insufficient to even partially satisfy the demand for these products. In connection with this fact, almost 3.8 million liters of plasma are now lacking in the EU for manufacturing purposes. Europe will require nearly eight million liters of plasma in 2025 in order to lessen its reliance on American plasma.[16] Even with the worldwide shortage of plasma products, the safety of blood donors and plasma products should be the major concern and must come first.

---

[12] Curling, Goss, Bertolini, 2013, p. 22.
[13] Weinstein, 2018, p. 1.
[14] WHO, 2021, p. 1–5.
[15] Strengers, 2023, p. 116–122.
[16] Simonetti A., Cees S. Europe needs two million extra donors of blood and plasma: How to find them? Vox Sanguinis. 2023;119(2), p. 122. https://onlinelibrary.wiley.com/doi/10.1111/vox.13540.

References

1. Bertolini J. Chapter 27. The purification of plasma proteins for therapeutic use. In: Simon TL, McCullough J, Snyder EL, Solheim BG, Strauss RG, editors. Rossi's principles of transfusion medicine. 5th ed. New York: Wiley Blackwell; 2016. p. 303.
2. Curling J, Goss N, Bertolini J. The history and development of the plasma protein fractionation industry—Chapter 1. In: Bertolini J, Goss N, Curling J, editors. Production of plasma proteins for therapeutic use. Hoboken, NJ: Wiley; 2013. p. 13.
3. Dooley J, Gallagher EA. Blood money: the financial implications of plasma sales for individuals and non-bank lenders. Federal Deposit Insurance Corporation; 2022. p. 1. https://www.fdic.gov/analysis/cfr/consumer/2022/papers/gallagher-paper.pdf. Accessed 6 Apr 2024.
4. Marketing Research Bureau. Introduction to the plasma industry. https://marketingresearchbureau.com/the-plasma-industry/. Accessed 6 Apr 2024.
5. Strengers PFW. Challenges for plasma-derived medicinal products. Transfus Med Hemother. 2023;50(2):116–22. https://pubmed.ncbi.nlm.nih.gov/37066053/.
6. Simonetti A, Cees S. Europe needs 2 million extra donors of blood and plasma: how to find them? Vox Sang. 2023;119(2):122. https://doi.org/10.1111/vox.13540.
7. Weinstein M. Regulation of plasma for fractionation in the United States. Ann Blood. 2018;3(1):1.

Image Source

Finnish Red Cross Blood Service. Plasma fractionation in the 1960s in Finland. https://www.veripalvelu.fi/en/history/. Accessed 10 Mar 2024.

COVID-19 Pandemic

Contents

References.. 257

Since the outbreak in 2019, more than seven million people have died due to COVID-19.[1] The COVID-19 pandemic has worldwide reduced the supply of blood and blood components and adversely affected the blood donation sector in many countries around the world.[2] Every coronavirus (CoV) has a zoonotic origin, meaning it spreads to several animal species and causes intestinal and respiratory infections. CoV is divided into four genera: alpha, beta, gamma, and delta. Mammals that are infected by alpha and beta include bats, cattle, domesticated animals, and humans. Birds and other mammals are more frequently infected by gamma and delta types. In 1937, a CoV was found to be the cause of a respiratory infection for the first time. Animals can easily contract coronavirus illness (COVID-19) from humans through aerosols, especially if they have been in close proximity or have shared common areas, such as confined or poorly ventilated rooms.[3] The first human

---

[1] Worldometer. Coronavirus Death Toll. 2024. https://www.worldometers.info/coronavirus/coronavirus-death-toll/. Accessed 7 Apr 2024.

[2] García-Erce J.A., Romón-Alonso Í., Jericó C., Domingo-Morera J.M., Arroyo-Rodríguez J.L., Sola-Lapeña C., Bueno-Cabrera J.L., Juárez-Vela R., Zalba-Marcos S., Abad-Motos A, Gea-Caballero V., Santolalla-Arnedo I, Quintana-Díaz M. Blood Donations and Transfusions during the COVID-19 Pandemic in Spain: Impact According to Autonomous Communities and Hospitals. International Journal of Environmental Research and Public Health. 2017;18(7), p. 3480. https://www.mdpi.com/1660-4601/18/7/3480.

[3] Zapatero Gaviria A., Barba Martin, R. What do we know about the origin of COVID-19 three years later? Revista clinica espanola. 2023;223(4), p. 240–243. https://www.ncbi.nlm.nih.gov/

coronavirus was discovered in 1965, and the name of this virus was created the same year.[4] It was established in 1965 that between 15% and 30% of human common colds were caused by CoV. In Wuhan, Hubei province (China), close to the Huanan market, the first case of pneumonia brought on by a new CoV, likewise belonging to the beta genus, was reported at the end of November 2019. China researchers first named it 2019-nCoV. It became known as SARS-CoV-2 and the disease COVID-19 on February 11, 2020.[5] Countries around the world have put in place a number of measures to ensure uninterrupted blood donation and to protect the health of blood donors. In the relentless global fight against COVID-19, in addition to vaccine production, experts have launched a program to collect plasma from COVID-19 patients.

Serotherapy[6] from recovering patients has really been utilized for a very long time. When poliomyelitis broke out in New York in 1916, for instance, it was tested as a medical treatment for acute paralysis. A small measles outbreak in Tunis was controlled in 1916 by the use of serotherapy by Nicolle and Conseil. The same therapeutic approach was employed by Hess in 1915 to treat the mumps and stop its testicular consequences. It was even used in the Spanish flu pandemic (1918—1919).[7,8] Last but not least, the Italian Francesco Cenci is credited with being the first to employ convalescent serum as a therapeutic tool, guarding against measles exposure in young children. Cenci collected 600 mL of blood from a 20-year-old male patient during an epidemic outbreak in 1901, 3 weeks after the patient had recovered from the measles. After blood coagulation, he collected serum in three sterile tubes and added phenic acid[9] solution as a protective measure. After receiving the convalescent serum vaccination, unlike their housemates' siblings, four children between the ages of 4 and 8 did not get the measles. It should be noted that a part of the serum was injected into Cenci's arm and the peritoneum of a rabbit 60 h before the product was administered to patients. Neither procedure caused any general or local reactions. There was another measles outbreak in December 1906, this time affecting roughly forty young patients. Through the convalescent serum injection,

---

pmc/articles/PMC10019034/.

[4] Rath L. What is the History of Coronavirus? WebMD. 2023. https://www.webmd.com/covid/coronavirus-history. Accessed 7 Apr 2024.

[5] Zapatero Gaviria A., Barba Martin R. What do we know about the origin of COVID-19 three years later? Revista clinica espanola. 2023;223(4), p. 240–243. https://www.ncbi.nlm.nih.gov/pmc/articles/PMC10019034/.

[6] Serotherapy is the administration of serum containing disease-specific antibodies during treatment.

[7] Stern A. M., Cetron M. S., Markel H. The 1918–1919 Influenza Pandemic in the United States: Lessons Learned and Challenges Exposed, Public Health Reports. 2010; 125(3), p. 6–8. https://www.ncbi.nlm.nih.gov/pmc/articles/PMC2862329/.

[8] Marson P., Cozza A., De Silvestro G. The true historical origin of convalescent plasma therapy. Transfusion and Apheresis Science. 2020; 59(5): 102847, p. 1–8. https://www.ncbi.nlm.nih.gov/pmc/articles/PMC7289739/.

[9] A phenic acid is an aromatic organic compound.

Cenci repeated prophylaxis effectively.[10] By 1949, convalescent plasma and serum were successfully used for treating measles, scarlet fever, mumps, whooping cough, anterior poliomyelitis, and other acute infections (virus pneumonia, epidemic keratoconjunctivitis, and infectious hepatitis).[11] The collection and therapy of plasma from COVID-19 patients started in February 2020 in China.[12] There have been numerous SARS-CoV-2 variations discovered in the US and around the world during the COVID-19 outbreak.[13] People who have recovered from COVID-19 develop natural defenses (antibodies) found in their plasma. The convalescent plasma can be donated through plasmapheresis or separated from the donated whole blood.

Currently, there are two ways in which plasma is used in the world to fight against COVID-19. The first is convalescent plasma, which contains antibodies that are transfused to sufferers whose immune systems are struggling to develop their own antibodies in the hope that it will have an impact on improving their condition. The second way is to transfuse hyperimmune immunoglobulin, which is more concentrated and therefore contains more antibodies.[14] There are also some antiviral medicines available on the market. Preventive measures from the basic care of hand hygiene, wearing masks, keeping physical distance, socializing outdoors, vaccination, and therapy with convalescent plasma or hyperimmune immunoglobulin, etc., have maintained COVID-19, but the threat still remains.

References

1. Alsever JB. Convalescent and hyperimmune plasma and serum. In: De Gowin EL, Hardin RC, Alsever BJ, editors. Blood transfusion. Philadelphia and London: W.B. Saunders; 1949. p. 420–7.
2. CDC. SARS-CoV-2 variant classifications and definitions. 2023. https://www.cdc.gov/coronavirus/2019-ncov/variants/variant-classifications.html. Accessed 7 Apr 2024.
3. García-Erce JA, Romón-Alonso Í, Jericó C, Domingo-Morera JM, Arroyo-Rodríguez JL, Sola-Lapeña C, Bueno-Cabrera JL, Juárez-Vela R, Zalba-Marcos S, Abad-Motos A, Gea-Caballero V, Santolalla-Arnedo I, Quintana-Díaz M. Blood donations and transfusions during the COVID-19 pandemic in Spain: impact according to autonomous communities and hospitals. Int J Environ Res Public Health. 2017;18(7):3480. https://www.mdpi.com/1660-4601/18/7/3480.

---

[10] Marson, Cozza, De Silvestro, 2020, p. 1–2.

[11] Alsever J. B. Convalescent and Hyperimmune Plasma and Serum. In: DeGowin E. L., Hardin R. C., Alsever B. J. Blood transfusion. W.B. Saunders Company Philadelphia & London, 1949, p. 3. 420–427.

[12] Ye M., Fu D., Ren Y., Wang F., Wang D., Zhang F., Xia X., Lv T., Treatment with convalescent plasma for COVID-19 patients in Wuhan, China, J. Med. Virol. 2020;92(10), p. 1890–1901. https://pubmed.ncbi.nlm.nih.gov/32293713/.

[13] CDC. SARS-CoV-2 Variant Classifications and Definitions. 2023. https://www.cdc.gov/coronavirus/2019-ncov/variants/variant-classifications.html. Accessed 7 Apr 2024.

[14] Piechotta V., Iannizzi C., Chai K.L., Valk S.J., Kimber C., Dorando E., Monsef I., Wood E.M., Lamikanra A. A., Roberts D. J., McQuilten Z., So-Osman C., Estcourt L. J., Skoetz N. Convalescent plasma or hyperimmune immunoglobulin for people with COVID-19: a living systematic review, Cochrane Database Syst. Rev., 2021;5(5):CD013600, p. 1–3. https://www.ncbi.nlm.nih.gov/pmc/articles/PMC8135693/.

4. Piechotta V, Iannizzi C, Chai KL, Valk SJ, Kimber C, Dorando E, Monsef I, Wood EM, Lamikanra AA, Roberts DJ, McQuilten Z, So-Osman C, Estcourt LJ, Skoetz N. Convalescent plasma or hyperimmune immunoglobulin for people with COVID-19: a living systematic review. Cochrane Database Syst Rev. 2021;5(5):CD013600. https://www.ncbi.nlm.nih.gov/pmc/articles/PMC8135693/.
5. Rath L. What is the history of Coronavirus? WebMD. 2023. https://www.webmd.com/covid/coronavirus-history. Accessed 7 Apr 2024.
6. Marson P, Cozza A, De Silvestro G. The true historical origin of convalescent plasma therapy. Transfus Apher Sci. 2020;59(5):102847. https://www.ncbi.nlm.nih.gov/pmc/articles/PMC7289739/.
7. Stern AM, Cetron MS, Markel H. The 1918–1919 influenza pandemic in the United States: lessons learned and challenges exposed. Public Health Rep. 2010;125(3):6–8. https://www.ncbi.nlm.nih.gov/pmc/articles/PMC2862329/.
8. Worldometer. Coronavirus Death Toll. 2024. https://www.worldometers.info/coronavirus/coronavirus-death-toll/. Accessed 7 Apr 2024.
9. Ye M, Fu D, Ren Y, Wang F, Wang D, Zhang F, Xia X, Lv T. Treatment with convalescent plasma for COVID-19 patients in Wuhan, China. J Med Virol. 2020;92(10):1890–901. https://pubmed.ncbi.nlm.nih.gov/32293713/.
10. Zapatero GA, Barba MR. What do we know about the origin of COVID-19 three years later? Rev Clin Esp. 2023;223(4):240–3. https://www.ncbi.nlm.nih.gov/pmc/articles/PMC10019034/.

Appendix A: History of Transfusion Medicine in Slovenia from 1875 to 1945

Abstract Similar to other cultures around the world, the Slovenian people have known throughout history that blood is of the utmost value. The humble beginnings of transfusion medicine in Slovenia date back to the second half of the nineteenth century, when the first successful blood transfusion was performed by Dr. Franz Fux. After his experiments, there is not any crucial evidence that the blood transfusions were performed until the 1920s. In the meantime, there were successful cases where doctors tried blood substitutes with saline and ether. The first doctor to have performed a blood transfusion with a new Rotanda syringe in the 1920s, based on evidence, was Dr. Adolf Ramšak. Although blood transfusions were uncommon at the time, they were still used in clinical settings. Despite the fact that blood donation in the twentieth century was based on a fee-paying system, there were parallel examples of altruistic, non-remunerated blood donation. Paid blood donation in Slovenia existed during a period of difficult living conditions. Blood donors used to be paid for their blood donations because it was almost, or in some cases, the only source of income available to them. Through the 1930s and 1940s, there were smaller groups of blood donors, but there wasn't any real Transfusion Medicine Organization until the Second World War ended.

Keywords First blood transfusion; Franz Fux; Adolf Ramšak; Professional blood donation; Other methods of blood loss replacement

History of Republic of Slovenia

The Republic of Slovenia is a country in Central Europe. Historically, it has been part of many different states, including the Roman Empire, the Byzantine Empire, the Carolingian Empire, the Holy Roman Empire, the Kingdom of Hungary, the Republic of Venice, the Illyrian Provinces of Napoleon's First French Empire, the Austrian Empire, and the Austro-Hungarian Empire. After World War I, on October 29, 1918, the Slovenes co-founded the State of Slovenes, Croats, and Serbs (SHS). This state lasted until January 1, 1918, when it merged with the Kingdom of Serbia and became the Kingdom of SHS (Serbs, Croats, and Slovenes). On October 3,

© The Editor(s) (if applicable) and The Author(s), under exclusive license to Springer Nature Switzerland AG 2024
Z. Kvržić, *History of Blood Donation and Transfusion Medicine*,
https://doi.org/10.1007/978-3-031-68715-0

1929, the country changed its name to the Kingdom of Yugoslavia. During this time, the Slovenian area was known as the Drava Banovina (Dravska Banovina). Named after the Drava River, this province included the majority of modern-day Slovenia. The Drava Banovina's capital was Ljubljana. The Kingdom of Yugoslavia collapsed during World War II in 1941. It officially ended, however, on November 29, 1945, when the monarchy was abolished by Yugoslavia's Communist Constituent Assembly. It was a part of the Democratic Federal Yugoslavia from August 10, 1945, to November 29, 1945. After this short period, it was part of the Federative People's Republic of Yugoslavia (29. 11. 1945–7. 4. 1963) and the Socialist Federal Republic of Yugoslavia (7. 4. 1963–25. 6. 1991). The Republic of Slovenia became an independent state on June 25, 1991. On January 15, 1992, Slovenia was officially recognized by the European Union. On May 22, 1992, Slovenia became a member of the United Nations; on March 29, 2004, it became a member of NATO (North Atlantic Treaty Organization); and on May 1, 2004, it became a member of the European Union (EU). The capital city of Slovenia is Ljubljana.

The First Blood Transfusion in 1875

The early, humble evidence of surgeons working in Slovenia can be traced back to the ninth century. The evidence was found on human bones with traces of some modest medical interventions. In 1530, we had surgeons based in the city of Ljubljana, and in 1569, in Novo Mesto. Until the end of the eighteenth century, surgeons were mostly foreigners. From the second half of the sixteenth to the end of the first half of the seventieth century, they were mostly Italians, and from the second half of the seventieth century to the end of the eighteenth century, they were mostly Germans. Toward the end of the nineteenth century, there were more surgeons who were Slovenians. They were mostly educated in Austria and Germany. The first serious school for surgeons (Medico-Surgical Center) in Ljubljana was formed in 1782. The first faculty of medicine was established in 1810, also in Ljubljana.[1] The pioneer of modern surgery in Slovenia was the surgeon and head or primarius of a surgical department, Dr. Edo Šlajmer (1869–1935). He introduced new surgical techniques, modern asepsis, new operative methods, X-ray diagnostics, chloroform narcosis, and lumbar and local anesthesia to Slovenian medicine. He became the head of the surgical department in Ljubljana in 1892.[2] From there, surgery in Slovenia developed extensively over time, and today it is performed with the most modern methods and equipment and with the rich professional and broad

---

[1] Borisov P. Od renocelništva do začetkov znanstvene kirurgije na Slovenskem. Ljubljana: Slovenska Akademija Znanosti in Umetnosti; 1977, p. 1–192.

[2] Zupanič Slavec Z., Goričar M. Prim. Dr. Edo Šlajmer, reformator kirurgije na Slovenskem (ob 150-letnici rojstva). Isis: Glasilo Zdravniške zbornice Slovenije., ISSN 1318-0193. 2015;24(1), p. 64–68. https://www.zdravniskazbornica.si/informacije-publikacije-in-analize/publikacije-zbornice-isis/isis-januar-2015.

knowledge of prominent, respected, hard-working, dedicated, and trained surgeons. Transfusion medicine is importantly connected to surgery.

Blood transfusions, among other professional reasons, are given in surgery in order to maintain hemodynamic stability and provide adequate oxygen delivery to tissues, resulting in a reduced risk of cardiac events, bleeding, and anemia in the post-operative period.[3]

Until the year 2021, it was believed that the first blood transfusion procedure was performed in Slovenia in the 1920s. With tireless searching, I found forgotten information about an even older case of blood transfusion, which was carried out in Ljubljana in 1875. In 2022, I published a few articles on the subject.

The first blood transfusion procedure was performed in Ljubljana by Austrian Primarius Dr. Franz Fux (Image A.1). He was born on December 2, 1822, in Steyr, Upper Austria. Dr. Fux attended the Gymnasium in Kremsmünster from 1834 to 1842. After finishing high school, he studied medicine at the Faculty of Medicine at the University of Vienna from 1842–43 to 1846–47. On July 22, 1848, he received his Doctor of Medicine degree. Dr. Fux had the ambition to become a surgeon. On July 22, 1848, he received his Doctor of Medicine degree.[4,5,6,7,8]

Dr. Fux started hospital practice in 1849 and became a surgeon on July 28, 1851. He worked in Graz and Vienna, and according to some accounts, he arrived in Ljubljana in 1854 and, according to others, in 1855. In the uncertain times following the outbreak of the cholera epidemic in 1855, Dr. Fux proved to be extremely successful in containing it.[9,10]

In 1856, following a decision of the provincial government of the city of Kranj, he took over the management of the eye ward of the local General hospital in Ljubljana. On September 1, 1858, the provincial government appointed him as a secondary because the increasingly frail head of the hospital, Dr. Leopold Nathan, needed help in his work. During this period, Dr. Fux performed most of the operations independently. When war broke out between the Austrian Empire and Italy in 1859, he was the chief physician of the surgical ward of the military garrison hospital. Dr. Fux took on the enormous challenge of caring for between 140 and 160 critically wounded soldiers. He performed 21 amputations, many minor operations, and

---

[3] Alamri A. A., Alnefaie M. N., Saeedi A. T., Hariri A. F., Altaf A., Aljiffry M. M. Transfusion Practices Among General Surgeons at a Tertiary Care Center: A Survey Based Study. Medical archives (Sarajevo, Bosnia and Herzegovina). 2018; 72(6), p. 418–424. https://www.ncbi.nlm.nih.gov/pmc/articles/PMC6340613/.

[4] Archiv der Universität Wien. Kassajournale, R77.59–R77.63.

[5] Archiv der Universität Wien. Studienkataloge MED 15.58.

[6] Archiv der Universität Wien. Rigorosenprotokoll, MED 16.36, p. 73–74.

[7] Herren P.T. Verzeichnis von ehemaligen Kremsmünster Studenten, Kremsmünster, Austria: Des k k Gymnasiums Druck von Jos Feichtingers Erben in Linz; 1877, p. 30.

[8] Kvržić Z. Dr. Franz Fux - imenitni zdravnik svojega časa, Revija za moje zdravje. - ISSN 2536-1791. 2022;9(64), p. 42–44. https://www.revijazamojezdravje.si/franz-fux/.

[9] Zgodovinski arhiv Ljubljana, SI_ZAL_LJU 10339, Pintarjeva Zbirka, TE 2.

[10] Keber K, Svetličič, A. Čas Kolere: epidemije kolere na Kranjskem v 19 stoletju. Ljubljana: Založba ZRC, ZRC SAZU. 2007, p. 102–104.

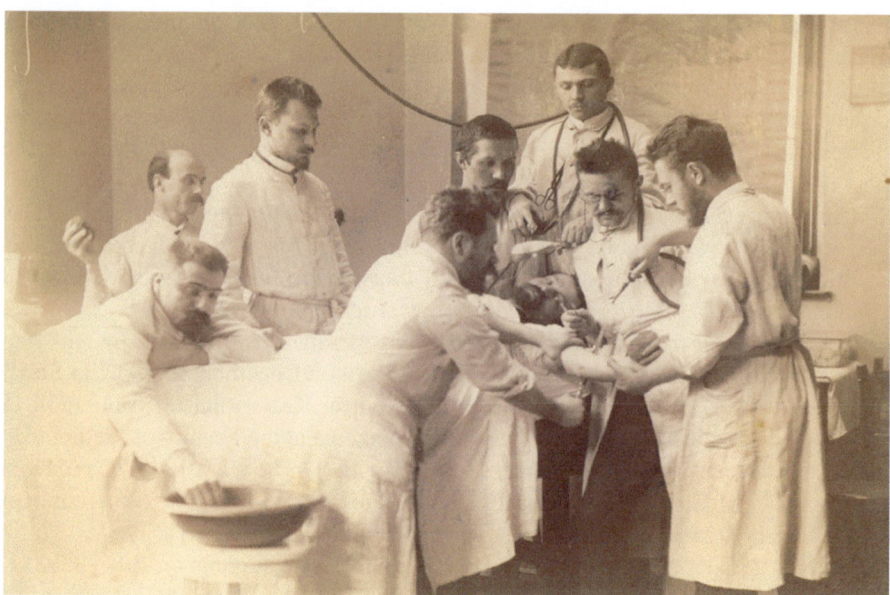

Image A.1 Dr. Franz Fux (first from the right) and his staff operating in the old surgical hospital in Ljubljana around 1885. (Source: Zupanič Slavec Z., Goričar M. Prim. Dr. Edo Šlajmer, reformator kirurgije na Slovenskem (ob 150-letnici rojstva). Isis: Glasilo Zdravniške zbornice Slovenije., ISSN 1318-0193. 2015;24(1), p. 64–68. https://www.zdravniskazbornica.si/informacije-publikacije-in-analize/publikacije-zbornice-isis/isis-januar-2015. The image of Dr. Franz Fux during surgery from around 1885 is the property of the Institute for the History of Medicine of the Faculty of Medicine in Ljubljana. The image in the book is published with the permission of Prof. Dr. Zvonka Zupanič Slavec. The permission was granted on April 2, 2021)

conservative surgery, which enabled a large number of soldiers to keep their limbs despite extensive injuries. During his career, he performed between 2000 and 3000 operations and treated around 30,000 patients. According to some accounts, the Imperial and Royal Ministry appointed Dr. Fux as the primarius of the surgical ward of the General Hospital in Ljubljana in 1859, and according to others, in 1861. He replaced the late Dr. Nathan (1790–1860).[11]

In 1861, together with Dr. Valenta and Dr. Vesel, he started a campaign to found a medical reading society, which was renamed the Society of Physicians in Ljubljana in 1862. The aim of the society was to cultivate medical science. The society held many successful scientific lectures. Dr. Fux was an exceptionally knowledgeable and intelligent physician who regularly educated himself and lectured. He gave many lectures and 67 case demonstrations. He established himself in the scientific field, publishing numerous articles in various journals and participating in scientific debates on cases in the profession. He published numerous articles in various

---

[11] Kvržić, 2022, 42–44.

journals on his cases of surgery, fractures, blood transfusion, replacement of bleeding loss with saline, etc.[12,13]

During the Austro-Prussian War in 1866, Dr. Fux performed many different operations on various wounded soldiers. He performed the operations simultaneously in private care and in the hospital. In 1887, he was made an Imperial Councilor and was also a Sanitary Councilor. He was a prominent doctor in academic circles, and many young doctors from the countryside and the city were trained by him to practice independently. He carried out his mission with the greatest joy and the greatest humanity toward his patients. Caring for the health and saving the lives of his patients was always his first priority. He carried out his mission tirelessly, even when he was seriously ill. Despite frequent fainting spells, he treated patients and took part in operations. He was forced to give up his practice when a serious illness left him bedridden. Dr. Fux died in Ljubljana of stomach cancer on a Saturday morning in early March 1892, at the age of 69.[14,15]

Dr. Fux briefly presented his only case of a successful blood transfusion in Ljubljana in a reputable Czech medical journal that I found, entitled *"Correspondenzblatt für Böhmen Organ des Vereines deutscher Aerzte in Prag Aerztliches"* (Correspondence Bulletin for Bohemia, Medical Organ of the Association of German Physicians in Prague). The entire right lower leg of the patient, a robust 37-year-old woodcutter, was shattered above the knee by a tree stump that tumbled over. After the leg was bandaged, the patient was advised to go immediately to the regional hospital in Ljubljana for treatment. Instead of following the advice, the patient allowed himself to be treated for a month and a half by a non-professional, a greaser. He left the patient after his relatives had unwound the wound and noticed an abscess[16] and maggots eating the injured leg. The leg had virtually amputated itself. The patient, in a serious condition, finally agreed to medical treatment and arrived at the hospital in Ljubljana in a half-dead state. Dr. Fux saved the patient's life with a human blood transfusion after the leg was finally amputated and the wound was successfully treated.[17,18]

The blood transfusion of Dr. Fux's blood was reported in the same year in the *"Laibacher Zeitung"* (a German newspaper on Slovenian soil) in an article from 1884 entitled *"Ein Beitrag zur Kochsalzblood transfusion als Prophylaktikum"* (Saline blood transfusion as a prophylactic), which was published in the Vienna In the medical journal *"Wiener medizinische Wochenschrift,"* Dr. Fux mentions that a

---

[12] Lbid.
[13] Meršol V., Sedemdeset let Slovenskega zdravniškega društva v Ljubljani. 1932;4(8-10), p. 131–138. https://www.dlib.si/details/URN:NBN:SI:DOC-23FDIHNG.
[14] Kvržić, 2022, 42–43.
[15] Zgodovinski arhiv Ljubljana, SI_ZAL_LJU 10339, Pintarjeva Zbirka, TE 2.
[16] Abscess is collection of pus.
[17] Fux F. Transfusion in Krain, Aerztliches Correspondenzblatt für Böhmen, 1875, p. 230. https://www.google.si/books/edition/Aerztliches_Correspondenzblatt_f%C3%BCr_B%C3%B6h/fTDRsb5cYQ0C?hl=sl&gbpv=1&dq=Transfusion+in+Krain&pg=PA230&printsec=frontcover.
[18] Kvržić, 2022, 42–43.

few years earlier he had carried out two blood transfusions, the first of which (1875) had been successful, but the second, which he carried out between 1875 and 1884, had unfortunately been fatal, and he had therefore abandoned blood transfusion therapy. In the book *"Gynaecology in Slovenia from the Beginning to the 1980s,"* the distinguished author mentions that in the past, researchers found an article by Dr. Fux in which he reported two blood transfusion attempts, the success of which was unknown. However, it is not known why the researchers who found Dr. Fux's 1884 article did not mention the real information that Dr. Fux had actually successfully carried out one of the two blood transfusions of human blood and that he had not merely attempted to carry out the blood transfusions. Whether this is due to a mistranslation or something else remains unexplained. The noble Dr. Fux is surely responsible for the modest beginnings of transfusion medicine in Slovenia, which are now at the highest professional level.[19]

Other Methods of Blood Loss Replacement in the 19th and Early 20th Centuries

In the nineteenth century, saline was employed for blood loss replacement, although some documented examples suggest that diethyl ether (Aether sulfuricus) or ether was an effective alternative in the early twentieth century.

Dr. Fux, in 1884, reported in his article a case where he successfully replaced blood loss with an infusion of saline.[20] A distinguished doctor from Ljubljana, Franc Derganc Senior (1877–1939), employed the use of ether during his operations. Dr. Derganc Sr. was introduced to this method at a conference in Paris in 1913. He used ether in an operation for peritonitis.[21] At the end of the operation, he infused 50–200 g of ether into the abdominal cavity. The ether boils at 34.6 °C, so it rapidly boils in the abdominal cavity and penetrates deep into all corners of the abdominal cavity. Dr. Derganc Sr. explained that the ether had a stimulating effect on the blood vessels of the intestine and that the ether constricted the blood vessels, causing blood to flow again to a large extent to the heart and into the bloodstream, so that the brain and its centers received sufficient blood again, respiration and pulse were corrected, the face turned yellow, and the patient's condition was visibly improved. As a result, the blue paralytic currents rapidly turned yellow, and peristalsis became apparent. Ether was the only bactericidal agent at that time that gave better results in peritonitis. Dr. Derganc Sr. used ether to wash the joints in severe infections, especially knee infections, which were a common cause of amputations at that time, and ether was used to prevent sepsis and the death of the patient.[22]

---

[19] Lbid.

[20] Fux F. Kochsalztransfusion als Prophylaktikum. Wiener medizinische Wochenschrift. Nr. 31. 1884, p. 1–2.

[21] Paritonis is an inflammation of the peritoneum.

[22] Florstchűtz V. Zgodovina kirurgije Slovenije od 1760 do 1928, Zusammenfassung P.o.: Acta chirurgica Yugoslavica; an. 6. 1959, 7, fasc. 2, p. 168–172.

The First Blood Transfusions in the 1920S

Except for Dr. Fux's experiments with blood transfusion, there are not any records that suggest that there were any performed until the 1920s. In this period, the first blood transfusions in Slovenia began in the 1920s, when the Slovenian territory was under the Kingdom of Serbs, Croats, and Slovenes. The first blood transfusions with human blood at that time were sensational news that was written about and discussed.

Dr. Pavel Lunaček, Dr. Zalokar's assistant, brought the blood transfusion technique from France to the Women's Hospital in Ljubljana in 1927.[23] The first blood transfusion supposedly was carried out on May 11, 1927, in the Women's Hospital, when a brave bank clerk saved his mother from probable death, according to a report in the local Ljubljana newspaper on May 12, 1927. Drs. Fink and Pehani performed the blood transfusion.[24] The next day, on May 13, there was a new announcement in another newspaper. It was reported that this actually was not the first blood transfusion, that the blood transfusion has been carried out for the past 6 years (1921), and that this was simply a blood transfusion with the newest equipment.[25] On May 14, an announcement from Dr. Mirko Černič from the city of Maribor was made. In it, he announced that exactly the same kind of blood transfusion from a healthy person to a sick person had been carried out at the surgical ward of the General Hospital in Maribor on April 23. The operation was carried out by his assistant, Dr. Adolf Ramšak, and the patient went home completely healthy on May 9.[26] In a letter written on January 31, 1956, to Dr. Eman Pertl, the distinguished Dr. Ramšak described, to the best of his recollection, the blood transfusion he and his surgical team had performed (Image A.2). The explanations is given as it follows: "*The female patient was extremely weak after hemorrhaging following childbirth or miscarriage. A Rotanda 100-cc syringe with glass cannulas and the direct blood transfusion technique were used to carry out the blood transfusion. The veins had to be prepared. Sodium citrate was used as an anticoagulant. The blood transfusion procedure was very difficult because the cannulas were repeatedly clogged, so they could not transfuse significant volumes. Nevertheless, the patient survived.*"[27]

The 3 days of contributions show that it was important for the academic community of surgeons to inform the public about the first new successes in blood

---

[23] Borisov P. Ginekologija na Slovenskem od nastanka do 80. let 20. Stoletja. Ljubljana: Slovenska akademija znanosti in umetnosti. 1995, p. 191.

[24] Anon. Prva transfuzija krvi v Sloveniji. Jutro. 1927;8(112), p. 3. https://www.dlib.si/details/URN:NBN:SI:DOC-KE7AUJ30.

[25] Anon. Senzacija, ki ni senzacija. Slovenski narod. 1927; letnik 60(108), p. 3. https://www.dlib.si/stream/URN:NBN:SI:DOC-AC6MWL9M/aed06c3a-a288-4445-b17e-4427d505671e/PDF.

[26] Černič M. Prva transfuzija krvi v Sloveniji.Jutro.1927;8(114), p. 4. http://www.dlib.si/?URN=URN:NBN:SI:DOC-48Q5USRH.

[27] Ramšak A. Personal letter from January 31, 1956. A copy of the letter is in the Maribor Regional Archives, Fond Eman Pertl, 1907–1987, AŠ 4, folder 6, personal letter of Adolf Ramšak, 31 January 1956. The letter for this book was obtained from Dr. Elko Borko's personal archive on March 19, 2021.

426
*

Črna, 31. 1. 1956.

Spoštovani gospod primarij!

Prav rad odgovarjam na Vaše vprašanje o podrobnostih in okolščinah v zvezi z našo prvo transfuzijo v mariborski bolnici. Bojim se le, da ne bom mogel povedati dosti kaj točnega, ker doba, ki je od takrat minula, je že dolga.

Kolikor se spominjam, je bila oseba, pri kateri smo delali transfuzijo, ženska, skrajno oslabela po krvavitvi po porodu ali splavu. Morala je biti že v izredno težkem stanju, da smo se odločila za ta, takrat izreden postopek. Uporabili smo metodo direktne transfuzije s pomočjo "Rotanda" brizgalke, 100 kubične, s steklenimi kanilami, tako da je bilo treba prim njej v vsakem slučaju veni izpreparirati. Kot anticoagulens smo vporabili natr. citr. Spominjam se, da potek ni bil preveč gladek, ker sta se kanili večkrat zamašili, tako da nismo mogli trasfudirati znatnejših množin, a spominjam pa se prav tako - in upam, da me spomin ne vara,-da je bil uspeh kljub temu popoln, to je, da je bolnica kmalu vzcvetela. Tako je bila ta transfuzija nam, ki smo bili direktno pri njej zaposleni in pa celotnemu kirurškemu oddelku v zadoščenje. - Verjetno sem ta poseg vpisal kot operacijo v operacijski protokol. Tako bi se morebiti iz oper. protokola dalo dognati ime pacijentke in najti morebiti še popis bolezni, kjer bi se dali eventuleno dobiti še bolj verodostojni podatki o vsej tej zadevi.

S tem v zvezi naj navedem, še to - kar pa Vam je verjetno itak že znano - da je nekaj časa po tem izšla v nekem ljubljanskem časopisu notica, da so dne tega in tega izvršili v ljubljanski bolnici prvo transfuzijo, ki da je tudi prva v Sloveniji. Prim. Dr Črnič pa je takoj poslal drugo notico - mislim da v lokalni mariborski dnevnik - da sem že pred tem na njegovem oddelku izvršil transfuzijo jaz in da je torej mariborska transfuzija prva v Sloveniji.-

V pozni jeseni 1927 sem se preselil iz Maribora v Črno. Seveda pa sem se še vedno zanimal za vse, kar se je v mariborski bolnici dogajalo.- Tako sem zasledil v nekem mariborskem časopisu članek, ki opisuje, da je Dr. Lutman na internem oddelku uspešno zdravil s transfuzijami nekaj primerov zastrupitve z benzolom. Kmalu pa je izšel drug članek, ki prvega popravlja v toliko, da je res, da so se ti pacijenti zdravili na internem oddelku, a transfuzije pa da je vršil kirurški oddelek.- Kdo pa je te transfuzije delal, ali primarij sam, ali kateri drugi zdŕvnik, pa ne vem.- Torej smo živeli takrat v dobi, ko še bila transfuzija še senzacija; manjkal je samo še "TT".-

Image A.2 Personal letter of Dr. Ramšak 1951. (Source: Ramšak A. Personal letter from January 31, 1956. A copy of the letter is in the Maribor Regional Archives, Fond Eman Pertl, 1907–1987, AŠ 4, folder 6, personal letter of Adolf Ramšak, 31 January 1956. The letter for this book was obtained from Dr. Gabrijel "Elko" Borko's personal archive on March 19, 2021)

transfusion and that it was important for a major achievement to be announced with at least the surname of the person credited with the blood transfusion. No information has been found on the alleged blood transfusions in Slovenia in 1921, despite an extensive search of sources that I conducted. If there is any truth to this story, there is a possibility that the data has been lost over time. In the present time, all the literature on the first blood transfusion attributes this credit to the eminent and accomplished surgeon Dr. Adolf Ramšak (Image A.3). The year in which Dr. Ramšak's first blood transfusion is mentioned is 1924, and the most common is 1926. This information is incorrect on both counts. Dr. Ramšak therefore performed the first blood transfusion in Maribor and in Slovenia with the most modern and completely new instruments of that period on April 23, 1927. Somewhere in the past, when writing the history of blood transfusions in Slovenia, there was an error in the description of the year of the first blood transfusion, which has been passed down through the generations as a fact and which has not been corrected up to now. The first historic blood transfusion in Slovenia, however, was performed, as mentioned before, by Dr. Fux.

Dr. Adolf Ramšak (1897–1968) was a physician and surgeon. He graduated in Graz, Austria, and in 1926 he specialized in surgery in Ljubljana. In 1927, he became the primarius of the Mining hospital in Črna na Koroškem, where he worked there until 1958 as a general physician and surgeon, and later in dispensaries in Maribor. He dealt with the occupational lead poisoning of miners and smelters. He also founded an anti-tuberculosis dispensary. His wife was Dr. Maria Štuhec. In

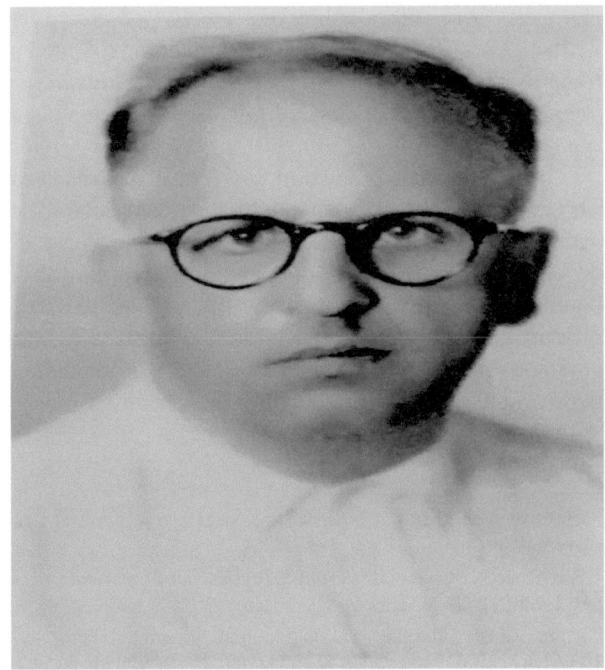

Image A.3 Primarius Dr. Adolf Ramšak 1938. (Source: Makarovič M., Modrej I., Primarius Dr. Adolf Ramšak 1938 in Črna in Črnjani. Črna na Koroškem: Občina Črna na Koroškem; 2013, p. 486–487. The mayor of the city of Črna na Koroškem, Madam Romana Lesjak, granted permission to use the image for this book on May 23, 2021)

1928, the Ramšaks were in charge of 14 patient rooms with 60 beds. Among the occupational ailments they already had to deal with was lead poisoning, a common illness among miners. They also treated various fractures and, above all, plucked aching teeth.[28]

The Great Depression and Impact on Blood Donation 1931–1941

The Great Depression, which began in the USA in 1929 and spread worldwide, had a negative impact on all types of economic activity. The crisis was felt in some countries until the early 1940s. The crisis reached the Kingdom of Yugoslavia, where it was felt strongly throughout its territory and, as a result, led to high unemployment and poverty. The difficult situation led people to look for various manual and hard jobs, both casual and professional, and many came to Ljubljana in search of a better life. Existing on the edge of survival, hunger, poor living conditions, and widespread misery created a new profession in the world: "professional blood donation," where people started to donate blood in exchange for money in the hope of surviving from 1 day to the next. With blood donations, they also wanted to help others in need. Professional-paid blood donation flourished in all the provinces of the Kingdom of Yugoslavia. In addition to the unemployed blood donors, who were the majority, it is mentioned that blood donations were also made by members of other professional economic strata. There were also cases where family members gave blood to each other, students, friends, hospital staff, etc. In the Kingdom of Yugoslavia, blood transfusions were seen as a great advance in medicine. The general public was enthralled by the new way of saving lives.

In 1935, primaries Dr. Robert Blumauer explained and commented on the blood transfusion: *"We used to read about these things in the newspaper; they were happening in the main centers of health science, in Vienna, in Berlin, in London, in America... Today, blood transfusions are just as common in Ljubljana."*[29]

The first Slovene blood donors lived harsh lives in extremely difficult conditions. They were mainly dissatisfied with the treatment and conditions for donating blood. This was also the situation in other parts of the world where paid blood donation had developed.[30] Some blood donors who had regular jobs had a telephone at home and could call the hospital to find out if they needed blood. Such blood donors were quicker to get in line to donate blood compared to unemployed blood donors, who could not live on blood donations alone. In order to survive, they had occasional and various jobs, such as bricklaying, delivering various shipments, and cutting down

---

[28] Makarovič M., Modrej I. Strokovno zdravstvo in Črna in Črnjani. Črna na Koroškem: Občina Črna na Koroškem; 2013. p. 486–487.

[29] Blumauer R. Provincialna kronika Jugoslovanske province hčera krščanske ljubezni (usmiljenk), leto 1935, I, p. 167–168.

[30] Anon. Cene človeške krvi v Ljubljani so precej različne, vendar pa precej nizke. Jutro. 1937;18(212), p. 3. http://www.dlib.si/details/URN:NBN:SI:DOC-I5Q49NOC.

trees.[31] More than half of them had families with many children. They lived in appallingly poor conditions, such as in tattered shacks and basement and attic dwellings on the periphery.[32] The living conditions were so harsh that Dinko Puc, the mayor of Ljubljana, urged the city's working population to donate at least 1% of their monthly salary to the hungry because there were more still employed people than there were jobless people in November 1931. Mayor Puc understood that winter was coming and that if aid was not provided, many people would suffer.[33] 33 blood transfusions were carried out by the surgical ward in the same year. As it was difficult to rapidly reach people in the surrounding area for emergency blood transfusions, 65 blood donors—mostly from the city of Ljubljana—responded to the first two appeals for blood donations. They thanked their blood donors for consistently responding as soon as possible to their appeal. One blood donor had his blood drawn nine times during this period. By 1931, minor blood transfusion reactions were seen in patients with fevers lasting up to 2 days. The Rotanda apparatus allowed whole blood to be transfused in 10–15 min.[34]

Before the Second World War, blood transfusions in the surgical ward in Ljubljana were a great and rare procedure. It was considered a major operation because two surgeons were involved. One was on the blood donor's side, and the other was on the patient's side. Before the procedure started, the blood donor was served cognac because it was believed that alcohol-enriched blood was beneficial for the blood transfusion patient. The surgical ward had a list of addresses of healthy blood donors who, when needed, would come to the hospital on call and, for a modest reward, donate a few hundred cubic centimeters of blood. The Rh blood group system was unknown before its discovery, and they were aware that a blood donor with blood group O was considered a universal blood donor.[35]

In 1933, the State Hospital for Women's Diseases reported an unfortunately fatal case of autotransfusion in a pregnant woman.[36] This is an early case of autotransfusion. No other mention of this method in sources from this period for Slovenia was found.

The second surgical ward in Ljubljana had performed 99 cases of blood transfusions by the year 1934, 66 on men and 33 on women. The indications for blood transfusion were mainly acute secondary anemia. Blood transfusions were performed for trauma, post-operative hemorrhage, and various operations, such as

---

[31] Anon. Ljudje, ki prodajajo svojo kri, še 30 let ni star (pa je dal že več kot 30 krat svojo kri bolnikom). Slovenski dom.1938; 3(276), p. 4. http://www.dlib.si/?URN=URN:NBN:SI:DOC-W7L5DSJC.

[32] Jutro, 1937, p. 3.

[33] Anon. Poziv župana Dinka Puca. Jugoslovan. 1931; 2(276), p. 3. https://www.dlib.si/stream/URN:NBN:SI:DOC-XY7133N6/d86618b3-71b2-4a9a-945b-34411edc767b/PDF.

[34] Bajc O. Kri za svojega bližnjega. Družinski tednik—Roman. 1932; 4(1), p. 3. http://www.dlib.si/details/URN:NBN:SI:DOC-IDI98SBA.

[35] Milčinski J. Transfuzija v partizanski bolnišnici. Delo. 1961;3(133), p. 7. http://www.dlib.si/details/URN:NBN:SI:DOC-LRXBNLOQ.

[36] Lunaček P. Sectio Caesarea. Zdravniški vestnik.1933;5(3), p. 90–117. http://www.dlib.si/?URN=URN:NBN:SI:DOC-GYDDEGCB.

those for stomach cancer, rectal cancer, the removal of the goiter, as a therapy for septic processes, etc.[37,38] They used the Rotanda apparatus and the Jüngling method; the syringe was flushed with a 3% sodium citrate solution, and no blood was observed to coagulate in the syringe. To stimulate the hemopoietic system (the system in the body that makes blood cells), 200 cc of blood was used for the blood transfusion. The average blood transfusion dose was between 400 and 500 cc. In severe cases, 700 cc of blood were transfused. Almost always, 100–200 cc of 25% glucose were added. They did not experience unpleasant complications because they always performed the biological test, according to Oehlecker. Blood donors were examined clinically, radiologically, and serologically and were constantly monitored.[39] Nevertheless, if the blood donor had developed syphilis at precisely this time, the transfused patient would also have contracted the disease.[40] It is possible that the reason for not noticing complications was because they did not pay enough attention to the unpleasant complications, or if they did occur, that they did not connect them to blood transfusions. It is also possible that they actually did not have any complications in the mentioned cases.

In 1932, a new regulation on payment for hospital treatment came out, and one of the many rulings was that to compensate for transfused blood, the patient had to pay only the blood donor and not the hospital administration. In the case of operations, medicines and other resources did not have to be paid for separately by the patients. Payment did not fully take off because patients cured by blood transfusions rarely thanked blood donors financially.[41] Financial rewards from the patients to blood donors were rare, small, and symbolic, e.g., 25 dinars, because most of the patients were poor. The hospital administration continued to pay blood donors the agreed-upon fee. In the Kingdom of Yugoslavia, the prices for donated blood varied. For comparison, blood donors from Belgrade were paid 600–800 dinars, those from Zagreb were paid 500–600 dinars, and those from Slovenia were paid 150–400 dinars.

From 1935 to 1938, blood donors in Slovenia could donate their blood every 1–3 months.[42,43,44] They donated 200–600 cc of blood. By 1937, blood donors in

---

[37] Venčeslav A. Transfuzije krvi v letu 1934. Zdravniški vestnik.1935;7(7—8), p. 291–292. http://www.dlib.si/?URN=URN:NBN:SI:DOC-AQ6MXYDG.

[38] Peršič I. Osteomyletis v letu 1934. Zdravniški vestnik. 1935;7(7–8) p. 285. http://www.dlib.si/?URN=URN:NBN:SI:DOC-AQ6MXYDG.

[39] Venčeslav, 1934, p. 292.

[40] Jerina Lah P. Novosti - izkušnje—pobude, Naše prve poti k organizirani transfuziološki službi. Obzornik zdravstvene nege. 1991;25(3/4),p. 229–234. https://obzornik.zbornica-zveza.si/index.php/ObzorZdravNeg/article/view/1904.

[41] Anon. Doma in po svetu, nov pravilnik o plačevanju lečenja v bolnicah. Delavska politika.1932; 7 (69), p. 2. http://www.dlib.si/?URN=URN:NBN:SI:DOC-T0RS64RE.

[42] Lavrič, 1935, p. 4.

[43] Anon. Ljudje, ki prodajajo svojo kri. Še 30 let ni star (pa je dal že več kot 30 krat svojo kri bolnikom. Slovenski Dom. 1938; 3 (276), p. 4. http://www.dlib.si/?URN=URN:NBN:SI:DOC-W7L5DSJC.

[44] Anon. Svojo kri prodajajo. Jutro.1936;17(88), p. 3. http://www.dlib.si/details/URN:NBN:SI:DOC-1P97ZI9H.

Slovenia were paid for the blood transfusion as follows: **Ptuj** (150 din.),[45]**Novo mesto** (200 din.),[46]**Ljubljana** (*Šlajmerjev dom 150 din., General State Hospital 250 din., Women's Hospital 300 din., Leonišče 400 din.*), **Celje**(*300–400 din.*), **Maribor** (200–400 dinars). Both sexes, ages 18–45, were invited to donate blood.[47,48,49,50,51,52]

The distinguished Primarius Dr. Božidar Lavrič from Ljubljana held a lecture in 1935 about blood transfusion. He mentioned that the modern apparatus for blood transfusion that they also used was Percy's apparatus.[53] Blood donors in 1935 were registered on a special list where information about their blood group, last medical examination, number of donations in general, and number of donations with positive and negative outcomes were entered.[54]

In May 1936, the administration of the General State Hospital in Ljubljana wanted to reduce the monetary reward for blood donors from 300 to 200 dinars. The blood donors opposed the administration's decision in vain. However, just then, the Minister for Social Policy and National Health, Dragiša Cvetković, came to Ljubljana for a visit. After visiting the General State Hospital in Ljubljana, a small group of impoverished blood donors stopped him at the gate and explained the desperate situation to the minister. Minister Cvetković listened to the representatives of the blood donor group and ordered, in the presence of the deputy manager of the hospital, that the current reward of 300 dinars will remain for donated blood. At the same time, he generously transferred another 200 dinars of extraordinary support to the blood donors, of whom seven out of 40 were in the hospital at the time. The money was immediately transferred to the administration of Dravska Banovina on the order of Cvetković's secretary. After this event, the administration of the hospital discontinued the midday and evening meals that the blood donors had received on the day of each blood transfusion. In July 1936, however, the administration of the hospital in Ljubljana reduced the reward for donated blood from 300 dinars to 200 dinars. Unemployed blood donors tried to improve their demands and conditions by protesting. Hospital employees had to donate blood instead of them. The blood donors' protest was unsuccessful, and in addition to reducing the monetary

---

[45] Jutro, 1937, p. 3.

[46] Anon. Novosti iz banovinske ženske bolnice. Jutro.1936;17(119), p. 9. http://www.dlib.si/?URN=URN:NBN:SI:DOC-9FF2AT15.

[47] Jutro, 1937, p. 3.

[48] Anon. Poziv dajalcem krvi. Delavska politika.1941;16(4), p. 3. http://www.dlib.si/?URN=URN:NBN:SI:DOC-N6NDNCAG.

[49] Lbid.

[50] Jutro 1936, p. 9.

[51] Anon. Ptujska bolnica vabi krvodajalce. Jutro.1937;18(207) p. 8. http://www.dlib.si/details/URN:NBN:SI:DOC-27OLOLAK.

[52] Anon. O oddaji krvi za transfuzije. Slovenski narod. 1936;69(98), p. 3. http://www.dlib.si/details/URN:NBN:SI:DOC-HXEU56M9.

[53] Lavrič B. Kri Se Preliva... Za Zdravje.1935;16(234), p. 4. http://www.dlib.si/?URN=URN:NBN:SI:DOC-8PIYAUM9.

[54] Blumauer, 1935, 167–168.

reward, the administration ordered blood donors to always be available for direct blood transfusions. There were cases when it was necessary to perform 3– 5 blood transfusions a day, and blood donors always had to wait for their turn. The wait was delayed deep into the night, and the blood donors had to lie on a hard bench in the waiting room until it was their turn to donate blood to a patient they did not know. The administration of the hospital referred to the lower reward because they interpreted the 200 dinars for donated blood as just a kind of tip because the blood donors were also paid by the patient who received their blood. In fact, blood donors rarely ever received additional rewards. This is confirmed by the case of an unemployed worker who donated blood 12 times in 1 year but received an additional financial reward only once. In the case in question, the blood donor stayed up all night in the hospital waiting room while the doctors decided minute by minute whether the patient would even need a blood transfusion. After the blood transfusion, the patient, if he could financially afford it, donated a few dinars to his blood donor so that the blood donor could afford a modest breakfast.[55,56] Regarding the meals, it has to be mentioned that in Slovenia, it is an obligatory tradition for blood donors to get a high-quality meal after the donation to boost their energy.

The group of blood donors had mainly disbanded by 1937 as a result of the administration of the Ljubljana General Hospital's financial issues and poor conditions. Blood donors were forbidden to wait in the waiting room in Ljubljana. When called to donate blood, they had to wait at the gate until the porter called an individual to donate blood on the doctor's orders. The blood donors had modest wishes: to wait for the call in the garden of the hospital and to no longer stay on the road outside the garden; and to have their order determined by the doctors and no longer by the porter. But all of this was unsuccessful. Healthy, strong, and abstinent people were invited. By raising the agreed fee from 200 dinars to 250 dinars, the administration of the General State Hospital tried to re-establish the blood donation group, but with poor results. This led to the fact that in cases of poisoning, severe blood loss, or other reasons where a blood transfusion was necessary, they advised that healthy and strong relatives come to the hospital with the victim, who could become his blood donors. If the patient had no relatives, the hospital found him a blood donor, which the patient himself had to pay for. In addition to the agreed fee, the hospital paid the blood donor additionally on behalf of the patient in the event that the patient was really poor and consequently unable to pay.[57] A price list for the General State Hospital in Ljubljana was approved by the administration of the General state hospital there and the Ministry of Social Policy and National Health in Belgrade. It included fees for the blood that doctors gave to specific patients as part of treatment, in addition to the usual costs of care. Poor citizens and all government, self-government, and government personnel were free from these levies. Private individuals who owned their own property were also assessed fees for their

---

[55] Anon. Dinar za gram krvi, krvodajalci, najznačilnejši »poklic' naše dobe, se bore za svojo nagrado. Jutro.1936; 17(162), p. 7. http://www.dlib.si/?URN=URN:NBN:SI:DOC-WT51C3SV.
[56] Jutro, 1937, p. 3.
[57] Lbid.

annual tax at the established rate, with consideration given to how frequently the patient in question received blood over the course of the same illness.[58] In this period, they were allowed to donate blood once every 4 weeks.[59] In 1937, the administration of the General State Hospital even prohibited women from donating their blood. This was due, as they referred to it, to medical reasons. However, no detailed explanation was given for this directive.[60]

In 1937, due to poor blood donation conditions in the Ljubljana General Hospital, the number of dedicated blood donors decreased from 50[61] to only 12 in 1 year. Extremely poor living conditions and the winter forced blood donors to ask the Slovenian people in 1938, through the newspapers, for modest gifts to make their lives a little better for the approaching Christmas and New Year holidays. Under the slogan "Little grows big," they asked the good-hearted people of Ljubljana for help. They emphasized that they wanted to have nice holidays with their families, that they could not help themselves much with the fee from donated blood, and that they were poorly dressed and badly shod. At the same time, the patients, who survived because of their blood, and the authorities were also asked for help.[62,63]

Blood groups were classified according to Moss[64] in 1938 and Landsteiner in 1940.[65] Interestingly, one of Landsteiner's close colleagues from the time of the discovery of blood groups was a Slovene, Dr. Janez Plečnik.[66] In 1938, it was reported that at General State Hospital Ljubljana, they had 12 blood donors from the blood group categories 2, 3, and 4.[67] This was equivalent to blood groups A, B, and O.

---

[58] Anon. Odškodnina za transfuzijo krvi. Jutro. 1937;18(269), p. 4. http://www.dlib.si/?URN=URN:NBN:SI:DOC-30T8CL1J.

[59] Anon.Transfuzija krvi v obči državni bolnišnici v Ljubljani. Slovenec.1937;65(12), p. 4 http://www.dlib.si/?URN=URN:NBN:SI:DOC-50VVQ2C5.

[60] Anon. Naš domači zdravnik. Slovenec. 1937; 115(65), p. 12. http://www.dlib.si/?URN=URN:NBN:SI:DOC-9AYHR2OB.

[61] Jutro, 1937, p. 3.

[62] Anon. Krvodajalci naslavljajo svojo prošnjo na dobra srca. Slovenski dom.1938;3(287), p. 3. http://www.dlib.si/?URN=URN:NBN:SI:DOC-DYQ9RGNJ.

[63] Anon.Tudi ti bi radi obhajali vesel Božič. Slovenec.1938;66(291), p. 7. http://www.dlib.si/?URN=URN:NBN:SI:DOC-QY4D5UUP.

[64] Anon. Krvodajalci naslavljajo svojo prošnjo na dobra srca. Slovenski dom. 1938;3(287), p. 3. http://www.dlib.si/?URN=URN:NBN:SI:DOC-DYQ9RGNJ.

[65] Lutman S. Transfuzija krvi v praksi. Zdravniški Vestnik. 1940;12(6—7), p. str. 213–215. https://www.dlib.si/stream/URN:NBN:SI:DOC-SUA1YXIK/e957e193-df10-484b-9b31-375de07d02e8/PDF.

[66] Potočnik M. Transfuziologija nekoč in danes. Zdravniški Vestnik. Vol 73 (2004): Supplement I, p. 3. https://vestnik.szd.si/index.php/ZdravVest/article/view/2411.

[67] Anon. Krvodajalci naslavljajo svojo prošnjo na dobra srca. Slovenski dom. 1938;3(287), p. 3. http://www.dlib.si/?URN=URN:NBN:SI:DOC-DYQ9RGNJ.

From this small group in 1938, three had blood group 2 or A, three had blood group 3 or B, and six had blood group 4 or O. Together, in two and a half years, they donated blood to 276 patients in the amount of around 118,000 cc of blood.[68]

Primarius Dr. Stane Lutman from the Maribor General Hospital introduced in the journal "Zdravniški Vestnik" the field of blood donation and blood transfusion in practice in 1940. He discussed the current issues with coordinating blood donation and said that, in reality, there should always be a universal blood donor available who could donate blood while being escorted by a doctor, even outside of Ljubljana in other locations throughout Slovenia. He promoted the idea that an organization dedicated to blood donation should be set up for this reason, with enough blood donors on hand to donate in the field. He proposed that the organization be created through the mutual cooperation of operative hospital departments, particularly the surgical and obstetric-gynecological departments, internal departments, hygiene institutes, medical centers, rescue stations, and the Red Cross.[69] In the same year, a lecture was organized in Maribor as part of the Red Cross week in the hall of the People's University on blood transfusion, which was mandatory for nursing assistants and volunteers. The public was invited to attend the lectures in as large a number as possible. The lecture was led by Dr. Kušar, a general hospital specialist.[70] In 1941, a special section of blood donors was established within the Red Cross Society in Maribor, and healthy people were invited to sign up for blood donation lists in the laboratory of the medical department of the General Hospital in Maribor, in the Health Center in Maribor, or in the Red Cross office.[71]

Blood transfusions in Slovenia saved many lives during the 1920s and 1940s. They were not as common as they are today, when blood is almost required every 5 min. But nevertheless, they were performed on their own terms quite often, when there was massive bleeding or when doctors believed that it might save lives in different health conditions, and that would help the body to recover. The direct blood transfusions from vein to vein were also a dramatic experience for the blood donor for several reasons. First, they were mostly poor and unprivileged with an unhealthy lifestyle, so when the procedure began, they really did not know if the procedure would be successful because of their poor physical condition, as they might have fainted. The patient next to the blood donor could have bled to death. This experience certainly left a psychological impact on the blood donor. Also, because of the surgical venesection, they had problems at work because their hands hurt after the procedure. A blood donor could also have been exhausted if he regularly donated blood. There was not any organization in the real sense of the word that promoted healthy lifestyles, organized safe blood donations, or made sure that there were always a sufficient number of blood donors on demand. There were, however, attempts and suggestions that, in the later years, led to organized transfusion medicine. The number of

---

[68] Lbid.

[69] Lutman S. Transfuzija krvi v praksi. Zdravniški vestnik. 1940;11(6–7), p. 213–215. http://www.dlib.si/?URN=URN:NBN:SI:DOC-SUA1YXIK.

[70] Anon. Predavanje v okviru Rdečega križa. Večernik.1940;14(213), p. 4. http://www.dlib.si/?URN=URN:NBN:SI:DOC-HFIB3I65.

[71] Delavska politika, 1941, p. 3.

blood donors who were part of a group through the 1930s that donated their blood regularly was about 50. Today, in Slovenia, to satisfy the needs for blood supply, we roughly need at least around 300 blood donors per day. It is also crucial to note that Slovenia is entirely self-sufficient in 100% blood component therapy and has more than 95,000 blood donors who each year faithfully donate their blood. It is also noteworthy to see how much was written in the 1930s on the struggles and triumphs of blood transfusion. Blood donors wrote about their lives, experiences, and motivations for donating blood in the press. Patients whose lives were saved by blood transfusions also expressed their gratitude in public letters to blood donors, physicians, and other hospital personnel. This demonstrates that they were all aware of how vital blood donation and blood transfusion were to mankind.

One of the most notable doctors who in Slovenia, at least until the end of the Second World War, performed blood transfusions and realized their importance were Ramšak, Fink, Pehani, Venčeslav, Bajc, Lavrič, Lutman, Hafner, Brezovnik, Janež, and others.

Blood Donation in Slovenia During World War 2 1941-1945

On April 6, 1941, Axis forces invaded the Kingdom of Yugoslavia, promptly took it over, and divided it up among Germany, Italy, Hungary, Bulgaria, and their client regimes. This marked the start of World War II in the country.

The Italian Occupier forbade night-time movement in Ljubljana, and blood donors, especially those with the desirable universal blood group O, had to be on duty at night on the benches in the surgical corridors.[72] In 1944, blood donors were paid 500 lire (Italian currency) for a single blood transfusion. Blood donors were entitled to an additional food voucher and were served lunch or dinner in the hospital.[73]

The first known documented blood transfusion was carried out by partisan guerrillas in the early spring of 1942. Nurses Bregant and Saveljev, by order of Professor Dr. Kanoni, smuggled two wounded partisans across the Italian blockade to Ljubljana for X-rays for a later operation. One of the wounded had to be operated on by Dr. Kukovec. They smuggled the wounded partisans with sterile and compulsory material across the river Sava at night to the Razore at Sostrem property, where the psychiatric hospital was kept. After examining the wounded partisan, Dr. Kukovec estimated that a blood transfusion would be necessary. The only person with the right blood group was Dr. Kalan from the psychiatric hospital. She decided to selflessly and courageously donate blood without hesitation. The brightest room and two tables for the operation were prepared. The wounded man was tied to one table, and Dr. Kalan lay down on the other. Dr. Kukovec operated on the wounded man. Nurses Bergantova and Saveljev were instrumentalists; Dr. Plesničar used two larger syringes with citrate to transfuse blood from the doctor's vein directly into the wounded partisan. She performed the procedure until the wounded partisan received enough blood and until his health condition improved. After the blood transfusion,

---

[72] Jerina Lah, 1991, p. 229.

[73] Anon. Sodobni pomočniki zdravniške znanosti. Slovenec. 1944;72(55), p. 2. http://www.dlib.si/?URN=URN:NBN:SI:DOC-5WBV4YZN.

he was observed for 3 days, and then he was moved from the room to the apiary with the other wounded. Every other day, both nurses dressed the wounded.[74,75] During the Second World War, the Partisan Diversionary Medical Service of Yugoslavia did not have blood grouping test serum, blood preservatives, or accessories in stock, or these rarely reached the Partisan hospitals, and it was even more difficult to reach the first surgical station when required for casualties.[76] The causalties that could have been saved with blood transfusion unfortunately, in many cases, died.

Due to all sorts of improvisation and objective post-war shortages, there was a high risk of transfusion to patients: blood was administered by syringes or from bottles into ampoules with needle attachments; bottles were not sterilized well, their surfaces peeled off; the same was true of rubber stoppers and various tubes for the blood transfusion and for collection systems; there was not enough sodium citrate, as imports were universally limited; and the same was for dextrose. The medical teams from the Anglo-American and Soviet armies had a considerable impact on the Yugoslavian doctors, who, with their professional help, were introduced to the use of preserved blood, plasma, and its fractions. The mass collection of blood and blood transfusion to the frontlines was introduced in cooperation with the fourth Transfusion Station of the III Ukrainian Army Division. Immediately after the liberation of Belgrade on 1 October 1944, the Medical Department of the Supreme Headquarters of National Liberation Army, in cooperation with the above-mentioned army division, established the War Blood Transfusion Service from the former Transfusion Department of the Hygiene Institute of Serbia. The war situation influenced that in the last months of the War of Liberation more transfusion stations were established to meet the needs of the front.[77]**Dr. Dimitrije Kalić organized this first blood transfusion service in Yugoslavia on October 24, 1944, in Belgrade, the capital city of Serbia. The name of the service was the Blood Transfusion Center of Serbia.**[78,79] According to the available literature, it is clear that the first call for blood donors was published in a Slovenian newspaper on May 22, 1945, a few weeks before the end of the war on Slovenian territory.[80] Female and male blood donors were invited to blood donations in newspapers by name and surname until 1948. In publicly available newspapers, it can be seen that from 1945 to 1952, invitations, requests, and benefits for donating blood were supplemented.

---

[74] Bregant Polak J. Transfuzija na Razorih. Delo. 1961;3(142), p. 7. http://www.dlib.si/?URN=URN:NBN:SI:DOC-1BIIDXUJ.

[75] T.P. Prva transfuzija v času IMOB na Razorih. Naša skupnost (Ljubljana Moste-Polje). 1986;27(16), p. 4 http://www.dlib.si/?URN=URN:NBN:SI:DOC-GZK7SQT3.

[76] Jerina Lah P. Razvoj službe transfuzije v Jugoslaviji. Transplantacija. 1988; 27(3) p. 80.

[77] Jerina Lah, 1991, p. 229–230.

[78] Sovdat Banič S. Pogovor z dr. Sonjo Sovdat Banič. Potočnik M., Levičnik-Stezinar S., Faganel J., Lukić L., Rožman P., Ulaga R., Vukovič-Dervišić B., 50 let organizirane transfuzijske službe v Sloveniji:1945-1995, Ljubljana: Zavod Republike Slovenije za transfuzijo krvi, 1995, p. 19.

[79] Institut za transfuziju krvi Srbije. Istorijat. https://itks.rs/istorijat.html#. Accessed April 10 2024.

[80] Anon. Poziv uprave Splošne Bolnišnice v Ljubljani. Slovenski poročevalec—glasilo osvobodilne fronte. 1945; 6(26), p. 3. http://www.dlib.si/?URN=URN:NBN:SI:DOC-JNSTO5DK.

Appendix B: History of Transfusion Medicine in Slovenia from 1945 to 2023

Abstract After the Second World War, a new transfusion service was established in Slovenia. The first bottles of blood were preserved and stored on June 4, 1945. That is why we celebrate this day as Slovenian Blood Donation Day. Indirect transfusions replaced direct transfusions, although these were, for a few years, still carried out on a small scale. At the beginning of the development, we, with the help of our military allies, learned new methods and approaches to transfusion medicine. The Blood Transfusion Center of Slovenia (BTCS) was founded initially as part of the Faculty of Medicine in Ljubljana in 1946, then became independent in 1955 and moved to a new building in 1958, where it is still operating at the same location. As the demand for blood increased, blood transfusion departments from 1949 slowly started to open in other parts of Slovenia. A major contribution to development and progress was the adoption of voluntary, non-remunerated, and anonymous blood donation in 1953 and the introduction of mobile blood donations. This helped to increase the number of blood donors who could respond quickly to blood donations in their hometowns. Advances in regulations and development ensured greater safety for the blood donor and the recipient. Since 1953, many advances have also been made in the field of transfusion medicine. Today, transfusion medicine in Slovenia is developed on a global scale, with a large number of altruistic blood donors who regularly donate whole blood or individual blood components.

Keywords Blood Transfusion Center of Slovenia; Blood donation in Slovenia; Transfusion medicine in Slovenia; Promotion of blood donation; Nurses in Slovenian transfusion medicine

The Organization of a Blood Transfusion Service in Slovenia After the Second World War

Yugoslavia's blood transfusion services experienced a number of difficulties after the war, including a lack of qualified personnel, supplies, and blood donors. There was a growing need for blood. Blood was used in a variety of risky, life-threatening circumstances. Much work was done in the years following the war to enhance blood transfusion medicine. The general public was being encouraged to donate blood voluntarily. Publicly available newspapers show that the organization, invitations, requirements, and rewards for blood donation were supplemented in the following decades because of the increasing supply and demand for blood and its components.

At the end of 1944, in Belgrade, Dr. Janez Milčinski (1913–1993) asked Sonja Sovdat Banič, a medical student at the time, if she would like to organize a transfusion service in the liberated territory of Slovenia. Dr. Sovdat Banič accepted the task without hesitation. The medical students Franc Fludernik and Marija Brus immediately agreed to go to Slovenia. All three worked at the Blood Transfusion Center of Serbia in Belgrade and were three of the pioneers of the blood transfusion service in Slovenia.[1] Besides Dr. Sonja Sovdat Banič and Franc Fludernik other notable doctors in transfusion medicine in the early following years after the war in Slovenia were Primarius Pavla Jerina Lah, Zlata Vašte Visenjak, Miran Hočevar, Ljerka Glonar, and others.[2] It has to be noted that in every generation in Slovenia, there are brilliant and dedicated doctors in transfusion medicine.

Doctor Sonja Sovdat Banič

Dr. Sonja Sovdat Banič (1922–2008), born in Ljubljana, first worked in 1944 as a medical student at the Blood Transfusion Center of Serbia (Image B.1). She oversaw the blood transfusion department after the Second World War. Between 1946 and 1948, she finished her medical education. She served as the director of the BTCS for 32 years (1948–1979). Dr. Sonja Sovdat Banič wrote professional publications in specialized journals and was in charge of many significant professional accomplishments in Slovenia's blood transfusion medicine.[3,4] Her maiden name was Sovdat. As a director and a doctor she was educated, capable, dedicated, hardworking, and highly professional.

Doctor Franc Fludernik

Franc Fludernik (1923–2013) was born in a town Črna na Koroškem in Slovenia (Image B.2). He began his medical studies in Ljubljana in 1941 and finished them in 1949. He worked at BTCS as a medical student, completing 2 years of his studies.

---

[1] Sovdat Banič S. Pogovor z dr. Sonjo Sovdat Banič. Potočnik M., Levičnik-Stezinar S., Faganel J., Lukić L., Rožman P., Ulaga R., Vukovič-Dervišić B., 50 let organizirane transfuzijske službe v Sloveniji:1945-1995, Ljubljana: Zavod Republike Slovenije za transfuzijo krvi, 1995, p. 19–20.

[2] Zupanič Slavec Z. Zgodovina zdravstva in medicine na Slovenskem-kirurške stroke, ginekologija in porodništvo. In. Jaunig S., editor. Razvoj tarnsfuzijske medicine Ljubljana: Slovenska Matica; 2018, p. 391–392.

[3] Potočnik, 2009, p. 269.

[4] Sovdat Banič, 1995, p. 19.

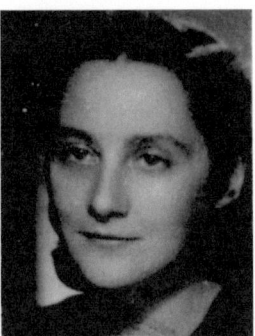

Image B.1 Doctor Sonja Sovdat Banič 1949. (Source: Doctor Sonja Sovdat Banič 1949. SI AS 1589/IV, Centralni komite Zveze komunistov Slovenije, šk. 3596 in 4345, članski dokumenti dr. Sonje Sovdat Banič. Permission to use the image was given by the Archives of the Republic of Slovenia on April 2, 2024)

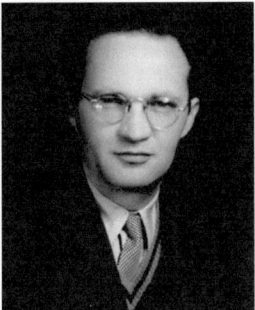

Image B.2 Doctor Franc Fludernik 1956. (Source: Doctor Franc Fludernik, 1956. Permission to use the image was given by Primarius Mr.Sc. Bogdan Fludernik, and the son of Dr. Franc Fludernik, on March 22, 2024)

He left BTCS in 1946 to continue his medical studies. He did his internship at the Maribor Hospital until 1952. After his internship, he wanted to specialize in surgery but did not get a specialization. He was a general practitioner in Velenje from 1952 to 1957, then Director of the Celje Health Center and Director of the Celje Hygiene Institute until 1971, and from 1971 until his retirement in 1988, he was employed at the Rače Health Station near Maribor. He was a double specialist. He was a specialist in occupational hygiene and a specialist in general medicine. As a doctor, he was a broad-minded individual with a keen sense of the needs of patients and a great deal of medical knowledge.[5]

---

[5] Interview with Dr. Bogdan Fludernik, son of Dr. Franc Fludernik. Written answers to the questions were obtained by Zdravko Kvržić on 14 September 2023.

Nurse Marija Brus

Marija Brus (1910–1999) was born in Sv. Peter Loka, near Zidani Most (Image B.3). Her maiden name was Vorina. She was the first and only nurse in Slovenia working in transfusion medicine. She worked at the BTCS from 1945 to 1946, where she was in charge of venipuncture in the operating theater. She is also mentioned in various written sources under the name Marjana, which was a conversational version of her name. She started attending the 4-year public folk primary school in Zidani Most on September 17, 1917. After finishing primary school, she continued her education at the three-class bourgeois school in Celje. After graduating from the bourgeois school in Celje, she decided to become a nurse. She studied in Belgrade at the 3-year Medical School in Nudilje, Belgrade. The term nudilja means caregiver. Maria Brus's professional title when she started working in the civil service was nurse assistant trainee, category IX. On 20.3.1943, she was transferred to the National Health Home in Užice. In 1944, she was employed at the Blood Transfusion Center of Serbia. After leaving the Blood Transfusion Center of the Faculty of Medicine in Ljubljana, she was employed for 1 year at the Hrastnik Health Center. She then worked at the Radeče Health Center. She retired in 1962. She was a professional, humane, and hard-working nurse.[6]

The first blood transfusion department in Slovenia was established in 1945, soon after their arrival in Ljubljana, as a part of what was then known as the Central Military Hospital (CMH) on Celovška Street.[7] With the ingenuity and

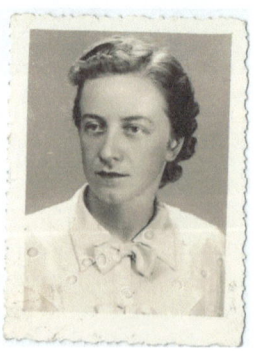

Image B.3 Marija Brus. (Source: Nurse Marija Brus. Permission to use the image was given by Miro Brus, son of nurse Marija Brus, on December 3, 2023)

---

[6] Kvržić Z. Marija Brus - prva medicinska sestra v transfuzijski medicini. Utrip: informativni bilten Zbornice zdravstvene nege Slovenije. ISSN 1318-5470. 2023;31(6), p. 16–18. https://www.zbornica-zveza.si/wp-content/uploads/2023/12/Utrip-December-2023-Januar-2024.pdf. Accessed 11 Apr 2024.

[7] Sovdat Banič S. Pogovor z dr. Sonjo Sovdat Banič. Potočnik M., Levičnik-Stezinar S., Faganel J., Lukić L., Rožman P., Ulaga R., Vukovič-Dervišić B., 50 let organizirane transfuzijske službe v Sloveniji:1945-1995, Ljubljana: Zavod Republike Slovenije za transfuzijo krvi, 1995, p. 19–20.

strong will of Dr. Sovdat Banič, she organized the blood transfusion department. She sought help from the Blood Transfusion Center of Serbia for the purchase of supplies and serums.[8] Via the publicity division, Dr. Sovdat Banič invited the first blood donors to Ljubljana, and on the second day, more than 150 people showed up at the gate to the blood transfusion department at Central Military Hospital in Ljubljana. All volunteers were registered and asked to be available when summoned because the location was not ready yet for blood donations. **On June 4, 1945, the first 19 bottles of blood were preserved and stored.** After the end of the Second World War, due to a shortage of nurses, the first blood collections, work in the laboratory, and preparation of blood-preserving materials were carried out by mobilized students and nurses, in addition to one official nurse. In 1946, a special course was organized to train orderlies for this work.[9]

The CMH management gave the blood donors lunch and flour, oil, and sugar as a gift.[10] The CMH Blood Transfusion Department supplied all military and civilian hospitals and clinics in Slovenia with preserved and stored blood, liquid plasma, and serums for blood grouping. After the disbanding of the CMH in September of 1945, the blood transfusion department did not come into the new formation. However, the increasing demand for preserved blood did not stop the department from working. **On January 15, 1946, it was taken over by the then Ministry of People's Health of the Federative People's Republic of Yugoslavia, which renamed it to the Blood Transfusion Center of the Faculty of Medicine in Ljubljana. The center became part of the Clinical Hospitals of the Faculty of Medicine.**[11] However, as it was not immediately possible to obtain premises for the center, it continued to work in the military hospital.[12] In May 1946, the center moved to emergency-adapted premises within the Clinical hospitals. Blood donors continued to give blood free of charge and were given special food vouchers for rationed food products and money to buy these food products[13,14] The aim of the establishment of the BTCS in Ljubljana, under the management of the distinguished Faculty of Medicine in Ljubljana, was to establish a modern transfusion service in Ljubljana and Slovenia. In some sources, it is differently stated when the center actually moved to new premises. Some sources claim that this was in May, while others say it was in June. The correct answer is in May. The evidence for this can be found in newspapers from May 1946.

---

[8] Potočnik M. Dr. Sonja Sovdat Banič: in memoriam, Zdravniški vestnik. 2009;78(5), p. 269. http://www.dlib.si/?URN=URN:NBN:SI:DOC-VEVY5U9Y.

[9] Sovdat Banič, 1995, p. 19–20.

[10] Lbid.

[11] Sovdat Banič S. Transfuzijska služba in krvodajalstvo v Sloveniji. Medicinski razgledi. 1971; 10(3), p. 339–343.

[12] Anon.Zahteva po popolni medicinski fakulteti uresničena. Ljudska pravica.1946;7(101), p. 12. http://www.dlib.si/?URN=URN:NBN:SI:DOC-MPJKFBDZ.

[13] Sovdat Banič, 1995, p. 19–20.

[14] Sovdat Banič S, 1971, p. 339–343.

In mid-May of 1946, the BTCS of the Faculty of Medicine in Ljubljana moved next to the general hospital into the former residential building of the Sisters of Mercy (nuns). The building had four main departments: a reception office, a laboratory, an operating room, and a plasma production room. Only seven people were employed at the institution. The blood was collected in bottles and sealed in a cabinet at a constant temperature. In hospitals, blood was warmed. The shelf life of stored blood was 3 weeks, and purified blood plasma was stored for up to 3 months. Blood was also sent to other parts of Slovenia. The hospital's microbiology institute tested a blood sample from each donation for syphilis. Blood compatibility testing between blood donors and patients, blood group identification, and creating test serums for blood grouping all received special attention. They recommended using stored blood rather than giving the patient directly donated blood. Radio and newspapers were used to advertise blood donations. Sodium citrate, whose content in the blood was 0.6%, was used to preserve the blood. Blood transfusions also faced complications, primarily due to a lack of personnel in the hospital departments who were fully trained in blood management procedures.[15,16,17]

The old Blood Transfusion Center of the Faculty of Medicine in Ljubljana was located by the river Ljubljanica in close proximity to today's Institute of Oncology Ljubljana (Images B.3 and B.4). It was the first building behind the entrance to the clinical hospital complex along the Ljubljanica River. Today, this building does not exist anymore. A newer building, which is the extension of the clinic of otorhinolaryngology and cervicofacial surgery of the Ljubljana University Medical Center, is located there (Image B.5).

In 1946, Dr. Sonja Sovdat Banič asked her superior, Dr. Lavrič, to release her from her duties of leading the center because she wanted to finish her schooling. Dr. Lavrič agreed with her decision and named Dr. Pavlo Jerino Lah, then a specialist in surgery, as the new head. Dr. Jerina Lah led the center from August 1946 to August 1948, when she left the center for work in Belgrade, the capital city of Serbia. In August 1948, after finishing her schooling, Dr. Sonja Sovdat Banič took the head position of the center once again.[18] Dr. Jerina Lah had important tasks in managing the center, controlling its development, coordinating the work with the management of other hospitals and other experts, educating the staff, and performing different organization tasks such as making sure that the material was prepared according to standards and that the work was done correctly. She had to ensure that, with regulations, both the blood donor and the patient were protected. She became the director of the Blood Transfusion Center of Serbia in 1951. As a doctor, she was highly motivated and professional.

In 1946, following a proposal by the Blood Transfusion Center of the Faculty of Medicine and the Ministry of National Health, the Ministry of Trade and Supply of the Government of the People's Republic of Slovenia decreed that from 1 May 1946 onward

---

[15] Jerina Lah, 1991, p. 231–232.

[16] Anon. V zavodu za transfuzijo krvi. Ljudska pravica.1946;7(301), p. 3. http://www.dlib.si/?URN=URN:NBN:SI:DOC-TNBL6JMX.

[17] Anon. Dragocena in požrtvovalna je pomoč krvodajalcev. Slovenski poročevalec. 1946;7(300), p. 3. http://www.dlib.si/?URN=URN:NBN:SI:DOC-C4POTL0X.

[18] Sovdat Banič, 1995, p. 19–20.

Appendix B: History of Transfusion Medicine in Slovenia from 1945 to 2023

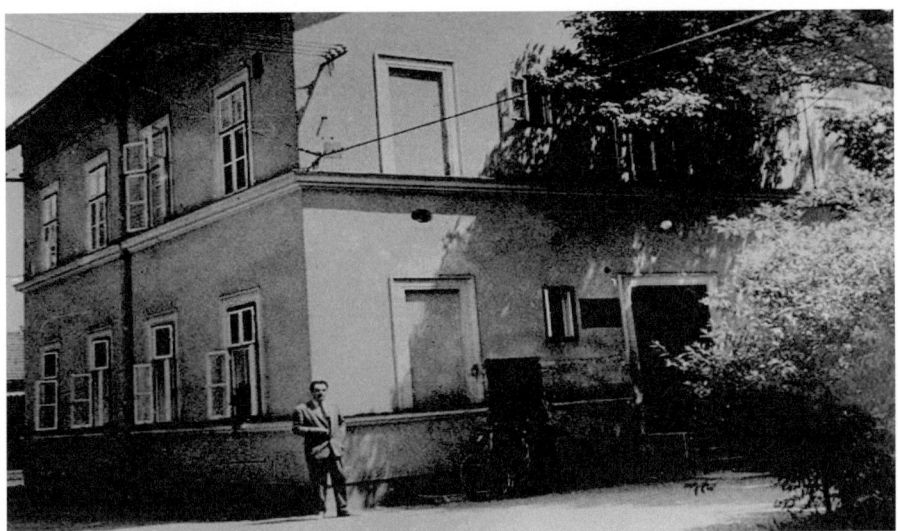

Image B.4 The old Blood Transfusion Center of the Faculty of Medicine in Ljubljana 1946–1958. (Source: The old Blood Transfusion Center of the Faculty of Medicine in Ljubljana 1946–1958. Archive of Blood Transfusion Center of Slovenia. Permission to use the image was obtained from the V.D. director of the Blood Transfusion Center of Slovenia, Peter Kavčič, M.Sc. business and economic. Science, on November 24, 2023. Permission to reuse the image from the article Zdravko Kvržić, Odvzem polne krvi pri krvodajalcu skozi različna zgodovinska obdobja (1875–2023). Utrip 31 (4), August–September, p. 17–21, was also given by the Nurses and Midwives Association of Slovenia on November 29, 2023)

all blood donors should receive, in addition to the additional rations ordered by Table K IV 1501/1 (dated 7 March 1946), an allowance in 500 g of sugar and 500 g of oil, namely, when donating 300 cc of blood and 750 g of sugar and 500 g of oil for over 300 cc of donated blood. On the day of the blood donation, the blood donors received a full day's food free of charge. After the meal, they received a basic food voucher from the hospitals where they donated blood. The hospitals declared the quantities of food consumed in their monthly food accounts. The District People's Committee billed the hospitals separately each month for the food for the blood donors. In addition, the blood donor was paid 1 dinar per 1 cc of blood drawn in order to ensure that the blood donor purchased supplements, oil, and sugar at the maximum price.[19,20] Blood donors had 300– 500 cc of blood drawn into bottles. The blood donors had free railroad transportation. The bottles of blood underwent chemical, bacteriological, and hematology tests before being released to the hospitals.[21] In 1947, the amount and type of food given to blood donors after donating blood were added to and increased.[22] In 1948, the blood

---

[19] Anon. Dodatki olja in sladkorja za krvodajalce. Ljudska pravica.1946;7(104), p. 8. http://www.dlib.si/?URN=URN:NBN:SI:DOC-JQ4CIHQH.

[20] Anon. Krvodajalci. Ljudska pravica.1946;7(180), p. 7. http://www.dlib.si/listalnik/URN_NBN_SI_doc-ZWZATNM4/8/index.html#zoom=z.

[21] Anon. Zavod za transfuzijo krvi medicinske fakultete v Ljubljani.Ljudska pravica.1946;7(162), p. 6. http://www.dlib.si/?URN=URN:NBN:SI:DOC-JEYNKOEC.

[22] Anon. Krvodajalci. Ljudska pravica. 1947;8(270), p. 6. http://www.dlib.si/?URN=URN:NBN:SI:DOC-ZEBZZQGC.

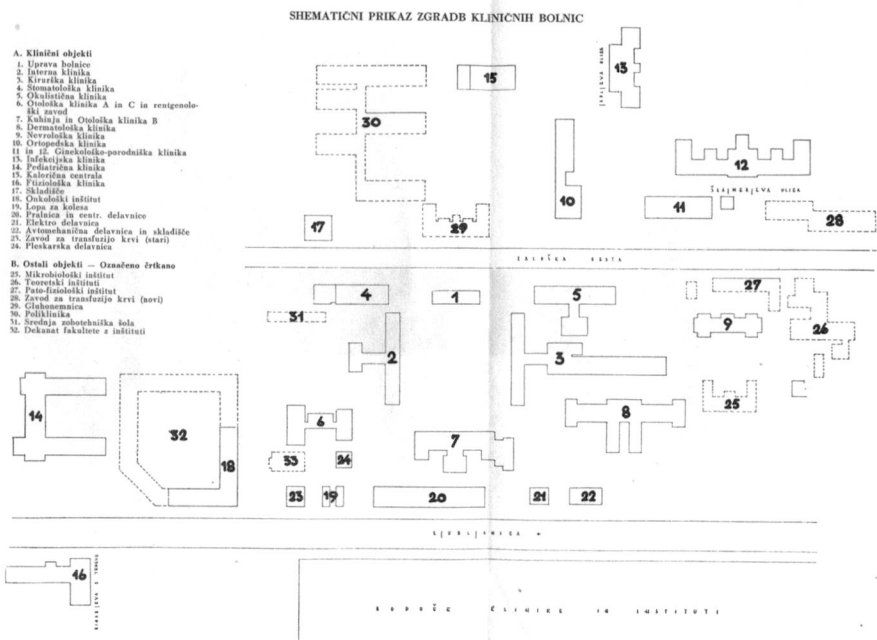

Image B.5 The image of the Clinical Hospitals of the Faculty of Medicine in Ljubljana. The old Blood Transfusion Center is listed under number 23. (Source: The image of the Clinical Hospitals of the Faculty of Medicine. The old Blood Transfusion Center is listed under number 23. This image is the property of the Institute for the History of Medicine of the Faculty of Medicine in Ljubljana. The image in the book is published with the permission of Prof. Dr. Zvonka Zupanič Slavec. The permission was granted on April 13, 2024)

donor was paid 1.5 dinars per cc for his blood.[23] In 1952, blood donors donated 500 cc of blood for 3500 dinars.[24] The award in food vouchers was not mentioned.

Blood grouping was done accurately by the tube method and on a slide. The laboratory of the center prepared test serums for ABO grouping. They were interested in acquiring serums for Rhesus (Rh) typing, but except for a few samples that they were successful in obtaining, they were not successful at providing larger quantities for everyday work. There were also problems with transporting the blood from the center to other places. They planned to get the thermostable containers, but they only got special containers for transporting blood, which only protected the blood bottles from breakage. Before the transportation of blood, they usually chilled the containers in the fridge. There were also problems with the preparation of the equipment for blood preservation. They worked with a glass factory in Hrastnik and a rubber factory in Kranj. For the first two and a half years, we had to take all the equipment and surgical linen to the surgical clinic in the septic ward to be sterilized. Because it was not possible to get our own autoclave.[25]

---

[23] Anon. Krvodajalci.Ljudska pravica. 1948;9(3), p. 8. Anon. Krvodajalci.Ljudska pravica.1948;9(3), p. 8. http://www.dlib.si/?URN=URN:NBN:SI:DOC-VJ8TMASP.

[24] Anon. Srednji vek napada. Slovenski poročevalec. 1952;13(129), p. 8. http://www.dlib.si/?URN=URN:NBN:SI:DOC-SPVANMPF.

[25] Jerina Lah, 1991, p. 233.

In 1947, the payment to blood donors increased from one dinar per cc donated to one and a half dinars per cc donated. The reimbursement of travel expenses from 100 to 150 dinars helped blood donors from outside Ljubljana come to donate blood.[26] During the same year, blood donors were allowed to donate blood as often as every 1.5 months, and on the day of the blood donation, fatty foods and white coffee were discouraged.[27] Blood donors must have been at least 21 years old.[28] Because of increasing demands, there was shortage of serum, plasma, and blood.[29] The need for stored blood increased in all hospitals. Blood donors traveled to Ljubljana from all over Slovenia. It soon became clear that the center could not cover the need for stored blood for all the hospitals in the country. It was therefore necessary to organize transfusion departments at the larger hospitals in order to attract those who were discouraged from donating blood, especially by the long journey to Ljubljana. The directors at the time were keen to set up blood transfusion departments, but there was a shortage of staff and facilities everywhere.[30] The blood transfusion department started to operate in Maribor in 1948.[31] In 1949, blood donors could also donate blood in the city of Celje.[32] Blood donors aged 21–50 could donate blood for indirect blood transfusions every 3 months, while those aged 50–60 could donate blood for indirect blood transfusions every 4 months.[33] Although blood donations in bottles for indirect blood transfusions dominated after the Second World War, some doctors still requested blood donors for direct blood transfusions, which were carried out at the Oncology Institute, the Pediatric Clinic, and especially the Internal Medicine Clinic. Although the first 2 years after the war saw an almost complete decline in the practice of direct blood transfusions, on February 3, 1952, it was the last time blood donors were invited for direct transfusions in Ljubljana. After this, I was not able to find any evidence in general in Slovenia that could suggest that there were any invitations for direct blood transfusions.[34] The

---

[26] Anon. Zavod za transfuzijo krvi poziva na darovanje krvi. Slovenski poročevalec, 1947;8(293) p. 6. http://www.dlib.si/?URN=URN:NBN:SI:DOC-SFTFJQOI.

[27] Anon. Krvodajalci. Ljudska pravica.1947;8(260), p. 6. http://www.dlib.si/?URN=URN:NBN:SI:DOC-C0NY6Z2I.

[28] Anon. Krvodajalci. Ljudska pravica.1947;8(198), p. 7. http://www.dlib.si/?URN=URN:NBN:SI:DOC-CZQUNZRZ.

[29] Anon. Zvišani obroki živil za krvodajalce. Ljudska pravica.1947;8(293), p. 6. http://www.dlib.si/?URN=URN:NBN:SI:DOC-WKNVYVIR.

[30] Sovdat Banič, 1995, p. 19–20.

[31] Potočnik, Levičnik-Stezinar, Faganel, Lukić, Rožman, Ulaga, Vukovič-Dervišić, 1995, p. 13–70.

[32] Anon. Dajalci krvi. Slovenski poročevalec. 1949;10(295), p. 6. http://www.dlib.si/?URN=URN:NBN:SI:DOC-280Y5TZC.

[33] Anon. Dajalci krvi. Slovenski poročevalec. 1952;13(29), p. 7. http://www.dlib.si/?URN=URN:NBN:SI:DOC-QPWXE62H.

[34] Kvržić Z. Zgodovina krvodajalstva in transfuzijske medicine v Sloveniji. 50 letučinkovitega sodelovanja: pomembna prelomnica ali izjemna priložnost? [Elektronski vir]:zbornik prispevkov z recenzijo: Zbornica zdravstvene in babiške nege Slovenije – Zveza strokovnih društev medicinskih sester, babic in zdravstvenih tehnikov Slovenije, Sekcija medicinskih sester in zdravstvenih tehnikov v anesteziologiji, intenzivni terapiji in transfuziologiji: 53. strokovni seminar: Rogaška

federal health authorities were committed to the revival, organization, and quality of the transfusion service in the country. In 1948, the first 6-month course in blood transfusion was held in Belgrade for participants from all the republics. In 1949, a special meeting was organized with representatives from all the Republican Health Committees, and conclusions were reached on the future transfusion service in all the Republics of Yugoslavia.[35]

The Introduction of Voluntary, Non-Remunerated, and Anonymous Blood Donation in 1953

Since 1953, Slovenia has seen significant improvements in blood donation and, in general, in the transfusion medicine process.

An effort to find blood donors for voluntary donation was launched by the Slovenian Red Cross as early as 1952.[36] In 1953, there were fewer blood donors and higher demands for blood, and many of those who did donate were giving too much whole blood in exchange for money and food vouchers, which was bad for their health. Even though safeguards were in place, improvements were needed because numerous blood donors were coming to the BTCS with borrowed ID cards in order to give blood repeatedly.[37] The decision for voluntary, non-remunerated, and anonymous blood donation began on January 1, 1953.[38] Understanding blood donors, medical professionals, and a sufficient blood supply in December 1952 made it possible for the transition to non-remunerated blood donation in the crucial early stages.[39] On January 27, 1953, a blood donation was organized by the main committee of the Slovenian Red Cross at the BTCS. On that day, at least 100 blood donors gave their blood free of charge in an exemplary way. Soon, Maribor and Celje followed this example, and later other places as well.[40] The first voluntary and non-remunerated blood donation in Maribor took place on February 2, 1953,[41] and in Celje at the beginning of April (till April 5) of the same year.[42] But the most significant blood

---

Slatina, 17. in 18. November 2023, p. 98–104. http://www.dlib.si/?URN=URN:NBN:SI:doc-JKK4AQKL. Accessed 25 March 2024.

[35] Jerina Lah, 1991, p. 231–232.

[36] Lad K. Kri za transfuziji, najplemenitejše darilo. Slovenski poročevalec. 1952;13(40), p. 4. http://www.dlib.si/?URN=URN:NBN:SI:DOC-LJWYRRFD.

[37] Bibič A. Kultura naroda in krvodajalstvo. Tovariš.1971;27(18), p. 12–13. http://www.dlib.si/?URN=URN:NBN:SI:DOC-CEZ50I9F.

[38] Kozinc Ž. Cena krvi. Tovariš. 1973;29(3), p. 3, 14–16. http://www.dlib.si/?URN=URN:NBN:SI:DOC-4VMSQVHF.

[39] Sovdat Banič, 1995, p. 21.

[40] Anon.Sledimo vsi prvim brezplačnim krvodajalcem. Slovenski poročevalec. 1953;14(23), p. 1. http://www.dlib.si/?URN=URN:NBN:SI:DOC-BLQOGO2W.

[41] Ferenčak T. Razvoj, pomen in organizacija transfuzijske službe. Ljubljana: Višja šola za zdravstvene delavce, Oddelek za medicinske sestre, diplomsko delo. 1962, p. 5.

[42] Anon. Prvi prostovoljni krvodajalci v Celju. Slovenski poročevalec.1953;14(81), p. 2. http://www.dlib.si/?URN=URN:NBN:SI:DOC-NSBLMKZR.

donation happened on March 9, 1953, in Zagorje at Savi. This occasion is significant for a number of reasons. This was the first mobile blood donation organized by the Slovenian Red Cross and conducted by the BTCS. With the help of mobile blood donations, the BTCS was able to address the shortage of blood donors at that time, since for a large population from a certain area, it was easier for them to donate their blood in their home place than to travel, for example, to Ljubljana. The same is true today.

Following this blood donation activity in Zagorje at Savi, Slovenia as a whole accepted voluntary, non-remunerated, and anonymous blood donation. The nationwide blood donation activity was overseen and promoted by the Slovenian Red Cross, which at the time was part of the Yugoslavian Red Cross.[43]

The iniciator of the first mobile blood donation in Zagorje at Savi was a Red Cross Volunteer Dr. Danilo Gomišček (1920–1974). The main committee of the Slovenian Red Cross, the Zagorje Red Cross, the unions organizing the blood donation, the BTCS, the Association of Communists of Yugoslavia, and the mine administration all organized and supported the mobile blood donation. The blood donors were not permitted to eat or drink anything except tea and bread for 6 h prior to the donation. Representatives of both sexes and of various ages, not just from this town but also from the larger surrounding area, gave blood. The blood was given by both day- and night-shift miners as well as individuals. All mine officials, the academic staff at the gymnasium, numerous other officials, housewives, and other workers donated blood in addition to the miners. There were 151 blood donors on that particular day.[44,45]

Doctor Danilo Gomišček

Dr. Danilo Gomišček (1920–1974) was a specialist in internal medicine (Image B.6). He was born in Bubnjarci, Croatia, and attended and completed primary and gymnasium school in Maribor. He started his medical studies in the school year 1939–1940 but did not finish them until after the Second World War, around 1947. He passed the internal medicine examination in 1958. During the Second World War, he supported the partisan resistance movement. After the war, he first worked as a doctor in Ljubljana, then moved with his family to Zagorje at Savi because the authorities at the time encouraged the relocation of medical personnel to smaller towns. He moved his family from Zagorje to Savi around 1956 in order to advance in his profession. Dr. Gomišček continued to receive professional training and improve his skills in his field. In Ljubljana, he worked at the Clinical Center at the Institute of Occupational, Traffic, and Sports Medicine. He was intelligent and kind,

---

[43] Kvržić Z. Zagorje ob Savi: zibelka prostovoljnega krvodajalstva. Savus. 2022;9(1) p. 20. https://savus.si/arhiv-tednika/.
[44] Lbid.
[45] L.K. Zgleden primer človekoljubne zavesti. Slovenski poročevalec.1953;14(62), p. 3. http://www.dlib.si/?URN=URN:NBN:SI:DOC-MX5WLNV4.

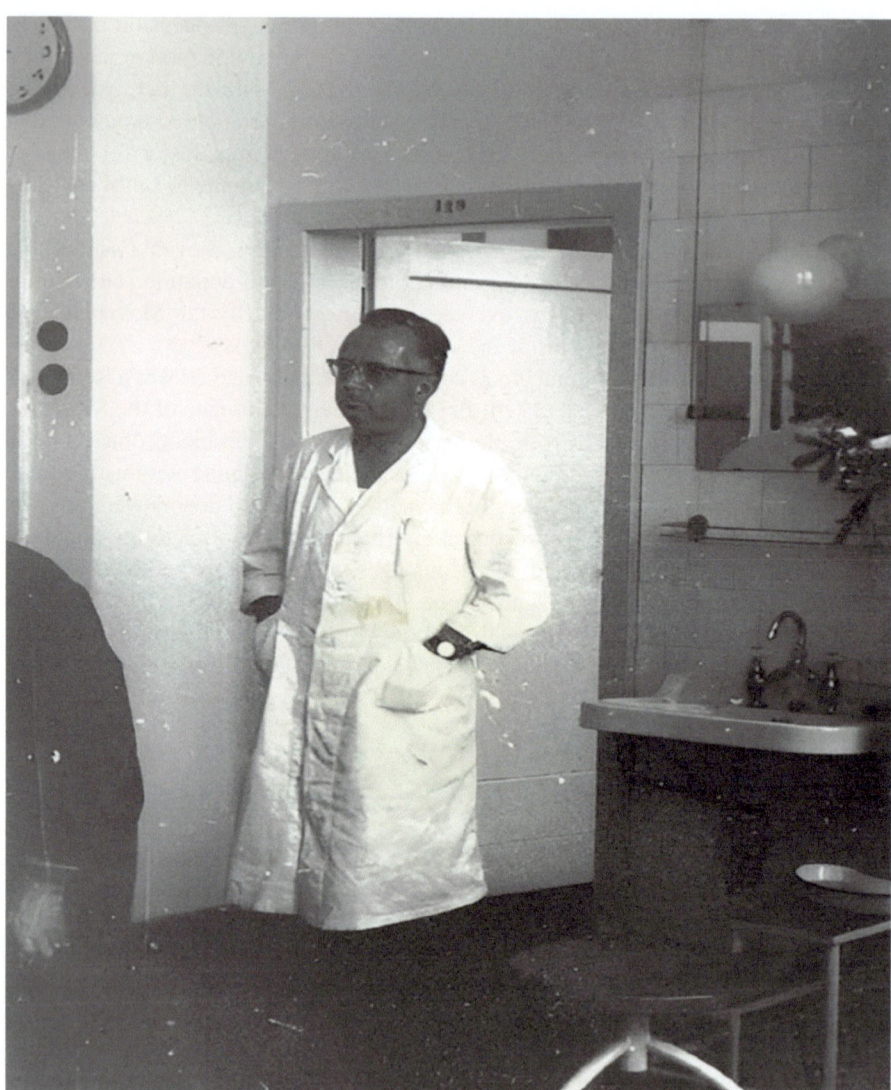

Image B.6 Dr. Danilo Gomišček. (Source: The image and permission to use it for this book were granted from the personal archive of Mr. Marko Gomišček on July 22, 2021. Permission for usage was also granted by Madam Alenka Kryštufek, the daughter of Danilo Gomišček, on July 16, 2021)

Appendix B: History of Transfusion Medicine in Slovenia from 1945 to 2023

and as a doctor, he was professional, responsible, and fully committed to his mission. He was very caring toward his patients and his family.[46,47,48,49,50]

Transfusion Medicine in Slovenia from 1953 to 2024

In 1953, blood donors could donate blood from the age of 18– 60. Healthy, physically fit individuals were welcome.[51] Blood donors were subjected before the donation to laboratory, X-ray, dermatological, veneral, and gynecological examinations.[52] Before donating blood, blood donors wore a coat, mask, cap, and galoshes, all white in color. The blood donor then lay down on a steel gurney, covered with a white sheet, and extended his arm through an opening into which a needle was inserted to draw blood. The blood flowed through a rubber tube and into a bottle. The blood-filled bottle was sealed, and a label with the date of collection and the exact details of the blood group was placed on it. The equipped bottle was taken to the refrigerator.[53] Using sodium citrate, the donated whole blood was usable for 2–3 weeks. The blood was stored in a refrigerator at +4 to +8 degrees.[54] A unique method was used to collect the plasma from donated blood. After collecting whole blood into bottles, the citrated blood's erythrocytes were allowed to sink to the bottom due to weight before the plasma was transfused to another bottle. As erythrocytes made up a significant portion of the total blood volume, this resulted in the loss of more than half of the blood. Plasma, on the other hand, was kept, used for several months, and more conveniently transported to hospitals from other locations. Small hospitals did not perform many blood transfusions, and entire blood that was not used within a specific amount of time would deteriorate.[55] In 1971, blood donors were still checked before their donation for X-rays of the lungs and heart and for laboratory tests. Fresh, whole blood that could later be processed into plasma or other

---

[46] Interview with Marko Gomišček, son of Dr. Danilo Gomišček. Written answers to the questions were obtained by Zdravko Kvržić on 22 July 2021.
[47] Kvržić Z. Ugleden zdravnik Danilo Gomišček. Savus. 2022;9(4), p. 22. https://savus.si/arhiv-tednika/.
[48] Lbid.
[49] Marko Gomišček, 2021.
[50] Interview with Alenka Kryštufek born Gomišček, daughter of Dr. Danilo Gomišček. Written answers to the questions were obtained by Zdravko Kvržić on 16 July, 2021.
[51] Anon. Krvodajalci. Slovenski poročevalec. 1953;14(204), p. 8. http://www.dlib.si/?URN=URN:NBN:SI:DOC-GGMTTQRR.
[52] Anon. V Zavodu za transfuzijo krvi v Ljubljani ustvarjajo dragocene rezerve krvi. Tovariš.1953;9(6), p. 140. http://www.dlib.si/?URN=URN:NBN:SI:DOC-6ZAIDI3C.
[53] T.G., Umrla bi če etc. Tovariš. 1953;9(6), p. 145. http://www.dlib.si/?URN=URN:NBN:SI:DOC-6ZAIDI3C.
[54] Tovariš, 1953, p. 140.
[55] Sovdat Banič S. O transfuziji krvi. Slovenski poročevalec.1953;14(21), p. 3. http://www.dlib.si/?URN=URN:NBN:SI:DOC-YCXXHBU1.

components was useful for 3 weeks.[56] Today, the testing of blood donors no longer involves X-ray examinations.

By the year 1973, the world standard for collecting blood was 420 mL. In Slovenia, 125–390 mL of blood was taken from the blood donor.[57] After the blood donation in at least mobile blood donations across Slovenia, blood donors would, in 1953, get a meal of sausage with bread, tea with rum, cognac, and Turkish coffee. Each blood donor received a written thank you note from the Red Cross.[58] Because of the constant encouragement of a healthy lifestyle, alcohol is no longer supplied to blood donors today. In Slovenia today, healthy blood donors who meet strict medical criteria for the protection of both the blood donor and the patient give 450 mL of their blood between the ages of 18 and 65, regardless of sex. Every 4 months, women donate blood; every 3 months, men.

The blood donation procedure is an important task in Slovenia, carried out by dedicated and hard-working registered nurses (Images B.7 and B.8). Nurses wore aseptic uniforms from 1945 until the end of the 1980s because collecting blood in glass bottles was an open system where contamination of blood was possible. The transition from aseptic uniforms to non-aseptic standardized uniforms that are still used today was done with the introduction of plastic blood bags with a closed system and with the expansion of blood component therapy. Today, even blood donors donate their blood in their everyday clothes. During the COVID-19 pandemic outbreak and later, it was mandatory for the staff and blood donors to wear protective masks.

Even though plastic bags replaced the glass bottles at the end of the 1980s, until 1997, blood was still collected in 500-ml glass bottles lined with silicone inside for heart surgery. Other blood donations were made in plastic bags.[59]

Since 1945 to the present, Slovenian nurses in transfusion medicine have consistently carried out their daily responsibilities in accordance with quality standards and the Slovenian Code of Ethics in Nursing in an exceptional professional, committed, safe, cautious, and efficient manner. In addition to many crucial professional duties, they perform laboratory work, whole blood and blood component procedures, blood processing, storage, and distribution of blood components.

Besides Ljubljana (1945), Maribor (1948), and Celje (1949), several smaller blood transfusion departments opened in Slovenian city hospitals from their humble beginnings in 1956 (Jesenice, Golnik, Nova Gorica, Koper, Murska Sobota, Ptuj, Slovenj Gradec) and 1957 (Novo mesto). The Novo Mesto transfusion department worked only for less than 8 months. It was once again opened in 1960. Although

---

[56] Bibič, 1971, p. 12.

[57] Kozinc, 1973, p. 15.

[58] Anon. Darujmo kri. Glas Gorenjske.1953;6(27), p. 1. http://www.dlib.si/?URN=URN:NBN:SI:DOC-KAH8SG95.

[59] Kvržić, Z. 2023. Odvzem polne krvi pri krvodajalcu skozi različna zgodovinska obdobja (1875–2023). Utrip: informativni bilten Zbornice zdravstvene in babiške nege Slovenije. ISSN 1318-5470.2023;31(4), p. 17–21. https://www.zbornica-zveza.si/wp-content/uploads/2023/08/Odvzem-polne-krvi-pri-krvodajalcu-skozi-razlicna-zgodovinska-obdobja-1875-2023-Kvrzic-Avgust-September-2023.pdf.

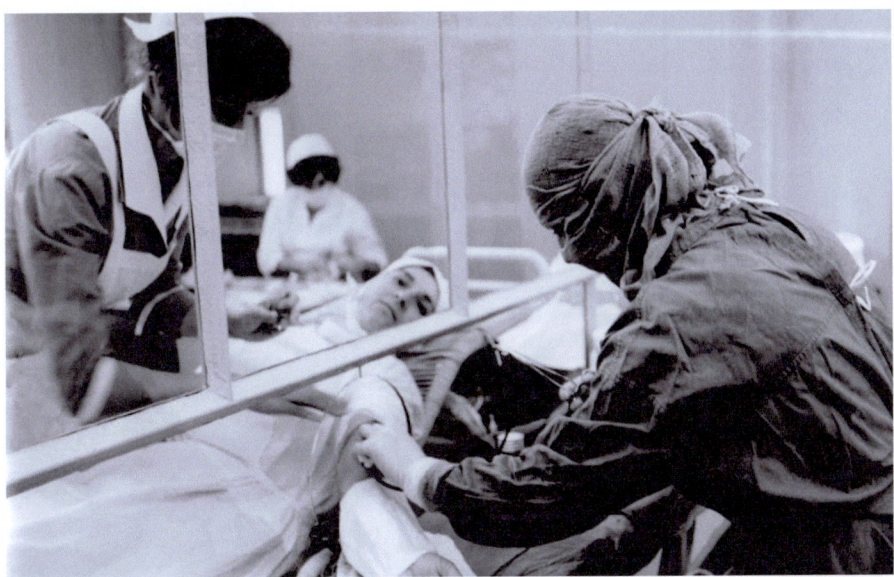

Image B.7 Blood donation procedure in Ljubljana around 1958–1960. (Source: Blood donation procedure in Ljubljana around 1958–1960. Archive of Blood Transfusion Center of Slovenia. Permission to use the image was obtained from the V.D. director of the Blood Transfusion Center of Slovenia, Peter Kavčič, M.Sc. business and economic science, on November 24, 2023. Permission to reuse the image from the article Zdravko Kvržić, Odvzem polne krvi pri krvodajalcu skozi različna zgodovinska obdobja (1875–2023). Utrip 31 (4), August–September, p. 17–21, was also given by the Nurses and Midwives Association of Slovenia on November 29, 2023)

officially established in 1956, the Slovenj Gradec hospital had a small blood transfusion cabinet as a part of a surgical department in 1954. In 1957, the transfusion departments of Jesenice, Nova Gorica, and Koper were canceled. In 1964, the transfusion department at Golnik was also canceled. In 1961, the transfusion department in Izola was established. The transfusion department in Trbovlje was opened in 1956, but it started to work in 1957. The transfusion department in Nova Gorica was opened once again in 1977. The transfusion department in Jesenice was again opened in 1992.[60,61] Interestingly, there was also a blood transfusion department that worked as a part of a Military Hospital and Military Medical Center in Ljubljana, at least from 1968 to 1991, until the entire operation of the hospital was canceled.[62,63]

Today, Slovenia is home to the BTCS located in Ljubljana, the Departments for Transfusion Medicine (Izola, Nova Gorica, Jesenice, Trbovlje, Novo mesto, Slovenj

---

[60] Potočnik, Levičnik-Stezinar, Faganel, Lukić, Rožman, Ulaga, Vukovič-Dervišić, 1995, p. 13–70.
[61] Sovdat Banič S, 1971, p. 339–343.
[62] Zupanič Slavec, 2018, p. 381.
[63] STA. Vojna bolnica Ljubljana in Vojaško medicinski center Ljubljana ne bosta več delovala.https://www.sta.si/797217/vojna-bolnica-ljubljana-in-vojasko-medicinski-center-ljubljana-ne-bosta-vec--delovala. Accessed 13 Apr 2024.

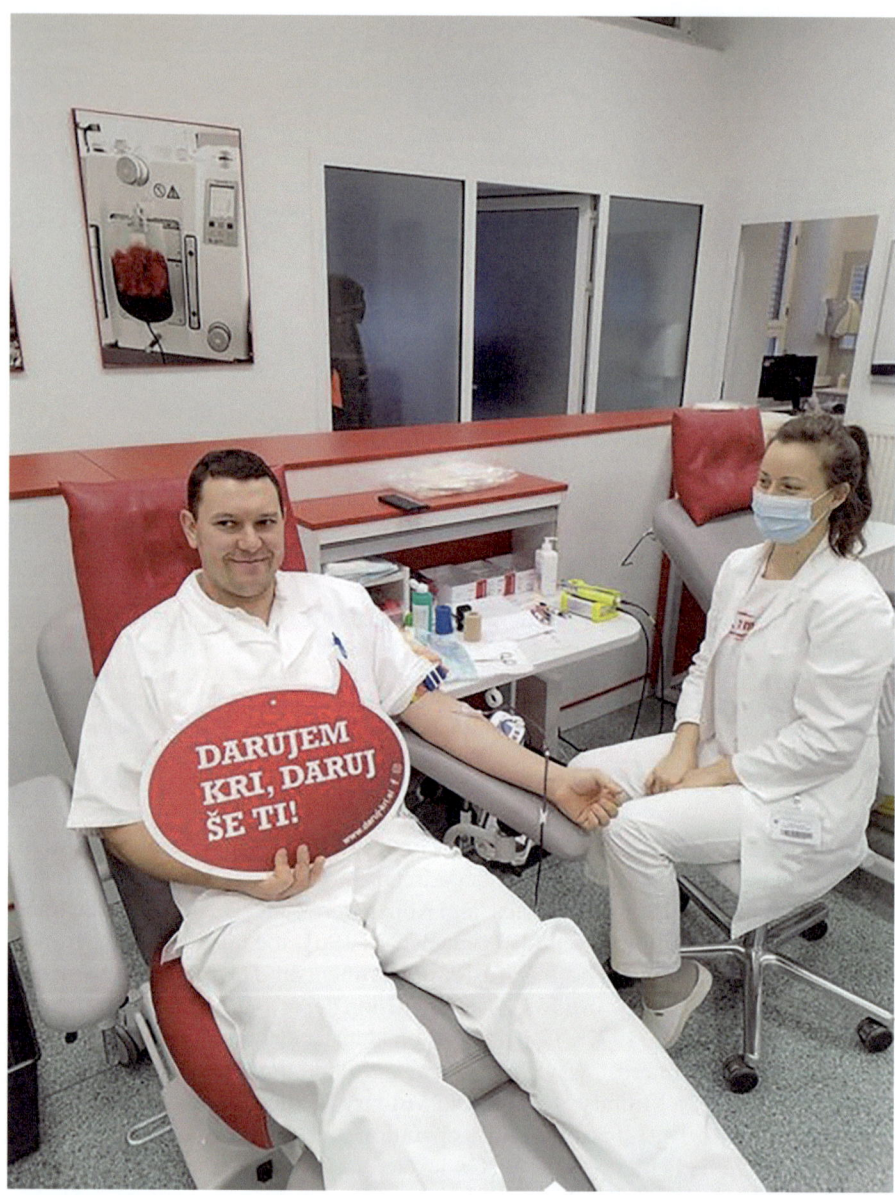

Image B.8 Modern blood donation procedure in Ljubljana 2023. (Source: Modern Blood donation procedure in Ljubljana in 2023. Archive of the Blood Transfusion Center of Slovenia. Permission to use the image was obtained from registered nurses on the image itself, Primož and Simona Hozjan, on November 23, 2023. Permission to reuse the image from the article Zdravko Kvržić, Odvzem polne krvi pri krvodajalcu skozi različna zgodovinska obdobja (1875–2023). Utrip 31 (4), August–September, p. 17–21, was also given by the Nurses and Midwives Association of Slovenia on November 29, 2023. The permission was also obtained from the V.D. director of the Blood Transfusion Center of Slovenia, Peter Kavčič, M.Sc. Business and Economic Science, on November 24, 2023)

Gradec), and the Units for Transfusion Medicine (Ptuj, Murska Sobota). The departments and units are located in hospitals. Then there is also the Center for Transfusion Medicine at the University Medical Center Maribor and the Transfusion Center at Celje General Hospital.

The Federal Commission for Blood Transfusion submitted to the Federal Institute of Public Health the Rules for the Operation of Blood Transfusion Institutions, Departments, and Stations, which went into effect in 1955. The bulletin included requirements for the standards for the equality and quality of blood transfusion equipment.[64]

The independent Federative People's Republic of Slovenia's Blood Transfusion Center was founded on December 25, 1955. The Center relocated to new and larger quarters at 6 Šlajmerjeva Street on October 25, 1958,[65] **and it continues to operate there independently under the name BTCS (Image B.9).**

On February 28, 1958, the Blood Donation Committee of the Slovenian Red Cross held a conference to report on the successes of blood donation and to adopt the program for the year. The conference decided to make June 4 "Blood Donors' Day," which would be the greatest recognition for the citizens who have given and continue to give blood for the patients. On this day, it was decided that celebrations and events would be held all over Slovenia to award special prizes to the most deserving organizers of blood donations and to the best work teams.[66] Slovenia continues to celebrate "Blood Donors' Day" on June 4 each year.

After the Second World War, there was no literature on transfusion medicine, so the doctors were supplied with literature from abroad (England, the Soviet Union, Switzerland, and Czechoslovakia) on a private initiative, and gaining experience abroad was not possible. In 1966, the first comprehensive domestic book, "Blood Transfusion," was published. "Bulletin Blood Transfusion" was an original source of information on novelties, experiences of this type of literature abroad, and current problems during the first years of the blood transfusion service. In 1967, the most important valid regulation of the Federal Law on Health was adopted: hygienic and technical conditions for the operation of institutions for blood transfusion, which was important for protecting the quality of work.[67]

As early as 1946, the Blood Transfusion Center of the Medical Faculty in Ljubljana tested every blood donation for syphilis.[68] All blood donations have been mandatory tested for syphilis: anti-Treponema pallidum since 1960; hepatitis B (HBsAg) since 1970; and HBV DNA since 2007. Aids: anti-HIV1/2 since 1986; and HIV 1 RNA from 2007; and hepatitis C: anti-HCV since 1993. The blood donor

---

[64] Jerina Lah, 1991, p. 231.
[65] Potočnik, Levičnik-Stezinar, Faganel, Lukić, Rožman, Ulaga, Vukovič-Dervišić, 1995, p. 13.
[66] Anon. Četrti junij dan krvodajalcev. Slovenski poročevalec.1958;19(50), p. 2. http://www.dlib.si/?URN=URN:NBN:SI:DOC-0QSVLA9N.
[67] Jerina Lah, 1991, p. 231.
[68] Lbid., p. 232.

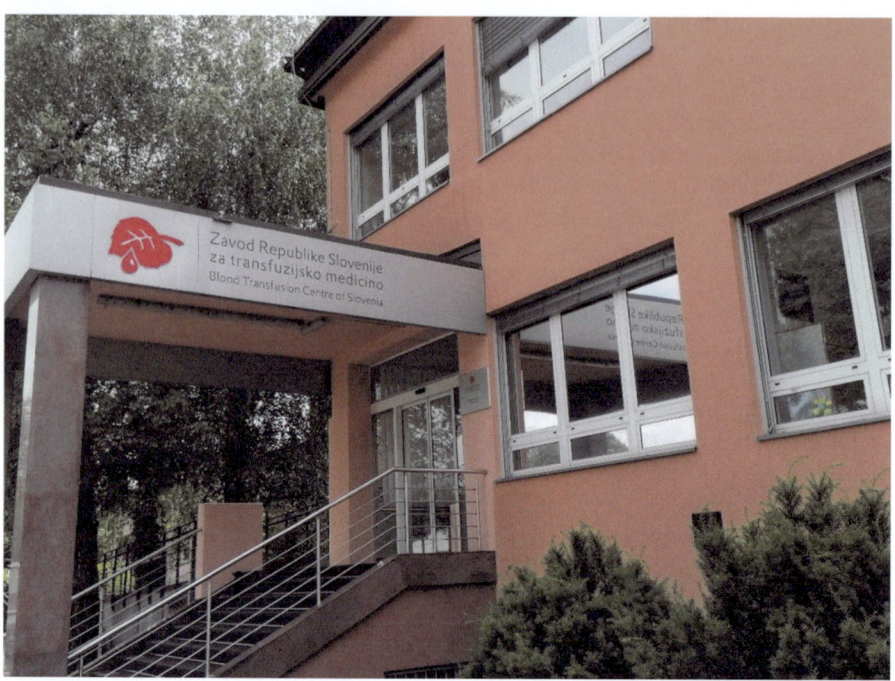

Image B.9 Blood Transfusion Center of Slovenia 2023. (Source: Blood Transfusion Center of Slovenia in 2023. Personal archive of the author Zdravko Kvržić. The permission was also obtained from the V.D. director of the Blood Transfusion Center of Slovenia, Peter Kavčič, M.Sc. Business and Economic Science, on November 24, 2023. Permission to reuse the image from the article Zdravko Kvržić, Odvzem polne krvi pri krvodajalcu skozi različna zgodovinska obdobja (1875–2023). Utrip 31 (4), August–September, p. 17–21, was also given by the Nurses and Midwives Association of Slovenia on November 29, 2023)

questionnaire was introduced in 1994.[69] In 1999, the EU's strict criteria for selecting blood donors required the introduction of a single medical questionnaire for blood donors. This allows a standardized format of questions for all blood donors before each blood donation.[70,71]

The first diagnosis of hemolytic disease of the fetus and newborn was made in Ljubljana in 1947, and the first exchange transfusion was carried out in 1952.[72]

---

[69] Majcen-Vivod B., Urlep-Šalinović V. Prevalenca hepatitisov A in B pri krvodajalcih z anamnezo zlatenice, Zdravniški vestnik: glasilo Slovenskega zdravniškega društva.2004;73(4), p. 227–230. https://vestnik.szd.si/index.php/ZdravVest/article/view/2287.

[70] Bricl I. Ogulin M. Življenje teče: letno poročilo transfuzijske službe v Sloveniji za leto 2007. Ljubljana: Zavod Republike Slovenije za transfuzijo krvi. 2008; p. 14. http://www.ztm.si/knjiznica/letna- porocila/ Accessed 13 Apr 2024.

[71] Bricl I. et al. Z vami življenje teče dalje: jubilejna publikacija ob 70. obletnici transfuzijske dejavnosti v Sloveniji, Ljubljana: Zavod Republike Slovenije za transfuzijo krvi; 2015, p. 15.

[72] Zupanič Slavec, 2018, p. 389.

Cross-matching before blood transfusion was introduced in 1963.[73] Manual plasmapheresis was introduced in 1969. Blood processing from a single bag started in 1979. Cytopheresis with a cell separator was first introduced in 1980, along with therapeutic plasmapheresis. Autotransfusion and automated plasmapheresis became routine work in 1987.[74] With plasmapheresis, BTCS collected plasma from recovered patients (convalescent plasma) as part of the European Emergency Support Instrument (ESI). We started the hyperimmune COVID-19 plasma (HCP) collection program in early July 2020, which lasted until 2021.[75]

The Federal Committee on Labor and Health published a draft rulebook for the selection of blood donors in 1988. It included products made from blood, plasma, and cellular components and established the requirements for manufacturing work zones.[76] In 1991, the principle of self-sufficiency of blood products was adopted in Slovenia.[77] The national organizer of blood donation campaigns is the Red Cross of Slovenia, which received national authorization from the state. This article is included in the Law on the Red Cross of Slovenia from 1993. It gives authorization to the Red Cross to recruit blood donors and organize blood donation campaigns.[78] On March 26, 1998, the Government of the Republic of Slovenia, on the basis of Decree No. 519-01/98-1, transformed the **BTCS as a public health center.**[79]

Some important achievements in the Slovenian transfusion medicine from 1953 to 1994:

- 1953—Anti-D serum and AHG serum were produced for determination of blood groups and Coombs test;[80]
- RhD started to be determined officially in 1953, and since 2006, other Rh antigens and antigen K have been determined in the blood donor. MAIPA and ELISA tests were introduced after 2001; ABO blood group serum was introduced in 1947; and monoclonal anti-A and anti-B antibodies were first produced in 1987;[81]
- 1957—Start of prenatal laboratory work to detect Rh-negative sensitized pregnant women;[82]

---

[73] Potočnik, Levičnik-Stezinar, Faganel, Lukić, Rožman, Ulaga, Vukovič-Dervišić, 1995, p. 13.
[74] Lbid.
[75] Kvržić Z., Mali P. Prikupljanje konvalescentne COVID-19 plazme sa plazmaferezom na Zavodu Republike Slovenije za transfuzijsku medicinu u Ljubljani. Liječnički vjesnik. 2021;143;2, p. 131. https://hrcak.srce.hr/file/386068.
[76] Jerina Lah, 1991, p. 231.
[77] Predlog zakona o preskrbi s krvjo, Republika Slovenija državni zbor, 21. 10. 1999. Available at: https://www.dz-rs.si. Accessed 18 Jun 2022.
[78] Zakon o Rdečem križu Slovenije (Uradni list RS, št. 7/93 in 79/10). https://pisrs.si/pregledPredpisa?id=ZAKO250. Accessed 13 Apr 2024.
[79] Republika Slovenije računsko sodišče. Revizijsko poročilo vzpostavitev enotnega transfuzijskega informacijskega sistema. 2017, p. 7. https://www.rs-rs.si/fileadmin/user_upload/revizija/1212/IS_ZTM.pdf. Accessed 9 Jun 2022.
[80] Potočnik, Levičnik-Stezinar, Faganel, Lukić, Rožman, Ulaga, Vukovič-Dervišić, 1995, p. 13–15.
[81] Zupanič Slavec, 2018, p. 389.
[82] Potočnik, Levičnik-Stezinar, Faganel, Lukić, Rožman, Ulaga, Vukovič-Dervišić, 1995, p. 13–15.

- In 1959, the first refrigerated bottle centrifuge for the preparation of washed erythrocytes and other blood components was introduced. In 1963, we obtained a lyophilization machine for drying plasma and later for cryoprecipitate;[83]
- 1960—The beginning of the production of antihemophilic plasma;
- 1963—Drying of human plasma;
- 1965—The beginning of the production of fraction 1 according to Cohn;
- 1965—Start of plasma collection with anti-D antibodies for processing into gammaglobulin;[84]
- 1967—The first cryoprecipitate, a concentrated preparation was produced for the treatment of patients with hemophilia A.[85] On March 1, 1967, the first doses of IgG anti-D were produced to prevent sensitization of Rh-negative women after childbirth.[86] In 1975, protection was extended to all RhD-negative women after an abortion. In 1977, protection was introduced systematically and made compulsory by law. At the end of 1993, protection for RhD-negative pregnant women at 28 weeks of pregnancy was introduced. The first intrauterine fetal blood transfusion in Slovenia and Yugoslavia was performed in 1968;[87]
- In 1969, the Immunology Laboratory, in agreement with clinical hospitals, introduced HLA typing for the purpose of matched kidney transplantation;[88]
- 1970—Beginning of protection of all Rh-negative women after childbirth;
- 1970—Preparation of lyophilized cryoprecipitate;
- 1972—Typing of HLA antigens of potential kidney donors;
- 1973—Start of plasma collection for anti-hepatitis B gammaglobulin;
- 1974—Introduction of the autoanalyzer as a sensitive method for determining erythrocyte antibodies;
- 1979—Blood processing, production of blood components from a single plastic bag;[89]
- At least since 1979, we have been guided by the rule that the patient should only receive the blood component that he requires;[90]
- 1980—Transition to component therapy, routine production of concentrated erythrocytes from double plastic bags;
- 1981—Planning and production of the albumin program;
- 1981—Collection of buffy coat for interferon production;
- 1982—Ambulatory care of hemophiliacs with cryoprecipitate;
- 1986—Routine anti-CMV testing as ordered;

---

[83] Zupanič Slavec, 2018, p. 389.
[84] Potočnik, Levičnik-Stezinar, Faganel, Lukić, Rožman, Ulaga, Vukovič-Dervišić, 1995, p. 13–15.
[85] Zupanič Slavec, 2018, p. 389.
[86] Potočnik, Levičnik-Stezinar, Faganel, Lukić, Rožman, Ulaga, Vukovič-Dervišić, 1995, p. 13–15.
[87] Zupanič Slavec, 2018, p. 389.
[88] Bricl I., Lampreht N., Potočnik M. Bricl I. Ogulin M. Življenje teče: letno poročilo transfuzijske službe v Sloveniji za leto 2004. Ljubljana: Zavod Republike Slovenije za transfuzijo krvi. 2005; p. 8. http://www.ztm.si/knjiznica/letna-porocila/. Accessed 13 Apr 2024.
[89] Potočnik, Levičnik-Stezinar, Faganel, Lukić, Rožman, Ulaga, Vukovič-Dervišić, 1995, p. 13–15.
[90] Zupanič Slavec, 2018, p. 389.

- 1987—Start of introduction of automatic data processing for blood donors;
- 1988—Introduction of micromethods in the blood donor typing laboratory;[91]
- In 1985, preparations for hematopoietic stem cell transplantation (HSCT) began at the Department of Haematology of the Ljubljana Clinical Center. The first bone marrow collection for autologous (HSCT) was performed on December 27, 1988, and the first autologous transplantation was performed on January 20, 1989. The first related allogeneic (HSCT) was performed on April 21, 1989;[92]
- 1990—Collection of stem cells from peripheral blood for transplantation;
- 1991—Management of the entire work process with the computer, introduction of the barcode system;
- In 1991, we set up a project for the self-supply and use of the state-of-the-art factor VIII and IX concentrates for the treatment of hemophilia;
- 1992—Establishment of the registry of unrelated bone marrow donors SLOVENIA—DONOR, inclusion in the international registry;
- 1992—Introduction of the gel technique for more demanding serological tests;
- 1993—Introduction of modern prenatal testing at 28 weeks of pregnancy, to protect against sensitization;
- 1994—Start of production of monoclonal anti-A, anti-B reagents for routine use;
- 1994—Adoption of GMP for transfusion medicine;
- 1994—The tissue typing center starts with HLA gene typing;
- 1994—The beginning of the introduction of a questionnaire for blood donors before blood collection.[93]

Slovenia started screening all collected units of donated blood for hepatitis C virus (HCV) RNA in 2000, utilizing NAT technology and the PCR method. In 2007, screening of donated blood was expanded to HCV, hepatitis B virus (HBV), and human immunodeficiency virus (HIV) detection.[94] The quality of blood components was improved by filtering whole blood in a closed in-line system in 2000 and by introducing automated blood processing and viral inactivation of platelet components in 2007. In 2003, we set up a laboratory for the final control of blood components as part of our quality system. In 2004, we also started to use commercial recombinant clotting factors for the treatment of hemophiliacs. In 2005, barcoding of patient blood samples and storage of frozen samples were introduced. In 2006, we started collecting hematopoietic stem cells for the treatment of patients with heart failure. We started collecting hemopoietic stem cells from the placenta for the public cord blood bank in 2008, in collaboration with obstetricians. In 2009, we restructured blood processing and started to prepare buffy coat platelets by fusion and filter erythrocytes before storage. Platelet gel for the treatment of surgical and

---

[91] Potočnik, Levičnik-Stezinar, Faganel, Lukić, Rožman, Ulaga, Vukovič-Dervišić, 1995, p. 13–15.
[92] Pretnar J. Petnajst let presajanja krvotvornih matičnih celic v Sloveniji. Zdravniški vestnik. 2004, Supplement I, p. 1–4.
[93] Potočnik, Levičnik-Stezinar, Faganel, Lukić, Rožman, Ulaga, Vukovič-Dervišić, 1995, p. 13–15.
[94] Levičnik Stezinar S., Nograšek P. Izplen presejalnega testiranja krvodajalcev s tehniko NAT v Sloveniji, Zdravniški Vestnik. Vol 81 (2012): Supplement II, p. 257–64. https://vestnik.szd.si/index.php/ZdravVest/article/view/764.

dermatological patients was launched in 2012. Extracorporeal photopheresis was introduced in 2012. [95]

According to Article 33 of the Act on Fundamental Rights in the Employment Relationship, which entered into force on October 14, 1989, blood donors were entitled to 2 consecutive days off after donating blood.[96] Article 169 of the Labour Relations Act, which entered into force on January 1, 2003, stipulated that one paid day be charged to health insurance. Wage compensation was transferred from the employer to the holder of the mandatory health insurance.[97] Article 167 of the Labor Relations Act, which entered into force on April 12, 2013, stipulates that blood donors have the right to be absent from work on the day they voluntarily donate blood. The employer pays the wage compensation to the employee at the expense of health insurance.[98]

According to the Blood Supply Act, the BTCS is responsible for supplying the population with blood and blood products on a national level as well as for connecting blood transfusion medicine with hospital activity. BTCS coordinates all activities related to the selection of blood donors, the collection, testing, processing, storage, and distribution of blood and blood products, the clinical use of blood, and the monitoring of serious adverse events or reactions related to blood transfusion. BTCS coordinates and connects the network of hospital blood transfusion departments and hospital blood banks at the national level, manages a unified information system, supports professional education and development, and conducts research activities. It also cooperates with international organizations, associations, and related institutes in other countries.[99]

Today, blood donation in Slovenia is promoted in many ways through all kinds of media: social networks, leaflets, brochures, lectures, courtesy invitations, billboards, events, and more. The most important way to promote blood donation is through mutual solidarity, which is constantly being strengthened and improved. Blood donors occasionally receive plaques, certificates of appreciation, and symbolic gifts as a token of their gratitude. The experience of blood donors who successfully donate blood and who share their positive experience among their social circle of people, which further spreads blood donation, is of great importance in the promotion of blood donation. Slovenian blood donors are altruistic, empathetic, and understanding. Time and again, they respond to appeals to help patients at risk. Many patients are immensely grateful to everyone who was involved in their treatment after they recovered. In Slovenia, the main reason for choosing to donate blood is still the desire to

---

[95] Zupanič Slavec, 2018, p. 389.

[96] Zakon o temeljnih pravicah iz delovnega razmerja (Uradni list SFRJ, št. 60/89, 42/90, Uradni list RS, št. 4/91, 97/01-ZSDP, 42/02-ZDR in 43/06-ZkoIP).

[97] Zakon o delovnih razmerjih (Uradni list RS, št.42/02, 79/06-ZZZPB-F, 103/07, 45/08-Zarbit in 21/13-ZDR-1).

[98] Zakon o delovnih razmerjih (Uradni list RS, št. 21/13, 78/13-popr., 47/15-ZZSDT, 33/16-PZ-F, 52/16, 15/17-odl. US, 22/19-ZPosS, 81/19, 203/20-ZIUPOPDVE in 119/21-ZČmISA).

[99] Zakon o preskrbi s krvjo (Uradni list RS, št. 104/06). https://zakonodaja.com/zakon/zpkrv-1. Accessed 13 April 2024.

help a fellow human being. There are cases where people decide to donate blood after they have received blood themselves and their health condition allows them to do so. All age groups of blood donors with different blood groups are welcomed and are role models, and each individual is valuable as a blood donor in his or her own way. In Slovenia, there are wonderful examples of entire families who are blood donors and who still carry on the tradition of blood donation in the footsteps of their ancestors. There are many beautiful stories of blood donation bringing people together to become friends as well as love stories of soul mates meeting at a blood donation. Slovenia can be proud of its blood donors because they are aware of the importance of healthy and safe blood and because they are always willing to selflessly respond to the needs of their blood groups. Blood donation in Slovenia has improved today compared to the past. The road to establishing altruistic, voluntary, non-remunerated, and anonymous blood donation as one of the greatest forms of interpersonal solidarity in the Republic of Slovenia has been long and steep. Today, we can be proud in Slovenia because we are self-sufficient in the supply of safe blood and safe blood products. The Republic of Slovenia has benefited from the tradition of voluntary, non-remunerated, and anonymous blood donation in many ways, and in general, we must continue to strive for higher goals in the field of blood donation and in general in transfusion medicine to save lives at risk and to recruit new and healthy blood donors.

Interesting Cases of Humanitarian Blood Donation from Slovenians Through Time

The Case of John Lovšin

The first known case of a Slovenian patient receiving a blood transfusion of human blood abroad occurred on June 15, 1921, in the USA. The patient of the blood transfusion was John Lovšin, from the town of Ribnica in Slovenia, who moved and lived in Tower, Minnesota, for 31 years. He was sick for a long time due to the weakening of the blood. A self-sacrificing compatriot gave him a few quarts of his own blood, which, unfortunately, failed to help the doctors treat the 60-year-old Mr. Lovšin.[100]

Humane Police Officer Andrej Galon

On November 20, 1928, the Jutro newspaper published an article about the self-sacrificing police officer Mr. Andrej Galon with the title "*A liter of blood for a wounded man on his deathbed. The noble sacrifice of a Slovenian police officer.*" Andrej Galon is the first Slovene known by name and surname who was reported to have selflessly donated blood for someone outside of Slovenia.

---

[100] Anon. Smrtna kosa. Glasilo K.S.K. jednote. 1921;7(24) p. 2. http://www.dlib.si/?URN=URN:NBN:SI:DOC-SDITIMC5.

The conductor Mr. Đuro Trbojević was particularly injured in the tram accident that took place in Belgrade on November 10, 1928. Despite the immediate transfer to the hospital and the quick help of doctors, his condition became more and more critical. His right leg had to be amputated, and the poor man lost a lot of blood. His brother Petar wanted to donate his blood to him, but he was anemic. The doctor suggested to Petar that he find someone else to donate blood for his brother. Petar remembered his comrade-in-arms, Andrej Galon, a native of the city of Ptuj from Slovenia, who at that time lived and worked in Belgrade and who, without hesitation, agreed to donate blood for the unfortunate Đura. *"I have enough blood, doctor!"* joked Galon when they put his hand next to the unconscious casualty for the blood transfusion. *"But if I ever need it, he will return the loan to me. The same amount—no more and no less! No profit!"* The heroic restraint of the cheerful Slovenian police officer aroused the admiration of all the doctors present. The police officer Galon donated over a liter of blood and saved Đura Trbojević's life. Mr. Galon left the hospital the same day.[101]

Slovenian Hero Alojzij Završnik

A young sailor in the Navy of the Kingdom of Yugoslavia, Mr. Alojzij Završnik from Ljubljana, sacrificed his blood to save the life of a Croat in 1930.

The doctors of the sanatorium Dr. Roić in Split were impressed by the self-sacrifice of the young wartime sailor Alojzij Završnik from the Ljubljana settlement Fužine, who saved the life of his sick Croatian comrade with his blood. A patient was lying in the sanatorium after a difficult operation. Due to massive blood loss, he needed a blood transfusion. The patient's family was looking for a blood donor themselves, and luckily they came across a young sailor, Alojzij Završnik, who happened to sense that they needed help. He immediately went to the hospital and donated a liter of his blood for the endangered patient, which saved his life. They wanted to pay him for the donated blood in the sanatorium, but Mr. Završnik proudly said:*"I don't need anything; I don't ask for anything; I gladly gave my blood to save my Croatian brother."* Everyone present was impressed by Mr. Završnik's statement and his selflessness.

A Few Examples of Noble Cases of Blood Donors from 1935 to 1952

Mr. Jakob Lovrec was a blood donor who started donating his blood in 1935. In 3 years, he donated blood to patients more than 30 times.[102] From 1936 to 1939, Mr. Lojze Ogorevc donated blood 45 times.[103] Franc Bužga had donated his blood 48

---

[101] Anon. Liter Krvi Za Ranjenca Na Smrtni Postelji. Plemenita požrtvovalnost slovenskega orožnika. Jutro. 1928;9(273) p. 3. http://www.dlib.si/?URN=URN:NBN:SI:DOC-7FLL88EZ.
[102] Slovenski dom, 1938, p. 4.
[103] Anon. Lojze Ogorevc, fant, ki je dal 45 krat svojo kri. Jutro.1939;20(37) p. 3. http://www.dlib.si/?URN=URN:NBN:SI:DOC-FQA4UNFC.

times by the year 1946.[104] A 60-year-old blood donor Katarina Baumgartner had saved 28 lives by 1949. She had blood group O and donated blood 20 times in the maternity ward and the rest elsewhere. In total, she donated 14 liters of blood.[105] Vekoslav Medvešček donated blood 175 times between 1943 and 1951.[106]

Valerija Zupan, First Woman Blood Donor at the First Slovenian Mobile Blood Donation in Town of Zagorje at Savi, 9/3/1953

Mrs. Valerija Zupan was the first woman to donate blood at the first Slovenian mobile blood donation in the town of Zagorje at Savi on March 9, 1953 (Image B.10). She was recognized for her noble act at the celebration of the 60th anniversary of voluntary blood donation in Slovenia in 2013, for which she is very happy. Mrs. Valerija Zupan, nicknamed Valči, was born on November 22, 1930, in the old Kingdom of Yugoslavia. In 2020, when I interviewed her, she was a proud 90-year-old. Her maiden name was Sajovic. As a young woman, during the first mobile blood donation, she worked in a local mine. Mrs. Zupan has been a native of Zagorje at Savi all her life. She has five great-grandchildren and a loving family. Mrs. Zupan's view of blood donation is very emotional and noble: *"Blood saves life, be it a child or an adult; everyone needs it; without it, many people would die. It couldn't be better for people to donate blood to each other. No one knows what awaits them in life; every person needs blood to live. If a person has good blood, he should donate it."* She herself says that she has donated blood many times because she was aware that there were always people who needed blood; she herself once needed blood. She thinks that it is unique that the Red Cross organizes blood donations, and she also generally praises the work of the Red Cross in Zagorje at Savi. She remembers that when she started donating blood, blood donors did not have a day off but drank cognac and went back to work.[107]

Rok Zabukovec A Noble Slovenian Blood Donor

Rok Zabukovec is a long-time blood donor who regularly and selflessly donates whole blood and blood components without hesitation (Image B.11). As a person and a blood donor, he is distinguished by a highly developed emotional empathy and concern for the health of his fellow citizens. He is also a Slovenian professional soldier who serves his country with pride and honor. "I first encountered blood donation when I was a child, when my father explained and presented to me what the blood donation procedure actually is. It is true that at that time the approaches were a little different than today, but I was nevertheless fascinated by the fact that a liquid is created in a person, in me: blood, which is of vital importance and which

---

[104] Slovenski poročevalec, 1946, p. 3.

[105] Anon. Katarina Baumgartner je dosedaj rešila že 28 življenj. Celjski tednik: glasilo osvobodilne fronte okrajev Celje - mesto, Celje-okolica in Šoštanj.1949;2(4), p. 3. http://www.dlib.si/?URN=URN:NBN:SI:DOC-AHY0RFTB.

[106] Anon. V osmih letih 80 litrov krvi za transfuzijo. Slovenski poročevalec.1952;13(25), p. 3. http://www.dlib.si/?URN=URN:NBN:SI:DOC-UOY8VDEC.

[107] Interview with Mrs. Valerija Zupan, Zdravko Kvržić conducted on September 12, 2020.

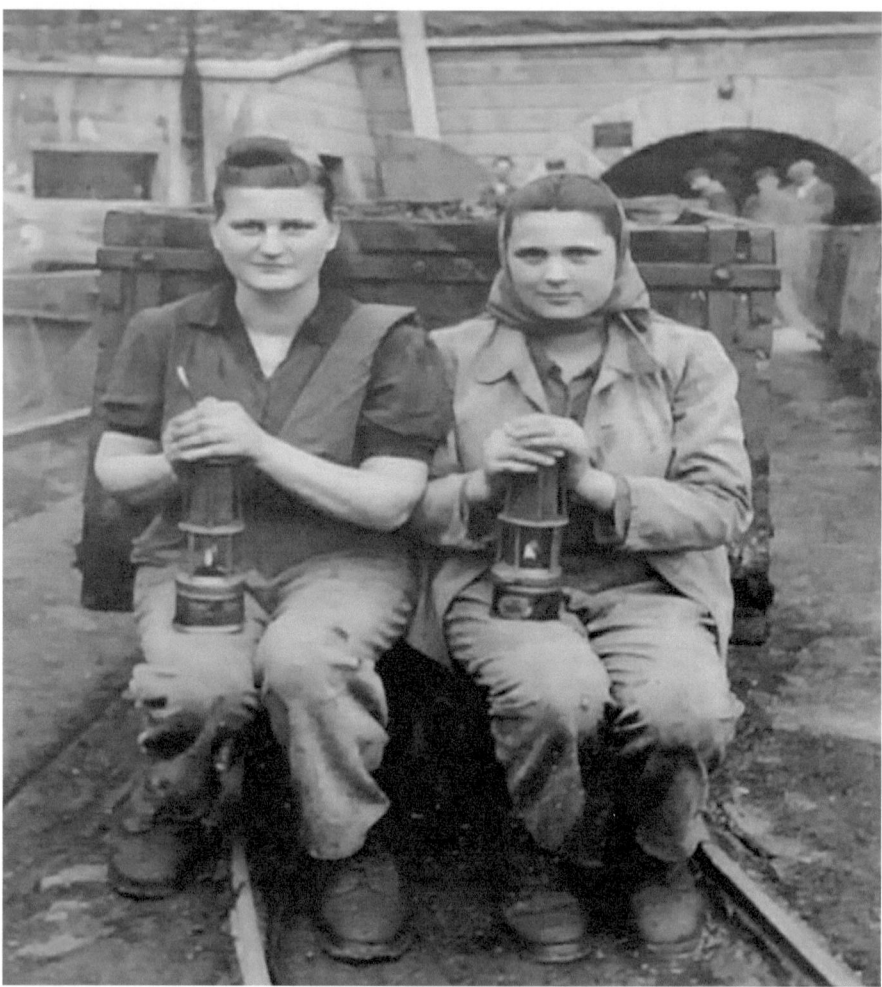

Image B.10 Valerija Zupan second from the right, around 1950s. (Source: Permission for usage of this image was granted for this book from the personal archive of Mrs. Valerija Zupan on January 4, 2021)

medicine can take from the blood donor, store, and then use for the purpose of saving the life of a person in distress. When I first donated those *'half liters'* of blood when I was 18, it felt great! By working in health care and then as a member of the Slovenian Army and by participating in various courses and missions, my awareness of the necessity of donating blood came to the fore even more. This feeling that your blood, plasma, or platelets will help someone is good—maybe even addictive—which is good in a way. You know in your heart that you have done something good for a fellow human being, and with all this, you hope that you yourself will never need blood. I will never forget the words of an elderly gentleman who sat next to me in the Izola hospital and donated blood just like me. His words were: *It's*

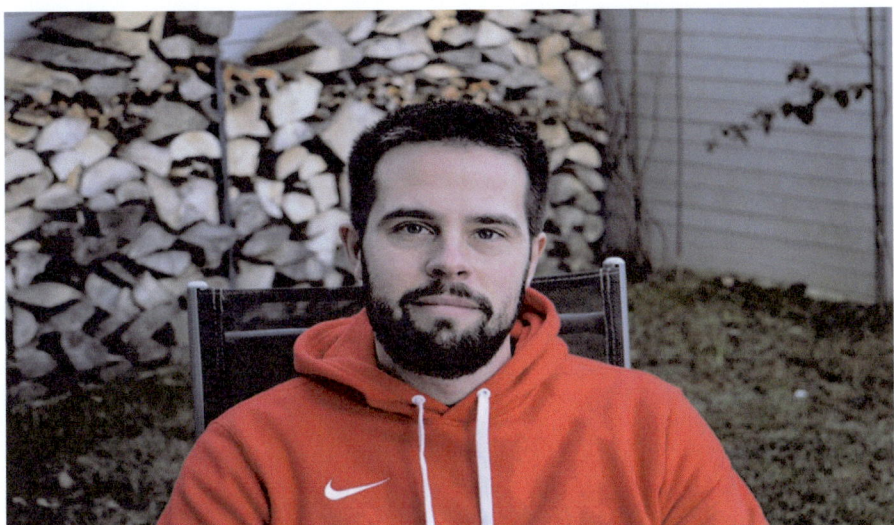

Image B.11 ROK ZABUKOVEC, 2021. (Source: Permission for usage of this image was granted for this book from the personal archive of Mr. Rok Zabukovec on January 18, 2021)

better to give than to receive. I say stick with it, and really, you can only hope that if the time does come and you need blood too, there will be someone there who will do this life favor for you. I know and am firmly convinced of this: *as long as I fulfill the conditions for donating blood, plasma, or platelets, I will be a blood donor! In my eyes, being a blood donor is not only about donating blood, talking to an excellent medical and nursing team, eating a good sandwich, and drinking coffee at the end; this is my life's mission."*[108]

Lev Arnejšek A Kind-Hearted Slovenian Blood Donor

Lev Arnejšek is a kind, knowledgeable, and socially responsible person with a big heart and a dedicated blood donor. He is a registered nurse by profession and worked for a few years at the BTCS in Ljubljana (Image B.12).

"When I started working at BTCS, I never thought about donating blood. But the more I worked, the more I came into contact with people who save lives through this noble act for various reasons. Despite my fear, I myself decided to take courage and donate blood. By doing this, I made it possible for a patient to survive. Despite feeling light-headed, I was happy. It is better that no one, including me and my loved ones, ever comes into a situation needing blood. But if it ever happens, there is a reassuring feeling that there are people (blood donors) who will help you. Blood donation is an honorable and courageous act that I am proud to have sometimes been able to participate in as a blood donor myself. To all this, I can add a story that marked my life. But not by me or anyone close to me needing blood. In 2014, as part of my regular work, I took part in a mobile blood donation. The participation of

---

[108] Interview with Mr. Rok Zabukovec was conducted on by Zdravko Kvržić on January 18, 2021.

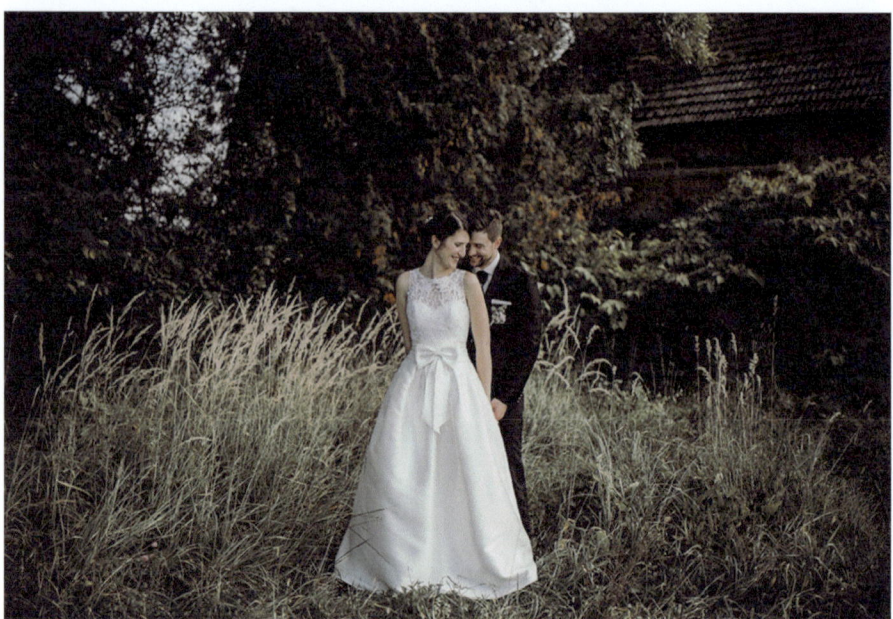

Image B.12 Zala and Lev Arnejšek, 2017. (Source: Permission for usage of this image was granted for this book from the personal archive of Mr. Lev Arnejšek on February 21, 2022)

blood donors that day was great. In between blood donations, a very nice girl named Zala came to donate blood. She laid down on my blood donor chair. The blood draw itself took much longer than the average time. Nevertheless, I enjoyed it immensely, and it felt like a spark had jumped between us. I dared to look up her phone number in the phone book and called her the next day. Despite the awkwardness, the feelings were mutual, and we went on a date after that. It has been quite a few years since then, and there have been many events, including marriage between us and the birth of our three wonderful children. I did not expect this to happen in any way, and these special and loving events that happened are the most pleasant and special for me in all this time."[109]

---

[109] Interview with Mr. Lev Arnejšek was conducted by Zdravko Kvržić on February 21, 2022.

References

1. Alamri AA, Alnefaie MN, Saeedi AT, Hariri AF, Altaf A, Aljiffry MM. Transfusion practices among general surgeons at a tertiary care center: a survey based study. Med Arch. 2018;72(6):418–24. https://www.ncbi.nlm.nih.gov/pmc/articles/PMC6340613/.
2. Archiv der Universität Wien. Kassajournale, p. R77.59–R77.63.
3. Archiv der Universität Wien. Studienkataloge MED 15.58.
4. Archiv der Universität Wien. Rigorosenprotokoll, MED 16.36, p. 73–74.
5. Borisov P. Od renoceluištva do začetkov znanstvene kirurgije na Slovenskem. Ljubljana: Slovenska Akademija Znanosti in Umetnosti; 1977. p. 1–192.
6. Blumauer R. Provincialna kronika Jugoslovanske province hčera krščanske ljubezni (usmiljenk), leto. 1935;1:167–8.
7. Anon. Prva transfuzija krvi v Sloveniji. Jutro. 1927;8(112):3. https://www.dlib.si/details/URN:NBN:SI:DOC-KE7AUJ30.
8. Anon. Senzacija, ki ni senzacija. Slovenski narod. 1927; letnik 60(108):3. https://www.dlib.si/stream/URN:NBN:SI:DOC-AC6MWL9M/aed06c3a-a288-4445-b17e-4427d505671e/PDF.
9. Anon. Cene človeške krvi v Ljubljani so precej različne, vendar pa precej nizke. Jutro. 1937;18(212):3. http://www.dlib.si/details/URN:NBN:SI:DOC-I5Q49NOC.
10. Anon. Ljudje, ki prodajajo svojo kri, še 30 let ni star (pa je dal že večkot 30 krat svojo kri bolnikom). Slovenski dom. 1938;3(276):4. http://www.dlib.si/?URN=URN:NBN:SI:DOC-W7L5DSJC.
11. Anon. Poziv župana Dinka Puca. Jugoslovan. 1931;2(276):3. https://www.dlib.si/stream/URN:NBN:SI:DOC-XY7133N6/d86618b3-71b2-4a9a-945b-34411edc767b/PDF.
12. Anon. Doma in po svetu, nov pravilnik o plačevanju lečenja v bolnicah. Delavska politika. 1932;7(69):2. http://www.dlib.si/?URN=URN:NBN:SI:DOC-T0RS64RE.
13. Anon. Novosti iz banovinske ženske bolnice. Jutro. 1936;17(119):9. http://www.dlib.si/?URN=URN:NBN:SI:DOC-9FF2AT15.
14. Anon. Svojo kri prodajajo. Jutro. 1936;17(88):3. http://www.dlib.si/details/URN:NBN:SI:DOC-1P97ZI9H.
15. Anon. Poziv dajalcem krvi. Delavska politika. 1941;16(4):3. http://www.dlib.si/?URN=URN:NBN:SI:DOC-N6NDNCAG.
16. Anon. Ptujska bolnica vabi krvodajalce. Jutro. 1937;18(207):8. http://www.dlib.si/details/URN:NBN:SI:DOC-270LOLAK.
17. Anon. O oddaji krvi za transfuzije. Slovenski narod. 1936;69(98):3. http://www.dlib.si/details/URN:NBN:SI:DOC-HXEU56M9.
18. Anon. Dinar za gram krvi, krvodajalci, najznačilnejši poklic' naše dobe, se bore za svojo nagrado. Jutro. 1936;17(162):7. http://www.dlib.si/?URN=URN:NBN:SI:DOC-WT51C3SV.
19. Anon. Odškodnina za transfuzijo krvi. Jutro. 1937;18(269):4. http://www.dlib.si/?URN=URN:NBN:SI:DOC-30T8CL1J.
20. Anon. Transfuzija krvi v obči državni bolnišnici v Ljubljani. Slovenec. 1937;65(12):4. http://www.dlib.si/?URN=URN:NBN:SI:DOC-50VVQ2C5.

21. Anon. Krvodajalci naslavljajo svojo prošnjo na dobra srca. Slovenski dom. 1938;3(287):3. http://www.dlib.si/?URN=URN:NBN:SI:DOC-DYQ9RGNJ.
22. Anon. Tudi ti bi radi obhajali vesel Božič. Slovenec. 1938;66(291):7. http://www.dlib.si/?URN=URN:NBN:SI:DOC-QY4D5UUP.
23. Anon. Predavanje v okviru Rdečega križa. Večernik. 1940;14(213):4. http://www.dlib.si/?URN=URN:NBN:SI:DOC-HFIB3I65.
24. Anon. Sodobni pomočniki zdravniške znanosti. Slovenec. 1944;72(55):2. http://www.dlib.si/?URN=URN:NBN:SI:DOC-5WBV4YZN.
25. Anon. Poziv uprave Splošne Bolnišnice v Ljubljani. Slovenski poročevalec—glasilo osvobodilne fronte. 1945;6(26):3. http://www.dlib.si/?URN=URN:NBN:SI:DOC-JNSTO5DK.
26. Borisov P. Ginekologija na Slovenskem od nastanka do 80. let 20. Stoletja. Ljubljana: Slovenska akademija znanosti in umetnosti; 1995. p. 191.
27. Bajc O. Kri za svojega bližnjega. Družinski tednik. 1932;4(1):3. http://www.dlib.si/details/URN:NBN:SI:DOC-IDI98SBA.
28. Bregant PJ. Transfuzija na Razorih. Delo. 1961;3(142):7. http://www.dlib.si/?URN=URN:NBN:SI:DOC-1BIIDXUJ.
29. Černič M. Prva transfuzija krvi v Sloveniji. Jutro. 1927;8(114):4. http://www.dlib.si/?URN=URN:NBN:SI:DOC-48Q5USRH.
30. Fux F. Transfusion in Krain, Aerztliches Correspondenzblatt für Böhmen; 1875. p. 230. https://www.google.si/books/edition/Aerztliches_Correspondenzblatt_f%C3%BCr_B%C3%B6h/fTDRsb5cYQ0C?hl=sl&gbpv=1&dq=Transfusion+in+Krain&pg=PA230&printsec=frontcover.
31. Fux F. Kochsalztransfusion als Prophylaktikum. Wiener medizinische Wochenschrift Nr. 1884;31:1–2.
32. Florstchűtz V. Zgodovina kirurgije Slovenije od 1760 do 1928, Zusammenfassung P.o. Acta Chirurgica Yugoslavica. 1959;7(2):168–72.
33. Herren PT. Verzeichnis von ehemaligen Kremsmünster Studenten. Kremsmünster, Austria: Des k k Gymnasiums Druck von Jos Feichtingers Erben in Linz; 1877. p. 30.
34. Jerina LP. Novosti - izkušnje—pobude, Naše prve poti k organizirani transfuziološki službi. Obzornik zdravstvene nege. 1991;25(3/4):229–34. https://obzornik.zbornica-zveza.si/index.php/ObzorZdravNeg/article/view/1904.
35. Lunaček P. Sectio Caesarea. Zdravniški vestnik. 1933;5(3):90–117. http://www.dlib.si/?URN=URN:NBN:SI:DOC-GYDDEGCB.
36. Lavrič B. Kri Se Preliva. Za Zdravje. 1935;16(234):4. http://www.dlib.si/?URN=URN:NBN:SI:DOC-8PIYAUM9.
37. Lutman S. Transfuzija krvi v praksi. Zdravniški vestnik. 1940;11(6-7):213–5. http://www.dlib.si/?URN=URN:NBN:SI:DOC-SUA1YXIK.
38. Peršič I. Osteomyletis v letu 1934. Zdravniški vestnik. 1935;7(7–8) 285. http://www.dlib.si/?URN=URN:NBN:SI:DOC-AQ6MXYDG.
39. Kvržić Z. Dr. Franz Fux - imenitni zdravnik svojega časa. Revija za moje zdravje. 2022;9(64):42–4. https://www.revijazamojezdravje.si/franz-fux/.
40. Keber K, Svetličič A. Čas Kolere: epidemije kolere na Kranjskem v 19 stoletju. Ljubljana: Založba ZRC, ZRC SAZU; 2007. p. 102–4.
41. Meršol V. Sedemdeset let Slovenskega zdravniškega društva v Ljubljani. 1932;4(8–10):131–138. https://www.dlib.si/details/URN:NBN:SI:DOC-23FDIHNG.
42. Makarovič M, Modrej I. Strokovno zdravstvo v Črna in Črnjani. Črna na Koroškem: Občina Črna na Koroškem; 2013. p. 486–7.
43. Milčinski J. Transfuzija v partizanski bolnišnici. Delo. 1961;3(133):7. http://www.dlib.si/details/URN:NBN:SI:DOC-LRXBNLOQ.
44. Ramšak A. Personal letter from 31 January 1956. A copy of the letter is in the Maribor Regional Archives, fond Eman Pertl, 1907–1987, AŠ 4, folder 6, personal letter of Adolf Ramšak, 31 January 1956. The letter for this book was obtained from Dr. Elko Borko's, personal archive on 19 Mar 2021.
45. Venčeslav A. Transfuzije krvi v letu 1934. Zdravniški vestnik. 1935;7(7-8):291–2. http://www.dlib.si/?URN=URN:NBN:SI:DOC-AQ6MXYDG.

46. T.P. Prva transfuzija v času IMOB na Razorih. Naša skupnost (Ljubljana Moste-Polje). 1986;27(16):4. http://www.dlib.si/?URN=URN:NBN:SI:DOC-GZK7SQT3.
47. Zupanič SZ, Goričar M. Prim. Dr. Edo Šlajmer, reformator kirurgije na Slovenskem (ob 150-letnici rojstva)., vol. 24. Isis: Glasilo Zdravniške zbornice Slovenije; 2015. p. 64–8. https://www.zdravniskazbornica.si/informacije-publikacije-in-analize/publikacije-zbornice-isis/isis-januar-2015.
48. Zgodovinski arhiv Ljubljana, SI_ZAL_LJU 10339, Pintarjeva Zbirka, TE 2.
49. Anon. V zavodu za transfuzijo krvi. Ljudska pravica. 1946;7(301):3. http://www.dlib.si/?URN=URN:NBN:SI:DOC-TNBL6JMX.
50. Anon. Dragocena in požrtvovalna je pomoč krvodajalcev. Slovenski poročevalec. 1946;7(300):3. http://www.dlib.si/?URN=URN:NBN:SI:DOC-C4POTL0X.
51. Anon. Dodatki olja in sladkorja za krvodajalce. Ljudska pravica. 1946;7(104):8. http://www.dlib.si/?URN=URN:NBN:SI:DOC-JQ4CIHQH.
52. Anon. Krvodajalci. Ljudska pravica. 1946;7(180):7. http://www.dlib.si/listalnik/URN_NBN_SI_doc-ZWZATNM4/8/index.html#zoom=z.
53. Anon. Zavod za transfuzijo krvi medicinske fakultete v Ljubljani. Ljudska pravica. 1946;7(162):6. http://www.dlib.si/?URN=URN:NBN:SI:DOC-JEYNKOEC.
54. Anon. Zavod za transfuzijo krvi poziva na darovanje krvi. Slovenski poročevalec. 1947;8(293):6. http://www.dlib.si/?URN=URN:NBN:SI:DOC-SFTFJQOI.
55. Anon. Krvodajalci. Ljudska pravica. 1947;8(260):6. http://www.dlib.si/?URN=URN:NBN:SI:DOC-C0NY6Z2I.
56. Anon. Krvodajalci. Ljudska pravica. 1947;8(198):7. http://www.dlib.si/?URN=URN:NBN:SI:DOC-CZQUNZRZ.
57. Anon. Zvišani obroki živil za krvodajalce. Ljudska pravica. 8(293):1947, 6. http://www.dlib.si/?URN=URN:NBN:SI:DOC-WKNVYVIR.
58. Anon. Dajalci krvi. Slovenski poročevalec. 1949;10(295):6. http://www.dlib.si/?URN=URN:NBN:SI:DOC-280Y5TZC.
59. Anon, Dajalci krvi. Slovenski poročevalec. 1952;13(29):7. http://www.dlib.si/?URN=URN:NBN:SI:DOC-QPWXE62H.
60. Anon. Sledimo vsi prvim brezplačnim krvodajalcem. Slovenski poročevalec. 1953;14(23):1. http://www.dlib.si/?URN=URN:NBN:SI:DOC-BLQOGO2W.
61. Anon. Prvi prostovoljni krvodajalci v Celju. Slovenski poročevalec. 1953;14(81):2. http://www.dlib.si/?URN=URN:NBN:SI:DOC-NSBLMKZR.
62. Anon. Krvodajalci. Slovenski poročevalec. 1953;14(204):8. http://www.dlib.si/?URN=URN:NBN:SI:DOC-GGMTTQRR.
63. Anon. V Zavodu za transfuzijo krvi v Ljubljani ustvarjajo dragocene rezerve krvi. Tovariš. 1953;9(6):140. http://www.dlib.si/?URN=URN:NBN:SI:DOC-6ZAIDI3C.
64. Anon. Darujmo kri. Glas Gorenjske. 1953;6(27):1. http://www.dlib.si/?URN=URN:NBN:SI:DOC-KAH8SG95.
65. Anon. Četrti junij dan krvodajalcev. Slovenski poročevalec. 1958;19(50):2. http://www.dlib.si/?URN=URN:NBN:SI:DOC-0QSVLA9N.
66. Anon. Smrtna kosa. Glasilo K.S.K. jednote. 1921;7(24):2. http://www.dlib.si/?URN=URN:NBN:SI:DOC-SDITIMC5.
67. Anon. Liter Krvi Za Ranjenca Na Smrtni Postelji. Plemenita požrtvovalnost slovenskega orožnika. Jutro. 1928;9(273):3. http://www.dlib.si/?URN=URN:NBN:SI:DOC-7FLL88EZ.
68. Anon. Lepa požrtvovalnost mladega mornarja. Jutro. 1930;11(260):5. http://www.dlib.si/?URN=URN:NBN:SI:DOC-3ROBW42F.
69. Anon. Junak. 1930;43(47):585. http://www.dlib.si/?URN=URN:NBN:SI:DOC-5D9BWSAR.
70. Anon. Lojze Ogorevc, fant, ki je dal 45 krat svojo kri. Jutro. 1939;20(37):3. http://www.dlib.si/?URN=URN:NBN:SI:DOC-FQA4UNFC.
71. Anon. Katarina Baumgartner je dosedaj rešila že 28 življenj Celjski tednik: glasilo osvobodilne fronte okrajev. Celje-mesto, Celje-okolica in Šoštanj. 1949;2(4):3. http://www.dlib.si/?URN=URN:NBN:SI:DOC-AHY0RFTB.
72. Anon. V osmih letih 80 litrov krvi za transfuzijo. Slovenski poročevalec. 1952;13(25):3. http://www.dlib.si/?URN=URN:NBN:SI:DOC-UOY8VDEC.

73. Anon. Naš domači zdravnik. Slovenec. 1937;115(65):12. http://www.dlib.si/?URN=URN:NBN:SI:DOC-9AYHR2OB.
74. Anon. Zahteva po popolni medicinski fakulteti uresničena. Ljudska pravica. 1946;7(101):12. http://www.dlib.si/?URN=URN:NBN:SI:DOC-MPJKFBDZ.
75. Anon. Krvodajalci. Ljudska pravica. 1947;8(270):6. http://www.dlib.si/?URN=URN:NBN:SI:DOC-ZEBZZQGC.
76. XXXX.
77. Anon. Krvodajalci. Ljudska pravica. 1948;9(3):8. http://www.dlib.si/?URN=URN:NBN:SI:DOC-VJ8TMASP.
78. Anon. Srednji vek napada. Slovenski poročevalec. 1952;13(129):8. http://www.dlib.si/?URN=URN:NBN:SI:DOC-SPVANMPF.
79. Bricl I, Lampreht N, Potočnik M, Bricl I, Ogulin M. Življenje teče: letno poročilo transfuzijske službe v Sloveniji za leto 2004. Ljubljana: Zavod Republike Slovenije za transfuzijo krvi; 2005. p. 8. http://www.ztmsi/knjiznica/letna-porocila/. Accessed 13 Apr 2024.
80. Bricl I, Ogulin M. Življenje teče: letno poročilo transfuzijske službe v Sloveniji za leto 2007. Ljubljana: Zavod Republike Slovenije za transfuzijo krvi; 2008. p. 14. http://www.ztmsi/knjiznica/letna-porocila/. Accessed 13 Apr 2024.
81. Bricl I, et al. Z vami življenje teče dalje: jubilejna publikacija ob 70. obletnici transfuzijske dejavnosti v Sloveniji. Ljubljana: Zavod Republike Slovenije za transfuzijo krvi; 2015. p. 15.
82. Bibič A. Kultura naroda in krvodajalstvo. Tovariš. 1971;27(18):12–3. http://www.dlib.si/?URN=URN:NBN:SI:DOC-CEZ50I9F.
83. Interview with Dr. Bogdan Fludernik, son of Dr. Franc Fludernik. Written answers to the questions were obtained by Zdravko Kvržić on 14 September 2023.
84. Interview with Marko Gomišček, son of Dr. Danilo Gomišček. Written answers to the questions were obtained by Zdravko Kvržić on 22 July 2021.
85. Interview with Alenka Kryštufek born Gomišček, daughter of Dr. Danilo Gomišček. Written answers to the questions were obtained by Zdravko Kvržić on 16 July, 2021.
86. Interview with Mrs. Valerija Zupan, Zdravko Kvržić conducted on September 12, 2020.
87. Interview with Mr. Rok Zabukovec was conducted on by Zdravko Kvržić on January 18, 2021.
88. Interview with Mr. Lev Arnejšek was conducted by Zdravko Kvržić on February 21, 2022.
89. Institut za transfuziju krvi Srbije. Istorijat. https://itks.rs/istorijat.html#. Accessed 10 Apr 2024.
90. Jerina LP, Pogovorzdr Jerino Lah P, Potočnik M, Levičnik-Stezinar S, Faganel J, Lukić L, Rožman P, Ulaga R, Vukovič-Dervišić B. 50 let organizirane transfuzijske službe v Sloveniji:1945-1995. Ljubljana: Zavod Republike Slovenije za transfuzijo krvi; 1995, p. 23.
91. TG. Umrla bi če etc. Tovariš 1953;9(6), 145. http://www.dlib.si/?URN=URN:NBN:SI:DOC-6ZAIDI3C.
92. Kozinc Ž. Cena krvi. Tovariš. 1973;29(3):3. http://www.dlib.si/?URN=URN:NBN:SI:DOC-4VMSQVHF.
93. Kvržić Z. Zagorje ob Savi: zibelka prostovoljnega krvodajalstva. Savus. 2022;9(1):20. https://savus.si/arhiv-tednika/.
94. Kvržić Z. Ugleden zdravnik Danilo Gomišček. Savus. 2022;9(4):22. https://savus.si/arhiv-tednika/.
95. Kvržić Z, Mali P. Prikupljanje konvalescentne COVID-19 plazme sa plazmaferezom na Zavodu Republike Slovenije za transfuzijsku medicinu u Ljubljani. Liječnički vjesnik. 2021;143(2):131. https://hrcak.srce.hr/file/386068.
96. Kvržić Z. Marija Brus—prva medicinska sestra v transfuzijski medicini. Utrip: informativni bilten Zbornice zdravstvene nege Slovenije. 2023;31(6):16–8. https://www.zbornica-zveza.si/wp-content/uploads/2023/12/Utrip-December-2023-Januar-2024.pdf. Accessed 11 Apr 2024.
97. Kvržić Z. Zgodovina krvodajalstva in transfuzijske medicine v Sloveniji. 50 letučinkovitega sodelovanja: pomembna prelomnica ali izjemna priložnost? [Elektronski vir]:zbornik prispevkov z recenzijo: Zbornica zdravstvene in babiške nege Slovenije – Zveza strokovnih društev medicinskih sester, babic in zdravstvenih tehnikov Slovenije, Sekcija medicinskih

sester in zdravstvenih tehnikov v anesteziologiji, intenzivni terapiji in transfuziologiji: 53. strokovni seminar: Rogaška Slatina, 17. in 18. November 2023, p. 98–104. http://www.dlib.si/?URN=URN:NBN:SI:doc-JKK4AQKL. Accessed 25 March 2024.
98. Kvržić Z. Odvzem polne krvi pri krvodajalcu skozi različna zgodovinska obdobja (1875–2023). Utrip: informativni bilten Zbornice zdravstvene in babiške nege Slovenije. 2023;31(4):17–21. https://www.zbornica-zveza.si/wp-content/uploads/2023/08/Odvzem-polne-krvi-pri-krvodajalcu-skozi-razlicna-zgodovinska-obdobja-1875-2023-Kvrzic-Avgust-September-2023.pdf.
99. Lad K. Kri za transfuziji, najplemenitejše darilo. Slovenski poročevalec. 1952;13(40):4. http://www.dlib.si/?URN=URN:NBN:SI:DOC-LJWYRRFD.
100. L.K. Zgleden primer človekoljubne zavesti. Slovenski poročevalec. 1953;14(62):3. http://www.dlib.si/?URN=URN:NBN:SI:DOC-MX5WLNV4.
101. Levičnik SS, Nograšek P. Izplen presejalnega testiranja krvodajalcev s tehniko NAT v Sloveniji. Zdravniški Vestnik. 2012;81(Supplement II):257–64. https://vestnik.szd.si/index.php/ZdravVest/article/view/764.
102. Lutman S. Transfuzija krvi v praksi. Zdravniški Vestnik. 1940;12(6-7):213–5. https://www.dlib.si/stream/URN:NBN:SI:DOC-SUA1YXIK/e957e193-df10-484b-9b31-375de07d02e8/PDF.
103. Jerina LP. Razvoj službe transfuzije v Jugoslaviji Transplantacija. 1988;27(3):80.
104. Majcen-Vivod B, Urlep-Šalinović V. Prevalenca hepatitisov A in B pri krvodajalcih z anamnezo zlatenice. Zdravniški vestnik: glasilo Slovenskega zdravniškega društva. 2004;73(4):227–30. https://vestnik.szd.si/index.php/ZdravVest/article/view/2287.
105. Republika Slovenije računsko sodišče. Revizijsko poročilo vzpostavitev enotnega transfuzijskega informacijskega sistema. 2017, p. 7. https://www.rs-rs.si/fileadmin/user_upload/revizija/1212/IS_ZTM.pdf. Accessed 9 June 2022.
106. Sovdat BS. O transfuziji krvi. Slovenski poročevalec. 1953;14(21):3. http://www.dlib.si/?URN=URN:NBN:SI:DOC-YCXXHBU1.
107. Sovdat BS. Transfuzijska služba in krvodajalstvo v Sloveniji. Medicinski razgledi. 1971;10(3):339–43.
108. Sovdat Banič S. Pogovor z dr. Sonjo Sovdat Banič. Potočnik M, Levičnik-Stezinar S, Faganel J, Lukić L, Rožman P, Ulaga R, Vukovič-Dervišić B. 50 let organizirane transfuzijske službe v Sloveniji:1945-1995. Ljubljana: Zavod Republike Slovenije za transfuzijo krvi; 1995, p. 19.
109. STA. Vojna bolnica Ljubljana in Vojaško medicinski center Ljubljana ne bosta več delovala. https://www.sta.si/797217/vojna-bolnica-ljubljana-in-vojasko-medicinski-center-ljubljana-ne-bosta-vec-delovala. Accessed 13 Apr 2024.
110. Ferenčak T. Razvoj, pomen in organizacija transfuzijske službe. Ljubljana: Višja šola za zdravstvene delavce, Oddelek za medicinske sestre, diplomsko delo; 1962, p. 5.
111. Potočnik M, Levičnik-Stezinar S, Faganel J, Lukić L, Rožman P, Ulaga R, Vukovič-Dervišić B. 50 let organizirane transfuzijske službe v Sloveniji:1945-1995. Ljubljana: Zavod Republike Slovenije za transfuzijo krvi; 1995. p. 19.
112. Potočnik MD. Sonja Sovdat Banič: in memoriam. Zdravniški vestnik. 2009;78(5):269. http://www.dlib.si/?URN=URN:NBN:SI:DOC-VEVY5U9Y.
113. Potočnik M. Transfuziologija nekoč in danes. Zdravniški Vestnik. 2004;73(Supplement I):3. https://vestnik.szd.si/index.php/ZdravVest/article/view/2411.
114. Predlog zakona o preskrbi s krvjo. Republika Slovenija državni zbor. https://www.dz-rs.si. Accessed 18 Jun 2022.
115. Pretnar J. Petnajst let presajanja krvotvornih matičnih celic v Sloveniji. Zdravniški vestnik. 2004;Supplement I:1–4.
116. Zakon o temeljnih pravicah iz delovnega razmerja (Uradni list SFRJ, št. 60/89, 42/90, Uradni list RS, št. 4/91, 97/01—ZSDP, 42/02-ZDR in 43/06-ZkoIP).
117. Zakon o Rdečem križu Slovenije (Uradni list RS, št. 7/93 in 79/10). https://pisrs.si/pregledPredpisa?id=ZAKO250. Accessed 13 Apr 2024.
118. Zakon o delovnih razmerjih (Uradni list RS, št.42/02, 79/06-ZZZPB-F, 103/07, 45/08-Zarbit in 21/13—ZDR-1).

119. Zakon o delovnih razmerjih (Uradni list RS, št. 21/13, 78/13-popr., 47/15—ZZSDT, 33/16—PZ-F, 52/16, 15/17-odl. US, 22/19-ZPosS , 81/19, 203/20—ZIUPOPDVE in 119/21-ZČmISA).
120. Zakon o preskrbi s krvjo (Uradni list RS, št. 104/06). https://zakonodaja.com/zakon/zpkrv-1. Accessed 13 Apr 2024.
121. Zupanič SZ. Zgodovina zdravstva in medicine na Slovenskem-kirurške stroke, ginekologija in porodništvo. In: Jaunig S, editor. Razvoj transfuzijske medicine. Ljubljana: Slovenska Matica; 2018. p. 379–92.

Image Sources

Zupanič Slavec Z, Goričar M. Prim. Dr. Edo Šlajmer, reformator kirurgije na Slovenskem (ob 150-letnici rojstva). Isis: Glasilo Zdravniške zbornice Slovenije., ISSN 1318-0193. 2015;24(1), p. 64–8. https://www.zdravniskazbornica.si/informacije-publikacije-in-analize/publikacije-zbornice-isis/isis-januar-2015. The image of Dr. Franz Fux during surgery from around 1885 is the property of the Institute for the History of Medicine of the Faculty of Medicine in Ljubljana. The image in the book is published with the permission of Prof. Dr. Zvonka Zupanič Slavec. The permission was granted on April 2, 2021.

Ramšak A. Personal letter from January 31, 1956. A copy of the letter is in the Maribor Regional Archives, Fond Eman Pertl, 1907–1987, AŠ 4, folder 6, personal letter of Adolf Ramšak, 31 January 1956. The letter for this book was obtained from Dr. Elko Borko's personal archive on March 19, 2021.

Makarovič M, Modrej I. Primarius Dr. Adolf Ramšak 1938 in Črna in Črnjani. Črna na Koroškem: Občina Črna na Koroškem; 2013, p. 486–7. The mayor of the city of Črna na Korokem, Madam Romana Lesjak, granted permission to use the image for this book on May 23, 2021.

Doctor Sonja Sovdat Banič 1949. (Source: Doctor Sonja Sovdat Banič 1949. SI AS 1589/IV, Centralni komite Zveze komunistov Slovenije, šk. 3596 in 4345, članski dokumenti dr. Sonje Sovdat Banič. Permission to use the image was given by the Archives of the Republic of Slovenia on April 2, 2024).

Doctor Franc Fludernik, 1956. Permission to use the image was given by Primarius Mr.Sc. Bogdan Fludernik, and the son of Dr. Franc Fludernik, on March 22, 2024.

Nurse Marija Brus. Permission to use the image was given by Miro Brus, son of nurse Marija Brus, on December 3, 2023.

The old Blood Transfusion Center of the Faculty of Medicine in Ljubljana. Archive of Blood Transfusion Center of Slovenia. Permission to use the image was obtained from the V.D. director of the Blood Transfusion Center of Slovenia, Peter Kavčič, M.Sc. Business and Economic Science, on November 24, 2023.

The image of the Clinical Hospitals of the Faculty of Medicine. This image is the property of the Institute for the History of Medicine of the Faculty of Medicine in Ljubljana. The image in the book is published with the permission of Prof. Dr. Zvonka Zupanič Slavec. The permission was granted on April 13, 2024.

The image and permission to use it for this book were granted from the personal archive of Mr. Marko Gomišček on July 22, 2021. Permission for usage was also granted by Madam Alenka Kryštufek, the daughter of Danilo Gomišček, on July 16, 2021.

Blood donation procedure in Ljubljana around 1958–1960. Archive of Blood Transfusion Center of Slovenia. Permission to use the image was obtained from the V.D. director of the Blood Transfusion Center of Slovenia, Peter Kavčič, M.Sc. Business and Economic Science, on November 24, 2023.

Modern Blood donation procedure in Ljubljana in 2023. Archive of the Blood Transfusion Center of Slovenia. Permission to use the image was obtained from registered nurses on the image itself, Primož and Simona Hozjan, on November 23, 2023. The permission was also obtained from the V.D. director of the Blood Transfusion Center of Slovenia, Peter Kavčič, M.Sc. Business and Economic Science, on November 24, 2023.

Blood Transfusion Center of Slovenia in 2023. Personal archive of the author Zdravko Kvržić. The permission was also obtained from the V.D. director of the Blood Transfusion Center of Slovenia, Peter Kavčič, M.Sc. Business and Economic Science, on November 24, 2023.

Permission for usage of this image was granted for this book from the personal archive of Mrs. Valerija Zupan on January 4, 2021.

Permission for usage of this image was granted for this book from the personal archive of Mr. Rok Zabukovec on January 18, 2021.

Permission for usage of this image was granted for this book from the personal archive of Mr. Lev Arnejšek on February 21, 2022.

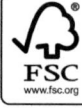

MIX
Papier aus verantwortungsvollen Quellen
Paper from responsible sources
FSC® C105338

If you have any concerns about our products,
you can contact us on
ProductSafety@springernature.com

In case Publisher is established outside the EU,
the EU authorized representative is:
Springer Nature Customer Service Center GmbH
Europaplatz 3, 69115 Heidelberg, Germany

Printed by Libri Plureos GmbH
in Hamburg, Germany